INTRODUCTION TO
AURAL REHABILITATION

Editor-in-Chief for Audiology
Brad A. Stach, PhD

INTRODUCTION TO AURAL REHABILITATION

RAYMOND H. HULL

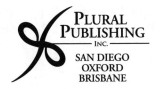

PLURAL
PUBLISHING
INC.

SAN DIEGO
OXFORD
BRISBANE

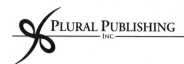

5521 Ruffin Road
San Diego, CA 92123

e-mail: info@pluralpublishing.com
Web site: http://www.pluralpublishing.com

49 Bath Street
Abingdon, Oxfordshire OX14 1EA
United Kingdom

FSC
Mixed Sources
Product group from well-managed
forests and other controlled sources

Cert no. SW-COC-002283
www.fsc.org
© 1996 Forest Stewardship Council

Typeset in 10½/13 Garamond book by Flanagan's Publishing Services, Inc.
Printed in the United States of America by McNaughton & Gunn, Inc.

Library of Congress Cataloging-in-Publication Data

Introduction to aural rehabilitation / [edited by] Raymond H. Hull.
      p. ; cm.
  Includes bibliographical references and index.
  ISBN-13: 978-1-59756-281-2 (alk. paper)
  ISBN-10: 1-59756-281-5 (alk. paper)
 1. Deaf—Rehabilitation. 2. Audiology. I. Hull, Raymond H.
 [DNLM: 1. Rehabilitation of Hearing Impaired. 2. Hearing Aids. WV 270 I651 2009]
 RF297.I58 2009
 617.8—dc22

                      2009018727

Contents

Preface

The book that you have just purchased is an introductory book on the nature and process of aural rehabilitation. As an introductory look at the processes involved in this exciting aspect of our field, it covers a broad range of topics considered to be the most important in preparing future professionals to serve children and adults with impaired hearing. It is a natural outgrowth of what previously became a popular text entitled *Aural Rehabilitation*, written and edited by this author, that resulted in four successful editions over a span of over 20 years. One of the reasons that those previous books were so popular among professors and students was not only the logical sequence in which the information was presented, but also the ease with which the book could be read. In other words, the book that you have purchased entitled, *Introduction To Aural Rehabilitation*, retains the readability and ease of understanding that the previous books by this author have maintained over the years, but also provides comprehensive information on the nature and process of aural habilitation and rehabilitation on behalf of children and younger and older adults who possess impaired hearing. Therefore, the information is presented in a readable fashion that has immediate theoretical and practical application.

The first page of each chapter provides a brief outline of the chapter for a quick content overview. Further, the examinations and answer sheets found at the conclusion of each chapter provide a ready-made opportunity for professors to quiz their students on a periodic basis, or to simply allow students to determine on their own whether they understood important points within each chapter.

This book is divided into four parts:

Part I: The Nature of Aural Rehabilitation presents information that is fundamental to the provision of services on behalf of all persons who possess impaired hearing, including an introduction to aural rehabilitation; an introduction to the nature and potential impact of hearing impairment and related terminology; an introduction to hearing aids and their components; and a psychosocial, educational, and vocational profile of persons with impaired hearing.

Part II: Introduction to Aural Rehabilitation: Children with Impaired Hearing concentrates on habilitative/rehabilitative services on behalf of children who possess impaired hearing. The information centers on the importance of family and its involvement in serving children who are hearing impaired; considerations regarding amplification for children; the development of auditory skills in children who are hearing impaired; language and speech development for children with impaired hearing; their educational management; and the issue of cochlear implantation on behalf of children.

Part III: Introduction to Aural Rehabilitation: Adults Who Are Hearing Impaired concentrates on matters that affect services on behalf of adults with impaired hearing. Chapters in this section address the impact of hearing impairment on adults, and procedures for counseling; hearing aid orientation; assistive listening devices for adults who are hearing impaired; and the history, theory, and application of aural rehabilitation for adults.

Part IV: Considerations for Older Adults with Impaired Hearing addresses special considerations for services on behalf of older adults who possess impaired hearing. The chapters in this section present information on psychosocial and physical factors of aging; the special nature of hearing loss in older adulthood; the impact of hearing loss on older adults; counseling the older adult who is hearing impaired; considerations for hearing aid use for older adults; techniques of aural rehabilitation for all adults who are hearing impaired; and programs for the hearing impaired elderly in health care facility environments.

Appendices: The Appendices of this book contain the most comprehensive compilation of assessments of communicative function in adults who possess impaired hearing found in any text on the topic of aural rehabilitation.

The topics for this book were by no means arbitrary. University professors and practitioners of audiology, speech-language pathologists, deaf educators, rehabilitation counselors, psychologists, otologists and otolaryngologists, along with upper-level undergraduate and graduate students across the United States, Canada, Europe, and other countries were consulted about the topics they felt were important in preparing audiologists and speech-language pathologists to work with children and adults who possess impaired hearing, and further, if they would prefer a term other than aural rehabilitation in this book. When a general consensus was reached, this book was designed, written, and prepared for you.

As an introductory look at the processes involved in aural rehabilitation, it covers a broad range of topics considered to be the most important in preparing future professionals to serve children and adults with impaired hearing. Therefore, a basic but diverse range of vocabulary and sophistication is acknowledged in regard to both the content of the chapters and the book's intended readership as an introductory book in this area of study. The book has been designed for use by a broad range of readers, primarily upper-level undergraduate students and early graduate students in audiology and speech-language pathology, and as a reference for professionals in audiology, speech-language pathology, deaf education, and other fields that serve children and adults with impaired hearing. Other interested readers include physicians, nurses, gerontologists, vocational rehabilitation counselors, teachers, psychologists, and sociologists.

Preparing this text has been an enjoyable and rewarding experience. It will prove to be a valuable source of information for serving children and adults who possess impaired hearing. Enjoy!

Contributors

R. Steven Ackley, PhD
Professor and Chair
Hearing, Speech and Language Sciences
Gallaudet University
Washington, DC
Chapters 3 and 12

Dale V. Atkins, MA, PhD
Psychologist, Author, Media Commentator
Greenwich, Connecticut
Chapter 5

William R. Hodgson, PhD
Professor Emeritus
Department of Speech, Language, and
    Hearing Sciences
University of Arizona
Tucson, Arizona
Chapter 6

Raymond H. Hull, PhD
Professor of Communicative Disorders and
    Sciences, Audiology/Neurosciences
Coordinator—Doctor of Audiology
    ProgramDepartment of Communication
    Sciences and Disorders
College of Health Professions
Wichita State University
Wichita, Kansas
Chapters 1, 11, 13, 17, 18, 19, 20

Jack Katz, PhD
Director
Auditory Processing Service
Research Professor
University of Kansas Medical Center
Clinical Professor

Touro Institute of Neurobehavioral Studies
Prairie Village, Kansas
Chapter 2

Thomas C. Kryzer, MD
Wichita Ear Clinic
Assistant Professor of Surgery and Family
    Medicine
University of Kansas School of Medicine
Wichita, Kansas
Chapter 9

Dawn Konrad-Martin, PhD
Research Investigator
VA RR&D National Center for
    Rehabilitative Auditory Research
    (NCRAR)
Portland VA Medical Center
Assistant Professor
Department of Otolaryngology, Head and
    Neck Surgery
Oregon Health and Science University
Portland, Oregon
Chapter 16

Daniel Ling, PhD (Deceased)
Professor Emeritus
Faculty of Applied Health Sciences
The University of Western Ontario
London, Ontario, Canada
Chapter 8

Michael R. Novotny, BA
The Ericksson School
University of Maryland Baltimore County
Baltimore, Maryland
Chapter 15

Molly Pottorf-Lyon, AuD, CCCA/SP
Adjunct Lecturer
Department of Communicative Sciences
    and Disorders
Wichita State University
Wichita, Kansas
Chapter 10

Judah L. Ronch, PhD
Professor and Undergraduate Academic
    Program Chair
The Erickson School
University of Maryland Baltimore County
Baltimore, Maryland
Chapter 15

Gabrielle H. Saunders, PhD
Investigator and NCRAR Deputy Director
    of Education Outreach and
    Dissemination
National Center for Rehabilitative Auditory
    Research
and
Assistant Professor
Department of Otolaryngology
Oregon Health and Science University
Portland, Oregon
Chapter 16

Joseph J. Smaldino, PhD
Professor and Chair
Department of Communication Sciences
    and Disorders
Illinois State University
Normal, Illinois
Chapters 4 and 14

Arlene Stredler-Brown, MA, CCC-SLP
Adjunct Faculty
University of Colorado
Adjunct Faculty
University of British Columbia
Boulder, Colorado
Chapter 7

Thomas P. White, MA, MBA
Professor Emeritus
State University of New York at Buffalo
Director Emeritus
Hearing Evaluation Services
Buffalo, New York
Chapter 2

*This book is dedicated to my wife, Lucinda,
and my daughter, Courtney.*

PART I

The Nature of Aural Rehabilitation

1

The Nature of Aural Rehabilitation

RAYMOND H. HULL

Introduction

Deafness is worse than blindness, so they say—it is the loneliness, the sense of isolation that makes it so, and the lack of understanding in the minds of ordinary people. The problem of the child deaf from birth is quite different from that of the man or woman who has become deafened after school age or in adult life. . . . But for all of them, the handicap is the same, the handicap of the silent world, the difficulty of communicating with the hearing and speaking world.
—Ballantyne, 1977

The aim of aural habilitative/rehabilitative efforts on behalf of children and adults with impaired hearing is to overcome the handicap. After discovering a hearing impairment and assessing its type and degree, medical referral by an audiologist is made, anticipating perhaps that the physician can correct the problem. The referral is made on the premise that the hearing impairment, per se, may be overcome.

If a hearing impairment cannot be medically treated, the audiologist then works with the patient to remediate the handicapping effects of the hearing loss and to help the child or adult overcome the communicative, social, and psychological effects of impaired hearing. A team of professionals may also become involved, perhaps including the physician, vocational rehabilitation counselors, educators, psychologists, sociologists, and speech pathologists, with the audiologist coordinating the team. The patient's family will also be involved in the aural rehabilitation treatment process. This task, in its totality, holds tremendous responsibility for all who are involved.

Why, then, is this important area in so many instances presented as a single chapter in books that deal with the subject of hearing impairment? Further, why are there so few published books that deal specifically with the effects of impaired hearing on children, adults, and aging persons, including approaches to counseling, the psychosocial and vocational impact of hearing impairment, and approaches for remediation, particularly when serving patients beyond audiologic assessment is among the most important services that audiologists provide?

The four parts of this book provide theoretical and practical information on serving children, adults, and the elderly who have impaired hearing. It addresses the issues and needs unique to each age group.

What Is Aural Rehabilitation?

What is aural rehabilitation? It has over the years been discussed from within the framework of speechreading, lipreading, visual communication, auditory training, and other subcategories so frequently that we have occasionally strayed from the totality of the habilitative and rehabilitative process.

Earlier, this chapter stated that the aim of aural habilitative/rehabilitative efforts for the hearing impaired is to overcome the handicap. What is the handicap? Impaired hearing may have a great impact on one person, but may not be as great a handicap to another. One person may remain despondent over his partial loss of hearing, but another may rebound and work with vigor to overcome the communication difficulties caused by the impairment. One person may encounter great social handicap from a relatively mild high-frequency hearing impairment, whereas another who possesses a more severe hearing loss may have only a mild occupational or social handicap. A child with a mild loss of hearing that is not detected until school age may suffer as great a handicap as one who has a greater loss of hearing that was discovered earlier. Two children with equal hearing loss may experience different degrees of impairment, because of the psychosocial and interactive/communicative environment in which they are raised.

If the catalyst for a psychosocial, educational, and/or occupational handicap resulting from either acquired or congenital hearing impairment could be pinpointed, it would probably revolve around its impact on "communication" and the interference either receptively, expressively, or both caused by a hearing impairment. A child with a severe congenital hearing loss, whether remediation is begun early or late, will have a language deficit to some degree that may impact upon educational and occupational successes, with language delay the primary basis for the communication deficit. An adult who acquires a hearing impairment that prevents adequate hearing of the speech of others may become despondent over his difficulties in maintaining an occupation or functioning socially. Again, the problem centers on an interference with communication as the result of the auditory deficit.

Aural rehabilitation and the strategies utilized in the process of aural rehabilitation center on the impact of impaired hearing on communication as experienced by adults who possess it. The majority has probably had normal hearing at some time in their lives and will probably have normal, or near normal, language function. In that regard, the impact of a hearing impairment on communicative function reveals itself from innumerable dimensions and avenues.

Children with impaired hearing may not have experienced normal language and will respond to their hearing loss, their environment, and communication in differing ways. Further, they also have parents, siblings, and other relatives who respond to them and their hearing loss in complex and varying ways.

In relation to acquired hearing loss, each adult no matter what age responds in different ways to a hearing impairment. Each has different demands, either self-imposed or externally imposed. Many have families or significant others who are also affected by the hearing deficit. For some individuals, their occupations may require precise and in-depth communication with other professionals or patients, whereas other persons' occupations require little communication with others. Some persons may have been greatly involved on a social basis, although others' social lives may have revolved around home and family. A university graduate whose spouse and parents have always had great expectations of him for success in the business world may feel a greater impact as the result of acquired hearing impairment than one who desires to be a good rancher and who is not required to communicate a great deal on his ranch in northern Montana.

Children with hearing impairment are born into families and environments that also differ. A child with profound hearing loss who is born into a family in which deafness has not previously occurred and whose parents become immobilized and noncommunicating out of self-pity and anger will not fare nearly as well as a child who is born deaf to parents who accept their child in a loving, nurturing, communicating environment.

Serving Children Who Are Hearing Impaired

Historical Background

Aural habilitation services on behalf of children have a much longer and more diverse history than services for adults who are hearing impaired. Even dating back to scholars in the 4th century BC and before, much of the history centers on education of children who are deaf, and then later the early oralism versus manualism debates. How-ever, a historical perspective is important in learning about the procedures utilized to serve children who have impaired hearing.

The recorded history of philosophical treatises on hearing impairment, children who are hearing impaired, their apparent ability to learn, and the "methods debate" on how hearing impaired children most efficiently learn language and speech began before the development of Hebrew law—that is, prior to 500 BC (Bender, 1981).

One of the first recorded philosophical opinions on the potential of children who are deaf to learn and to speak was rendered by Aristotle (355 BC). His theories and philosophies on most topics carried so much weight in his day that others not only hesi-tated questioning them, but even venturing into the topic areas at all. This situation was particularly disastrous for the hearing im-paired, because Aristotle's declaration regard-ing the "deaf" was: "Those who are born deaf all become senseless and incapable of reason. Men who are born deaf are in all cases dumb; that is to say, they can make vocal noises, but they cannot speak" (Gian-greco, 1976, p. 72). Unfortunately, the Greek words *kophoi*, meaning "deaf," and *eneos*, meaning "speechless," had at the time taken on the additional local meanings of "dumb," and even "stupid" in some instances. There-fore, a misinterpretation of Aristotle's state-ments could have become the interpreta-tion that cast the mold for children and adults who were deaf or hearing impaired for centuries.

By the 16th century, some prominent individuals, primarily priests and physicians, began to challenge the opinions of Aristotle. For example, Giralamo Cardano (1501-1576) of Italy braved the opinion that he could see no reason why people who are deaf could not be taught. In "De inventione dialectica," Cardano wrote that he had observed a man

who was born deaf who had learned to read and write, and in that manner could learn and could communicate with others. From that Cordano ventured the opinion that people who are deaf were capable of reason (Farrar, 1923).

During the 17th century, rapid advance-ments occurred in many areas, particularly in the development of educational philoso-phy, intellectual growth, political theory, and scientific thought. In relation to people who were deaf, such names as Lock (1632-1704), Francis Bacon (1561-1626), Bonet (1579-1629), Bulwer (1614-1684), and others dominated the scene. The quarrel between John Wallis (1617-1703) and William Holder (1616-1698) concerning the best method for teaching people who were deaf sparked a beginning of public interest in the area of deafness (Bender, 1981; Giangreco & Gian-greco, 1976; Hodgson, 1953).

During the 18th century, great growth occurred in services on behalf of the indi-viduals who were deaf. Jacob Pereira (1715-1780) was recognized as the first teacher of the deaf in France who, with de l'Epée (1712-1789), also of France, was among the first to make deaf education a matter of public concern. He wrote about his work and brought positive attention to the learning potential of children who are deaf (Bender, 1981; Giangreco, 1976), as did his contemporary Samuel Heinicke (1727-1790) of Germany (Hodgson, 1953). Jean Itard (1774-1838) of France conducted research into the hereditary nature of deaf-ness. He concluded that, indeed, deafness can be inherited, although it can skip gen-erations (Bender, 1981).

In the 19th century, other significant strides were made in the detection and understanding of hearing loss and education of people who are deaf. Some were impor-tant to the future of services on behalf of individuals in America who were deaf. The

Braidwoods and the Watsons were the operators of nearly all of the schools for the deaf in England, both adhering to an oral method of teaching, emphasizing oral speech (Bender, 1981; Deland, 1931). At the same time, deaf education in France was under the direction of Sicard, who emphasized a manual approach to teaching language to children who are deaf (Bender, 1981).

In America, the first school for the deaf, the American Asylum, was begun by Thomas Gallaudet (1781–1851), a proponent of manualism who is considered to be the father of deaf education in America (Bender, 1981; Giangreco, 1976). So the first school for the deaf in America was manual in orientation.

In an effort to begin an oral school in this country, on March 16, 1864, Gardiner Green Hubbard, a concerned and influential citizen, and Samuel Howe, superintendent of the Massachusetts School for the Blind, petitioned the Massachusetts General Court to incorporate an oral school for the deaf in that state. Governor Bullock of Massachusetts listened to them. After receiving a letter from philanthropist John Clarke offering $50,000 to establish an oral school for the deaf, Governor Bullock persuaded the state legislature to approve the establishment of a school. It was later named the Clark School for the Deaf and was established in October 1867 (Bender, 1981).

Alexander Graham Bell strongly influenced the future of services on behalf of children with impaired hearing in the United States. Bell's mother became deaf because of illness. Further, Alexander married Mabel Hubbard, who was deaf from scarlet fever in early childhood. When he invented the telephone, Bell also saw its potential for electronically amplifying sound for the hearing impaired. He was also moved by the impressive way that his mother and wife were able to communicate without using manual signs. So he openly differed with Gallaudet's manual approach to teaching the deaf. With $200,000 that he received from the Volta prize for his work with electricity, Bell initiated the Volta Bureau in Washington, DC, in 1867. Out of the Volta Bureau arose the Alexander Graham Bell Association for the Deaf.

The debates between Gallaudet and Bell about manualism and oralism continue today. However, those involved in the debates have as their goal the best and most efficient method for language development and communication for children who are deaf.

Current Theory and Practice

The 20th century brought more eclectic approaches for the development of language among children who are hearing impaired. Generally, the various approaches had as their goal the utilization of the most efficient sensory avenues available to children with impaired hearing. Although there are sometimes vast differences between the individual philosophies, they are all believed by adherents to be in the best interest of hearing-impaired children. Approaches are generally structured around six primary philosophies or methodologies (Boothroyd, 1982). Those include:

1. Emphasis on Speech. This philosophy centers on speech as the avenue for communication to provide a person with the requisite independence that we strive for on behalf of the deaf (Bader, 2001; Calvert & Silverman, 1975; Fry, 1978; Hochberg, Levitt, & Osberger, 1983; Kretschmer & Kretschmer, 1978; Ling, 1978, 1981, 1984a, 1984b; Ling & Milne, 1980; Osberger, Johnstone, Swarts, & Levitt, 1978; Pollack, 1970; Sanders, 1993; Vorce, 1974).

2. Emphasis on Hearing. This primarily unisensory approach emphasizes the earliest possible identification of hearing impairment in children and the earliest uses of amplification, so that the child's auditory system can play its natural role in the enhancement of auditory perceptual skills and, thus, the development of speech and language (Boothroyd, 1982). The goal is for hearing to play as great a role as possible in the development of speech and language (Bader, 2001; Boothroyd, 1982; Calvert & Silverman, 1975; Chase, 1968; Hirsh, 1966; Ling, 2001; Ling & Milne, 1980; Markides, 1983; Pollack, 1970, 1985; Simmons-Martin, 1977).

3. Manual Supplements to Speech. Cued speech is a manual supplement to lipreading. It is used as a manual supplement to an oral approach to the development of communicative competence (Berg, 2001; Cornett, 1967; Ling & Ling, 1978).

4. Emphasis on Language and Communication. This philosophy emphasizes that the mastery of language, no matter what the mode, is critical for the cognitive, emotional, and social growth of child. It supports total communication and the simultaneous use of hearing, speech, and manual communication. It is believed that the use of manual communication will provide a base for communication and that speech will emerge out of it as communicative competencies become more highly developed (Boothroyd, 1978; Fry, 1978; Groht, 1958; Harris, 1963; Kretschmer & Kretschmer, 1978, 1984; Ling, 1981; Simmons-Martin, 1977).

5. Cognitive Emphasis. With this philosophy, a specific modality for language stimulation is deemphasized. The primary concern is placed on providing children who are hearing impaired with optimal opportunities for cognitive skills development. However, proponents generally had their own personal preference about the modality emphasized (e.g., manual, auditory, total) (Blank, Rose, & Berlin, 1978; Boothroyd, 1982; Grammatico & Miller, 1974; Moeller & McConkey, 1984; Stone, 1980; Taba, 1962).

6. Emphasis on the Child and His Parents. Successful intervention on behalf of children who are hearing impaired depends, at least to a more than moderate degree, on the emotional well-being of the child, which, in turn, depends on the emotional well-being of the parents (Atkins, 2001; Boothroyd, 1982). No matter how great the expertise of the clinician, parents exert the greatest impact on the social, communicative, and emotional growth of their child (Bader, 2001; Boothroyd, 1982; Lillie, 1969; Luterman, 1987; Mindel & Vernon, 1987; Moses, 1985; Phillips, 1987).

These philosophies are individual approaches that are found to one degree or another throughout the last century. However, it is seldom that one observes a professional who employs a single approach to the exclusion of others. It is, thankfully, most common to observe a wise clinician utilizing the best of several approaches to the benefit of a child and his family.

The Potential Impact of Impaired Hearing

In discussing aural habilitation services for children, we are in most instances referring to children who possess hearing losses that are prelingual. These children generally possess a primary impairment of hearing that will, if left untreated, result in other impairments secondary to the hearing loss. An insightful treatise by Boothroyd (1982) describes the potential impact of a severe congenital hearing loss on a child if the hearing loss is left unattended. The result may include any or all of the following:

1. A Perceptual Problem. A child may have difficulty identifying objects and events by their sounds.
2. A Speech Problem. A child does not learn the connection between the movements of his speech mechanism and the resulting sounds. Consequently, the child has difficulty acquiring control of speech.
3. A Communication Problem. A child may not learn his native language. The child has difficulty understanding what people say and cannot participate in conversational exchange.
4. A Cognitive Problem. Therefore, a child has difficulty acquiring auditory/oral language. Children without language must learn about their world only from concrete aspects, not the elements that normally hearing children use, for example, the abstract elements of language.
5. A Social Problem. A child who has hearing impairment as a toddler does not hear the verbal signals signaling that he is about to transgress parental limits. At a later age, this child cannot have social rules explained to him, unless alternative avenues for communication have been established.
6. An Emotional Problem. If a child is unable to satisfy his evolving needs through spoken language, unable to make sense of the seemingly precipitous and capricious reactions of parents and peers, and constantly feeling acted upon rather than feeling in charge, the child may

become confused and angry, and may develop a poor self-image.
7. An Educational Problem. A child with limited language derives minimal benefit from formal education.
8. An Intellectual Problem. A child will be deficient in general knowledge and language competence—both of which are included in a broad definition of intelligence.
9. A Vocational Problem. Lacking in verbal skills, general knowledge, academic training, and social skills, the hearing-impaired child will reach adulthood with limited possibilities for gainful employment.
10. Parental Problems. The instinctive reactions of parents to a baby's failure to develop language are to withdraw language input and to reduce interaction. When they discover the true nature of the deficit, they may well enter a state of denial and confusion, which reduces their general effectiveness as parents and further undermines the social and emotional development of their child.
11. A Societal Problem. The withdrawal of interaction by the parents will be repeated later by society.

The Process of Aural Rehabilitation

To reduce the potential negative outcomes of a prelingual hearing loss to the extent possible, a comprehensive program of aural habilitation will need to be introduced. In fact, all children with impaired hearing will require habilitative intervention in some form. The differences lie in the degree of hearing loss, time of onset of the hearing loss, and the impact of the hearing loss and the child's environment on language development. The components will include some or all of the following:

1. Parental Guidance. It is critical that the child with hearing impairment have well-adjusted parents, in other words, parents who have overcome the anger, anxiety, and apprehension that they may have felt on diagnosis of their child's hearing loss; who have accepted their child as a child, not as a burden; and who have accepted their role in the development of their child. This requires continuity of support from the day of diagnosis and every step along the way (Sanders, 1993; see pp. 228–259).

2. Audiologic Services. Early audiological management is extremely important for both the child with hearing impairment and his parents. For the child, it is critical that amplification be offered as early as possible. Each day that amplification is not provided is a day lost in the child's auditory development. A hearing aid or hearing aids should be fit and hearing aid performance must be evaluated by the audiologist who will be involved in services for the child on a long-term basis. The clinician should do all that can be done to make the fitting of the hearing aid(s) a happy occasion. The joy is in observing a child respond and attend to sound perhaps for the first time, and to celebrate this first day in the hearing life of the child. On the other hand, a solemn and ceremonious atmosphere surely will be reflected in both the child's and the parent's acceptance of the hearing aid(s).

3. Auditory Development. This aspect of service involves providing the child the opportunity to develop an awareness of sounds in his environment and to develop the ability to recognize people and objects by the sounds they make; to make judgments about what is heard; to make judgments about where sounds come from; and to use hearing not only for recognizing speech, but for understanding and producing speech.

4. Cognitive/Language Development. Even though auditory development cannot be separated from cognitive development, and even though much of what we do in helping a child develop auditorily also involves cognitive/linguistic development of the child, the components involved in language development must be at least discussed separately. As Boothroyd (1982) observed, we are not only assisting the child to develop a "world model," or a conceptual model of his world—the raw materials from which to construct his internal world models —but also the language required to interact with it and those within it. The child must have access to a rich linguistic environment to not only learn to understand language, but to also express it (Figure 1–1).

5. Speech Development. A child should also have the opportunity for access to speech, no matter what earlier expressive mode for communication was used. Of course, if the child has no access to auditory sensitivity because of the severity of the hearing loss, the child should not be forced to use a form of communication that is doomed to failure. However, if a child appears to have access to the hearing and motor skills that will permit speech development, it should be encouraged in a natural and interactive way. If it is forced and drilled, speech training may become a dreaded and punishing experience for the child, and progress will be delayed.

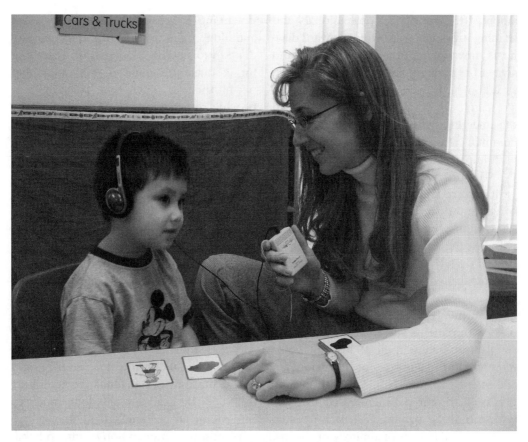

Figure 1–1. A child is involved with listening and language therapy.

Aural Rehabilitation for Adults

Historical Background

It has been interesting to note the progress of the field of audiology as an aural rehabilitation service following its advent during World War II. Its history is important as we study the process of aural rehabilitation services on behalf of adults.

Military aural rehabilitation programs provided the birthplace for the field of audiology in the 1930s. The Veterans Administration expanded the role of the audiologist and the standards for professionals and equipment in the 1930s and 1940s. The first training program for audiologists was developed at Northwestern University in the 1940s and programs expanded rapidly through the 1950s and 1960s. As a young profession, growing pains were experienced. As instrumentation became more elaborate during the 1950s and particularly the 1960s and the field became more sophisticated through research, there was a shift of emphasis toward pure and applied research and toward diagnosis of site of the lesion causing an auditory disorder. It was apparent that the emphasis among the majority of professionals and training programs was turning toward diagnosis, instrumentation, and research and away from aural rehabilitation. Results from an automated piece of equipment or from a research project were more tangible than the emerging signs of improvement in social communication observed in an adult patient with impaired hearing.

The process of working with patients with impaired hearing on the improvement of communication skills can be difficult. Interaction with younger or elderly adults with hearing impairment and helping them to deal with the emotional impact of hearing impairment along with their frustrations and fears require that the audiologist become involved on a close professional basis with patients and their families.

Unfortunately, in the 1950s and 1960s, research and diagnostics became popular, and interest in aural habilitation/rehabilitation of hearing impairment faded. Courses within training programs in the areas of differential diagnosis of auditory problems, speech and hearing sciences, instrumentation, and experimental audiology expanded rapidly and new faculty were hired to teach them. Amid the array of those courses and the blinking lights of the equipment, training programs generally offered a course titled "aural rehabilitation." When it came to finding a faculty member to teach the course, often the lowest ranking faculty member or a doctoral assistant would submit to the task. Students generally reflected the same passive response, not only in regard to the course or courses, but also to aural rehabilitation practicum experiences with children and adults who possessed hearing impairment. However, in most instances, that attitude does not prevail today. A more humanistic approach to services on behalf of people with impaired hearing is becoming predominant among practicing professionals and professors of audiology training programs and their students. Prospective students are searching for graduate programs in audiology that permit them to concentrate on learning to provide restorative services, including the fitting and dispensing of hearing aids and other nonhearing assistive listening devices, counseling, and other such professional services. So our field appears to be achieving a healthy balance.

Academy of Rehabilitative Audiology

One of the positive steps taken during the past four decades toward strengthening the professional stature of aural rehabilitation, the professionals who provide those services, and students in training who desire to provide them after graduation was the origin of the Academy of Rehabilitative Audiology in 1966. The academy has done much to bring about an awareness of the importance of professional preparation in aural rehabilitation and services on behalf of children and adult patients with impaired hearing.

As procedures for providing aural rehabilitative services for children, adults, and aging persons with hearing impairment become more sophisticated, along with increased emphasis on the need for professional involvement in the fitting and dispensing of hearing aids and subsequent follow-up, the professional prominence and stature of the rehabilitative/restorative aspects of audiology continue to expand. But as a primary health care profession, both the diagnostic and habilitative/rehabilitative aspects of audiology must carry an equal share of the responsibility in serving children and adults with impaired hearing. This is also true in conducting research to discover new and more effective ways of providing those services.

The Process of Adult Aural Rehabilitation: Definitions and Considerations

What are aural rehabilitation and the provision of aural rehabilitation services on the behalf of adults with hearing impairment? Aural rehabilitation is defined as an attempt to reduce the barriers to communication that result from hearing impairment and facilitate adjustment to the possible psychosocial, educational, and occupational impacts of that auditory deficit. In discussing aural rehabilitation, we are generally referring to serving those who had normal to near-normal hearing post-lingually but have sustained hearing loss that, if left untreated, may impede social, occupational, and educational functioning. The persons who possess impaired hearing vary in age, gender, and social status as greatly as the type, audiometric configuration, and degree of their hearing loss. If viewed from the provision of aural rehabilitation services, services on their behalf may include the following.

Assessment of Hearing

Assessment of an individual's hearing, per se, and the determination of his ability to hear and understand speech are the first important steps in the aural rehabilitation process. In the past, this step may have been the first and last, except for possible referral for a hearing aid if one appeared warranted. Often other avenues for remediation of an auditory impairment were not taken. For example, according to Rosen (1967) in an early treatise on aural rehabilitation,

> As he [the patient] takes leave of the audiologist, he knows that he has a hear-

ing loss. . . . It is true that the audiologist may have mentioned lipreading, auditory training, or training in the use of a hearing aid, but probably did not offer those services himself. Furthermore, the advice was likely offered half-heartedly, as if the audiologist was really not aware of or convinced of its value. (p. 42)

This attitude is not as widespread as it appeared to be in the early 1960s, but it is still with us to some degree. If the attitude of the audiologist who conducts an audiologic evaluation is such that he is not convinced of the value of aural rehabilitative/restorative services, two things are possible. The individual with the auditory deficit may either not be referred for rehabilitative services, or the patient may become so discouraged as a result of the audiologist's attitude that even though a referral is made, the patient may not keep the appointment. It is discouraging to find audiologists who apparently entered the field of audiology because it is a helping profession, but who feel uncomfortable when they must interact with people with impaired hearing on a face-to-face basis. Nevertheless, the accurate assessment of the extent of a hearing deficit, per se, is the first step in the process of aural rehabilitation. With that information, (a) assessment of the handicapping effects of the hearing loss, (b) the initiation of a hearing aid fitting, (c) counseling, and (d) the other steps involved in the aural rehabilitation program can begin including family involvement and the development of strategies for communication in spite of the hearing loss.

Assessment of the Benefits of Amplification

Discussion of the benefits of amplification for individual patients should be the second step in the aural rehabilitation treatment process, along with, if indicated, the fitting and dispensing of the instruments. Correspondingly, along with the fitting and dispensing of hearing aids, assessment of the handicapping effects of the hearing loss should be made. In that regard, steps a, b, and c in this sequence must go hand in hand.

An accurate determination of a patient's candidacy for hearing aids can be made by a skilled audiologist who will sift through the patient's audiometric configuration, speech recognition results, and dynamic range and will also assess or discuss the specific emotional and social consequences of each patient's hearing loss and his communicative needs. The hearing aid evaluation and/or evaluation for other assistive listening devices is only one part of the total aural rehabilitation program, but it is an important part.

Assessment of the Impact of the Hearing Deficit

Assessment of the impact of the hearing deficit on individual patients is again important for formulating a viable aural rehabilitation program based on individual patients' communicative needs. The assessment may include attempts at determining the impact of the hearing loss on the individual emotionally, socially, occupationally, and educationally. In most instances, when dealing with younger and older adults with impaired hearing, the potential impact of the hearing deficit on the educational aspects of life may not be the most important. For young adults of school age, it becomes extremely important, as it is for younger or older adults who desire to be involved in continuing education programs for occupational advancement or simply for the enjoyment of learning.

There are at present a number of scales and procedures that have been out-lined for the assessment of the handicap of hearing impairment in adult patients, some of which are found in the Appendices of this book. In light of the probability that they had normal to near-normal communicative function before onset of the hearing loss, the impact of the hearing loss on the personal lives and their occupational or educational goals is, in many ways, a personal thing. Everyone is affected differently.

The results of the audiometric evaluation provide an audiologist with information regarding the possible communicative impact resulting from the hearing loss, particularly when observing the shape of the audiogram notations, the degree and configuration of hearing loss, and a patient's ability to hear and understand speech. A patient's response to that specific hearing loss can be evaluated and taken into consideration as his treatment program is being developed, including the possible fitting and dispensing of hearing aids. The perceptive audiologist will be able to observe patient behaviors and respond appropriately to them.

Evaluation of the impact of the hearing impairment on adult patients, then, is an important part of an ongoing aural rehabilitation program. It is, however, a task that is probably never finished, because as patients face new situations, their responses to them will differ. As physical, occupational, and personal environments change, so do the responses of persons to their hearing impairment. Evaluation, therefore, is ongoing and patients must also be taught to evaluate themselves and their reactions to new communicative environments.

Perhaps the most important component of the evaluation process prior to the initiation of services and affecting the decision to terminate them is the patient's own opinion, or self-assessment of his ability to function communicatively in his own communicating world. We can administer sophisticated scales of communication, but probably the most important measure is the response we receive when we ask our patient to describe the situation in which he has his greatest difficulty hearing, and the one that is the least difficult. Scales for evaluating communicative ability are found in the Appendices of this book.

The Treatment Program

A formal aural rehabilitation treatment program is, of course, not separated in any way from the procedures previously discussed, but rather it is an extension of them. It involves (a) ongoing counseling to facilitate adjustment to the hearing loss, (b) facilitating increased efficiency in communication including establishment of priorities in communication, and (c) developing a treatment program that targets each individual patient's communicative needs, if a "formal" treatment program is warranted. The procedures used may involve efforts toward greater efficiency of the use of a patient's residual hearing, greater awareness and use of visual clues in communication, modification of the patient's frequented communicative environments, and other specific tasks. Of course, the patient's family and significant others are important elements in the total process of aural rehabilitation, and it is important that they be involved to the extent possible from the beginning (Figure 1–2).

Formal treatment programs may not be the most important aspect of the aural rehabilitation effort, but for many patients who can benefit from treatment strategies that

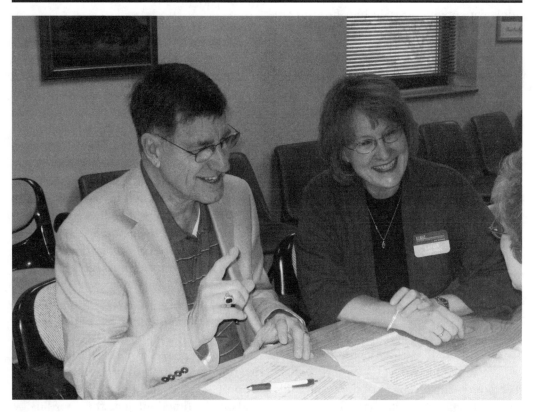

Figure 1–2. An adult and his spouse are both involved in learning communication strategies.

may enhance communication in their most difficult environments, they are a critical aspect of the total process. The process, for example, may involve problem solving of difficult listening situations. The most successful aural rehabilitation treatment programs are those in which information sharing, counseling, and hearing aid orientation are involved.

Involvement of Other Professionals

Involvement of other professionals, perhaps including the vocational rehabilitation counselor, the social worker, educational personnel, the speech/language specialist, and the psychologist, is important to the ongoing aural rehabilitation program for individual patients who require those services. For older adult patients who reside in a health care facility, involvement of facility personnel is critical. Included may be the activity director, occupational therapist, social worker, nurses, nurses' aides, and others who are in close contact with the patients. It is incumbent on the audiologist to call on other professionals to facilitate the rehabilitation process. It is also important to know when the problems an adult is facing are beyond the scope of an audiologist's knowledge and skill, and to be aware of proper referral sources. As a team leader in the aural rehabilitation process, the audiologist can function as a catalyst in the development of a truly comprehensive rehabilitation process for those patients who require additional services.

Involvement of the Family

The positive involvement of the family and/ or significant others in a patient's life can be one of the most strengthening aspects of the aural rehabilitation program, both for the younger and older patient. The words *positive involvement* are stressed here because involvement by a non-understanding family member, or a friend who in the end decides that he "does not have the time" or who otherwise does not desire to become involved, can be damaging. If a spouse, another family member, or another significant other is to be a part of a patient's aural rehabilitation program, it is important that he be involved from the time of the initial evaluation, particularly during the period of discussion of the communicative impact of the hearing loss on the patient. As the significant other becomes aware of the impact of the hearing deficit, with appropriate guidance that person can become an important catalyst in facilitating adjustment and enhancing the communication abilities of the patient.

Summary

What is aural rehabilitation? According to Costello et al. (1974), in an early classic paper developed by members of the Committee on Rehabilitative Audiology of the American Speech-Language-Hearing Association, "Audiologic rehabilitation is designed to assist individuals with auditory disabilities to realize their optimal potential in communication regardless of age, or the age of the person at the onset of the disability" (p. 68). Even though this statement was developed over 30 years ago, the philosophy still holds true. It is a rewarding process that has as its goal the reduction of barriers to communication that may have resulted from the hearing loss. Within the process, a number of professionals may be involved, with the audiologist functioning as the coordinator, or facilitator, of the team. A patient's family will be a critical element in the process.

The process is as complex as the patient and the impact of the hearing impairment on communication and, unquestionably, it carries great responsibility. Only those audiologists who are willing to accept that responsibility should provide those services. That means coming face-to-face with people—children, younger adults, older persons, the patient's siblings, and his family—who require a close professional relationship and a service that will enhance their ability to function communicatively in their individual communicating world.

References

Atkins, D. V. (2001). Family involvement and counseling in serving children who are hearing impaired. In R. H. Hull (Ed.), *Aural Rehabilitation* (pp. 79-96). San Diego, CA: Singular.

Bader, J. L. (2001). Language development for children who are hearing impaired. In R. H. Hull (Ed.), *Aural rehabilitation* (pp. 121-134). San Diego, CA: Singular.

Ballantyne, J. (1977). *Deafness.* New York: Churchill Livingstone.

Bender, R. E. (1981). *The conquest of deafness.* Danville, IL: Interstate.

Berg, F. S. (2001). Educational management of children who are hearing impaired. In R. H. Hull (Ed.), *Aural Rehabilitation* (pp. 169-186). San Diego, CA: Singular.

Blank, M., Rose, S., & Berlin, L. (1978). *The language of learning: The preschool years.* New York: Grune & Stratton.

Boothroyd, A. (1978). Speech perception and sensorineural hearing loss. In M. Ross & T. Giolas (Eds.), *Auditory management of hearing-impaired children* (pp. 92-101). Baltimore: University Park Press.

Boothroyd, A. (1982). *Hearing impairments in young children.* Englewood Cliffs, NJ: Prentice Hall.

Calvert, D., & Silverman, S. (1975). *Speech and deafness.* Washington, DC: Alexander Graham Bell Association for the Deaf.

Chase, R. A. (1968). Motor organization of speech. In S. J. Freeman (Ed.), *The neuropsychology of spatially oriented behavior* (pp. 132-144). Homewood, IL: Dorsey Press.

Cornett, R. (1967). Cued speech. *American Annals of the Deaf, 112*, 3-13.

Costello, M. R., Freeland, E. E., Hill, M. J., Jeffers, J., Matkin, N., Stream, R. W., et al. (1974). The audiologist: Responsibilities in the habilitation of the auditorily handicapped. *ASHA, 16*, 68-70.

Deland, F. (1931). *The story of lipreading.* Washington, DC: The Volta Bureau.

Farrar, A. (1923). *Arnold on the education of the deaf.* London: Francis Carter.

Fry, D. B. (1978). Language development in the deaf child. In F. Bess (Ed.), *Childhood deafness: Causation, assessment and management* (pp. 123-142). New York: Grune & Stratton.

Giangreco, C. J. (1976). *The education of the hearing impaired.* Springfield, IL: Charles C. Thomas.

Grammatico, L., & Miller, S. (1974). Curriculum for the preschool deaf child. *The Volta Review, 79*, 19-26.

Groht, M. A. (1958). *National language for deaf children.* Washington, DC: Alexander Graham Bell Association for the Deaf.

Harris, G. (1963). *Language for the preschool deaf child.* New York: Grune & Stratton.

Hirsh, I. J. (1966). Teaching the deaf child to talk. In F. Smith & G. A. Miller (Eds.), *The genesis of language* (pp. 129-138). Cambridge, MA: MIT Press.

Hochberg, I., Levitt, H., & Osberger, M. J. (Eds.). (1983). *Speech of the hearing impaired.* Baltimore: University Park Press.

Hodgson, K. (1953). *The deaf and their problems.* London: Watts.

Kretschmer, R., & Kretschmer, L. (1978). *Language development and intervention with the hearing impaired.* Baltimore: University Park Press.

Kretschmer, R., & Kretschmer, L. (1984). Habilitation of language of deaf children. In W. H. Perkins (Ed.), *Current therapy of communication disorders: Hearing disorders* (pp. 212–235). New York: Thieme-Stratton.

Lillie, S. M. (1969). *Management of deafness in infants and very young children.* Paper presented at the 47th Annual International Convention of the Council for Exceptional Children, Denver, CO.

Ling, D. (1978). Auditory coding and recording: An analysis of auditory training procedures for hearing-impaired children. In M. Ross & T. Giolas (Eds.), *Auditory management of hearing-impaired children: Principles and prerequisites for intervention* (pp. 98–120). Baltimore: University Park Press.

Ling, D. (1980). Early speech development. In G. T. Mencher & S. E. Gerber (Eds.), *Early management of hearing loss* (pp. 128–142). New York: Grune & Stratton.

Ling, D. (1984). *Early intervention for hearing-impaired children: Oral options.* Boston: College Hill Press.

Ling, D. (1984). *Early intervention for hearing-impaired children: Total communication options.* Boston: College Hill Press.

Ling, D. (2001). Speech development for children who are hearing impaired. In R. H. Hull (Ed.), *Aural rehabilitation* (pp. 145–168). San Diego, CA: Singular/Thomson Learning.

Ling, D., & Ling, A. (1978). *Aural habilitation: The foundations of verbal learning in hearing-impaired children.* Washington, DC: Alexander Graham Bell Association for the Deaf.

Ling, D., & Milne, M. M. (1980). The development of speech in hearing-impaired children. In F. Bess, B. A. Freeman, & J. S. Sinclair (Eds.), *Amplification in education* (pp. 245–270). Washington, DC: Alexander Graham Bell Association for the Deaf.

Luterman, D. (1987). *Deafness in the family.* Boston: College Hill Press.

Markides, A. (1983). *The speech of hearing-impaired children.* Manchester, UK: Manchester University Press.

Mindel, E. D., & Vernon, M. (1987). *They grow in silence: The deaf child and his family.* Silver Spring, MD: National Association for the Deaf.

Moeller, M. P., & McConkey, A. J. (1984). Language intervention with preschool deaf children: A cognitive/linguistic approach. In W. H. Perkins (Ed.), *Current therapy of communication disorders: Hearing disorders* (pp. 287–302). New York: Thieme-Stratton.

Moses, K. L. (1985). Infant deafness and parental grief: Psychosocial early intervention. In F. Powell et al. (Eds.), *Education of the hearing-impaired child* (pp. 223–231). San Diego, CA: College Hill Press.

Osberger, M. J., Johnstone, A., Swarts, E., & Levitt, H. (1978). The evaluation of a model speech training program for deaf children. *Journal of Communication Disorders, 11,* 293–313.

Phillips, A. L. (1987). Working with parents. A story of personal and professional growth. In D. Adkins (Ed.), Families and their hearing-impaired children. *The Volta Review, 89*(5), 131–146.

Pollack, D. (1970). *Educational audiology for the limited hearing infant.* Springfield, IL: Charles C. Thomas.

Pollack, D. (1985). *Educational audiology for the limited hearing infant and pre-schooler.* Springfield, IL: Charles C. Thomas.

Rosen, J. (1967). *The role of the audiologist in aural rehabilitation.* Unpublished manuscript, University of Denver.

Sanders, D. A. (1993). *Management of hearing handicap: Infants to elderly.* Englewood Cliffs, NJ: Prentice Hall.

Simmons-Martin, A. (1977). Natural language and auditory input. In F. Bess (Ed.), *Childhood deafness: Causation, assessment and management* (pp. 111–128). New York: Grune & Stratton.

Stone, P. (1980). Developing thinking skills in young hearing-impaired children. *The Volta Review, 82*(6), 345–353.

Taba, H. (1962). *Curriculum development: Theory and practice.* New York: Harcourt, Brace and World.

Vorce, E. (1974). *Teaching speech to deaf children.* Washington, DC: Alexander Graham Bell Association for the Deaf.

End of Chapter Examination Questions

Chapter 1

1. **According to the author, the primary objective of aural rehabilitation is to:**
   a. assist hearing-impaired persons to overcome the handicap of hearing impairment.
   b. diagnose the hearing impairment.
   c. treat the hearing impairment.

2. **Which of the following problems might a child who possesses a severe congenital hearing loss experience?**
   a. social problems
   b. cognitive problems
   c. emotional problems
   d. all of the above

3. **Auditory development is generally defined as:**
   a. the physical maturation of the auditory system.
   b. the ability of the patient to be aware of and recognize sounds in his environment.
   c. structuring an auditory intervention plan for the patient.

4. **Assessment of an individual's hearing is generally thought of as the first step in the process of aural rehabilitation. According to the author, that assessment should begin with:**
   a. the fitting of an amplification device.
   b. determining the extent of a high-frequency hearing loss.
   c. determining the ability to hear and understand speech.
   d. determining the impact of one's hearing loss on social issues.

5. **The second step in aural rehabilitation should be:**
   a. assessment of the type of hearing loss.
   b. assessment of amplification benefits.
   c. assessment of the impact of hearing loss on the individual.

6. **Besides the audiologist, another professional (other professionals) who might be involved in the aural rehabilitation process is (are):**
   a. the vocational counselor.
   b. the social worker.
   c. the speech-language pathologist.
   d. all of the above.

7. **In aural rehabilitation programs, the audiologist generally functions as the team leader. What role(s) might he or she play?**

8. (True/False) According to the information presented in this chapter, an aural rehabilitation program focuses exclusively on increasing the efficiency of communication.

9. (True/False) All individuals experience an equal degree of handicap from equal degrees of hearing loss.

10. (True/False) Aural rehabilitation programs with all ages of patients are equally enhanced by positive family involvement.

End of Chapter Answer Sheet

Name _____   Date _____

Chapter 1

    1. Which one(s)?   a   b   c

    2. Which one(s)?   a   b   c   d

    3. Which one(s)?   a   b   c

    4. Which one(s)?   a   b   c   d

    5. Which one(s)?   a   b   c

    6. Which one(s)?   a   b   c   d

    7. _____

    _____

    _____

Circle one:

    8. True or False?

    9. True or False?

    10. True or False?

2

Introduction to the Handicap of Hearing Impairment: Auditory Impairment versus Hearing Handicap

JACK KATZ AND THOMAS P. WHITE

Chapter Outline

Introduction

To understand the aural rehabilitative needs of a patient, a careful interview should be carried out as well as a battery of audiometric procedures. An in-depth interview or questionnaire and specialized diagnostic tests are required to obtain the broadest understanding of the hearing level and habilitative/rehabilitative needs. In the end, however, there will always be an element of uncertainty. This limitation in precise prediction is due to variations in each patient's mental and physical abilities, motivation, alertness, and other factors. Even when accurate audiometric data are obtained, the specialist is left with many questions regarding a person's hearing and communicative needs. For example, audiologists do not know with whom the person communicates and if it is within a large lecture hall, an elementary school classroom, or over a taxicab CB radio. Auditory tests do not tell clinicians if a child has a well-developed vocabulary and language system or if she has optimal classroom conditions. Unless audiologists test further, they will not know how well individuals are able to use visual information to supplement auditory information. Responses to questionnaires can often help the audiologist in gaining a patient's perspective and other insights (Kaplan, Bally, & Brandt, 1990; Lamb, Owens, & Schubert, 1983).

It is helpful to begin with a discussion of terminology. For example, sometimes cause and effect are confused with measurement and function.

Functional Terminology

Some individuals, even professionals, may use the terms *hearing loss*, *hearing level*, *hearing impairment*, and *hearing handi-* cap interchangeably. This is not helpful in understanding the needs of each individual. The following sections delineate these terms.

Hearing Level versus Hearing Loss

Hearing level (HL) is a measurement made on an audiometer and reported in decibels (American National Standards Institute [ANSI], 2004). Hearing levels obtained in a controlled acoustical environment compare a patient's performance to the responses of individuals in a standard population, that is, a population with normal hearing. In essence, it is the dial reading on an audiometer at which an individual responds in a specified manner. Hearing loss is used to indicate the type of problem (e.g., conductive versus sensorineural), or the amount of hearing that has been lost (Davis & Silverman, 1978). If a person's 40 dB threshold is labeled as a 40 dB HL (hearing level), but it was previously known to be 25 dB, then it could also be said that it is a 45 dB hearing loss.

It should be noted that the criteria for significant hearing loss for children is often lower than for adults. This is, because they cannot rely on the linguistic and world knowledge of adults to help them make sense of what they hear and because of the demands to learn new vocabulary and concepts and terms, hearing levels over 15 dB may be considered significant (Stredler Brown, in press).

Hearing Impairment versus Hearing Handicap

Hearing impairment is closely associated with hearing level and the terms are sometimes used interchangeably. Hearing impairment can also relate to measures that are not in dB, such as word recognition scores. Hearing impairment implies that performance is poorer than normal. It is generally categorized as mild, moderate, or severe. Hearing handicap refers to the interference in communication/hearing that results from a hearing loss. Thus, the negative influence of a hearing impairment on the person's ability in life situations is the hearing handicap. For example, an individual with a hearing level of 30 dB HL may have more difficulty in her communicative environment than another individual with a 50 dB HL, because the first person may have greater communicative demands in her occupational or personal life.

Relationship of Terms

The terms just described can best be understood as they relate to individual cases. Two case presentations may clarify their use.

Case 1

A 42-year-old woman was seen by an audiologist following a sudden onset of tinnitus and hearing loss. The audiometric results revealed a flat sensorineural hearing loss. The pure-tone speech-frequency average was 45 dB HL in each ear. According to a pre-employment audiogram, the patient had normal hearing with an average of 8 dB HL in each ear. Thus, there was a 37 dB hearing loss associated with the incident. Her hearing impairment is classified as moderate. The actual hearing handicap is greater than this because the patient reports considerable difficulty in communicating. The problem is more acute in this case, because the patient works as a librarian and people tend to speak softly in libraries.

Case 2

A 5-year-old child attends a regular kindergarten class. He has normal hearing up to 1000 Hz in each ear, but at this point his thresholds fall off markedly. The hearing level at 2000 Hz is 35 dB poorer than his 0 dB HL at 1000 Hz. Although there is a mild hearing impairment according to standard classifications, this child has major difficulties in distinguishing high-frequency consonants from one another and in developing age-appropriate verbal concepts. This problem is increased because the child has been placed in a relatively noisy classroom with a teacher who has never had a child with a hearing impairment in her class. In addition, she does not know the special accommodations that should be made for this particular youngster. Thus, the level of difficulty is underestimated when simply looking at the hearing level. These concepts are discussed further by Weinstein, Richards, and Montano (1995).

Congenital versus Acquired Hearing Loss

One factor that influences the effect of a hearing loss is when it occurred. Severe congenital or prelingual hearing losses (losses prior to the development of aural speech and language) have a great impact on language, voice, and articulation, because the individual may not develop these skills normally. Such an individual generally does not have constant language stimulation or accurate feedback of her own speech production. As an adult, the person may continue to have limitations in language, as well as in voice and articulation. Prelingual hearing disorders also have a more deleterious effect on social, educational, and vocational aspects of a person's life, than if the hearing loss occurred after oral speech and language developed.

The same type of loss at an older age, especially a sudden catastrophic loss of hearing, will likely have a profound influence on an individual, but of a much different type. There will be no diminution of the person's language ability and relatively little change in her voice quality. However, over a period, articulatory movements will tend to become less precise, typically affecting the high-frequency sibilant sounds first. Because the individual is not able to monitor articulation and voice effectively, she may compensate for this by increasing speech volume.

A sudden catastrophic loss is usually more devastating than one of gradual onset in two ways. First, the psychological impact of isolation is much greater because of the suddenness of the onset. Second, the person who has a sudden onset of hearing loss will tend to have difficulty utilizing her residual hearing to make fine distinctions among, for example, the sounds of speech. Patients with progressive hearing loss have been able to alter their auditory perceptions in a gradual manner. The person with a sudden loss may not know how to listen for clues to distinguish, for example, the singular form of a word from the plural, whereas the person whose hearing has diminished over time may have developed strategies for doing so.

Obviously, the complex interactions of people, their needs and environments, and the various test indicators provide infinite possibilities about a person who has a hearing loss. Audiometric results give us guidance and general knowledge about a patient's hearing, but in the end, they fail to reveal things that the patient or the patient's family can tell an audiologist. The contribution of audiometric test results in predicting hearing handicap is discussed in the following section.

Types of Hearing Loss

Conductive Loss

Knowing the type of hearing loss can help in predicting the handicap that a patient has. For example, conductive losses, particularly when the patient possesses normal to near normal bone conduction, are associated with good discrimination ability for speech. Patients with conductive hearing loss may achieve very good speech discrimination simply from increased volume. Although the communicative effects of conductive loss in an adult are not as severe as an equivalent sensorineural loss, there is growing evidence that a mild conductive loss early in life may have significant long-term effects (Dalzell & Orwid, 1976; Holm & Kunze, 1969; Secord, Erickson, & Bush, 1988). Furthermore, in some cases, earmold drainage may contraindicate the use of an earmold for the hearing aid, and a conductive overlay on top of a sensorineural problem can complicate the use and types of amplification. Figure 2–1 is an example of an audiogram that reveals a conductive hearing loss.

Cochlear Loss

Most cochlear (sensory) losses reveal some diminished word recognition ability. There is usually a direct relationship between hearing level and the ability to discriminate speech (Thompson & Hoel, 1962). Generally speaking, the more depressed the hear-

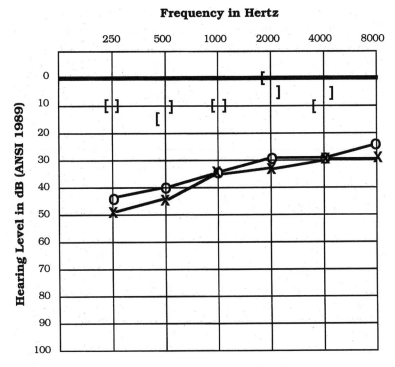

Frequency in Hertz

Figure 2–1. Example of a conductive hearing loss.

ing level, the poorer the word recognition score. Disorders of the cochlea produce a variety of audiometric patterns that provide clues to their etiology. Detection of these problems can lead to preventative measures and, thus, minimize any further hearing loss. Most cochlear hearing losses are greater in the high frequencies than in the low frequencies. This is because presbycusis (hearing loss due to aging) and noise-induced hearing loss, the most common causes of sensorineural disorder, primarily affect the higher frequency region of the cochlea. On the other hand, cochlear losses associated with Ménière's disease, for example, are generally greater in the low frequencies than in the high frequencies. A flat audiometric configuration may be seen in ototoxic-related disorders. These patterns are not mutually exclusive and, thus, may overlap one another.

Another characteristic commonly seen in sensory losses is intolerance for loud sounds (often associated with recruitment). Consequently, this factor must be considered in the use of amplification. In patients with extremely small dynamic ranges, the use of amplification could be challenging. That is, some individuals with sensory losses have an intolerance for sounds only slightly above their threshold levels. This might make effective use of amplification more difficult.

Cochlear losses may also affect the speech and voice of the individual. Because inner ear functioning is decreased, the internal feedback loop is reduced to the extent that the patients are unable to monitor their own speech and voice patterns properly.

This can lead to articulation disorder as well as to reduced vocal inflection and quality. This effect is related to the extent and duration of the hearing loss. Figure 2–2 is an audiogram that shows a typical sensory (cochlear) hearing loss.

Cochlear Implants

Generally, those who benefit most from cochlear implants are those who have cochlear impairment. Cochlear implants essentially bypass the defective cochlea and stimulate fibers of the auditory nerve. These devices play an important role in the rehabilitation of patients with severe or profound hearing losses. Because cochlear implants can produce normal or near-normal thresholds, it is important to recognize that these individuals still function as hard of hearing persons and that they need more, rather than less, help from audiologists in maximizing their skills to benefit fully from their implants. Despite good sensitivity to sounds, in most cases brain reeducation is needed to enable the individual to be effective in group communications as well as in using the telephone (Katz, 1998).

Neural Loss

The effects of a neural hearing loss, which is caused by a decline in function of the auditory nerve (cranial nerve VIII) and beyond, are generally more a problem of clarity than

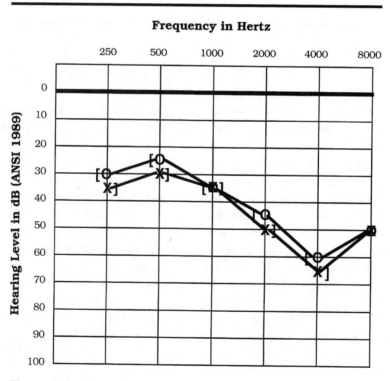

Figure 2–2. Example of a sensorineural hearing loss.

of sensitivity. Consequently, audiometric findings will usually show more significantly depressed word recognition scores than in cochlear cases with equal pure-tone thresholds. This, in turn, may complicate not only normal communications, but also the use of a hearing aid that is designed to alleviate the communicative breakdown.

Another characteristic of neural losses is the presence of reflex, or tone, decay or the inability to maintain the audibility of pure tones. For example, Costello and McGee (1967) discussed patients who appeared as either being deaf or aphasic, although their pure-tone thresholds were quite good. These cases were found to have severe discrimination losses and rapid tone decay. It should be noted that many persons with brainstem dysfunction, as well as those with CN VIII losses, have poor discrimination for speech and significant tone decay.

Central Dysfunction

Peripheral hearing disorders may be due to disease at the conductive, cochlear, or eighth nerve levels of the auditory system. Dysfunction in the brain or brainstem results in a central disorder. Although it also might produce a hearing loss, central dysfunction is generally associated with more subtle changes, including figure-ground processing and localization problems. These difficulties may compound the problems associated with a concomitant or coincidental hearing loss; however, central auditory dysfunction, by itself, can produce sufficient difficulty to cause a person to seek evaluation by an audiologist.

Stach (1989) points out that a high percentage of people who fail to benefit from hearing aids, at least among the elderly, have central processing problems. Thus,

the audiologist should consider this possibility when an individual does not receive the expected degree of benefit from amplification, or when the amount of auditory disability far outweighs the person's hearing loss as shown on the standard audiometric tests.

Unilateral versus Bilateral Hearing Loss

The problems produced by hearing loss may be increased or minimized, depending on whether the loss involves one or both ears. The difficulties associated with unilateral hearing impairments generally are not limited to the amount of loss alone. Although the thresholds in the affected ear are lowered, one would think that if either ear could hear a sound, the individual would benefit fully by its presence. In this way, the better ear would be expected to dominate and greatly reduce the adverse influence of the poorer ear. However, the handicap resulting from a unilateral loss is due not only to the loss of sensitivity, but even more likely to the imbalance between the ears, which tends to disable important central processes (Jerger, Silman, Lew, & Chmiel, 1993).

Individuals who have unilateral losses often experience some listening problems. One obvious difficulty is the lack of hearing when someone is speaking on the person's impaired side. Two other problems are not as closely linked with the severity of the loss. For one thing, people with unilateral losses can be expected to have trouble in localizing the source of a sound. But perhaps the most important problem associated with this type of loss is difficulty understanding speech in a background of noise or when the acoustical conditions are poor. Similarly, a person with a bilateral hearing loss who wears a monaural hearing aid tends to lose the benefits she might derive from the binaural system. Thus, that person cannot benefit fully from her central functions. For example, the person may be unable to separate foreground from background and to locate sounds in space.

Unilateral losses in children, although perhaps not as devastating as hearing lost suddenly in adulthood (Bardon, 1986), have potentially important consequences. A complete journal issue was devoted to the work of Bess and his colleagues, dealing with unilateral hearing loss in children (Bess, 1986). Their work confirms that unilateral losses are associated with poor localization of sound in space, as well as with difficulty on speech-in-noise tasks. The greater the loss in the poorer ear, the greater the difficulty.

What Audiometric Data Reveal

In their simplest form, hearing disorders can be viewed as changes in sensitivity, frequency range, and fidelity. Sensitivity can be likened to the decibel (intensity) variations produced by an attenuator. A reduced frequency range is similar to the effects of an acoustic filter that selectively impedes the passage of some frequencies and permits others to pass. A lack of fidelity is the distortion caused by the nonlinear transmission of a sound because of the breakdown of either peripheral or central structures.

The influence of sensitivity (degree of loss) and frequency range (configuration) are described first, because they provide the most reliable audiometric information. The disorders of fidelity (clarity), although vitally important, are not as quantifiable. Fidelity and other factors that are less precise reduce a clinician's ability to predict the handicap from the pure-tone information. The audiologist and the patient will be best served when all of the available information is used.

Degree of Loss

One of several things that audiometric data reveal is the degree of loss. This information is important, because it provides a general indication of the handicap an individual may experience. To put hearing threshold levels into perspective, general classifications are shown along with their predicted handicaps in Table 2-1. This permits an audiologist to make general statements about a person's hearing function and probable needs. However, the clinician cannot state with great certainty the specific effects of a loss. Thus, this table should be used only as a guideline, not as an absolute.

Many methods of categorization have been proposed, including those of Davis and Silverman (1978), Green (1978), and Hodgson (1978). The emphasis of each method varies, according to its purpose. These purposes include medical-legal definitions, handicapping effects, rehabilitative needs, and the impact on children versus adults.

The influence of the degree of loss may not be as obvious as it might appear. Generally, the rule of thumb is the greater the hearing level the greater the handicap. However, the actual handicap, when compared to the degree of hearing loss, may vary considerably. Important factors contributing to these differences include personality, intelligence, motivation, occupation, and environmental conditions. Individuals who rely heavily on communicative function for their work, such as salespersons, attorneys, and teachers, who possess relatively mild hearing loss may notice significantly greater handicap than those whose jobs are not as

TABLE 2–1. Relationship of Three Frequency Speech Averages to Typical Hearing Difficulties and Amplification Considerations*

ANSI (1989) Levels in Decibels	Classification	Approximate Discrimination (%)	Typical Speech Understanding (Unaided)	Typical Adult Amplification Considerations	Typical Child Amplification Considerations
0–24	Essentially normal	92	No significant limitations	Generally none but depends on configuration; high-frequency loss may benefit; possible special fittings may be warranted	Generally none but preferential seating is recommended; mild gain FM system optional on case-by-case basis for classroom
25–39	Mild	82	Difficulty with faint speech especially from a distance	Recommended based on reported degree of difficulty; mild gain canal and in-the-ear units are appropriate	Preferential seating required; mild gain hearing aid may be considered; in-the-ear or behind-the-ear units recommended based on degree of difficulty; FM systems can be considered
40–54	Moderate	70	Frequent difficulty with normal speech	Frequent to full-time hearing aid use; canal aids useful; in-the-ear and behind-the-ear instruments are more effective; assistive listening devices may be considered	Full-time use of amplification; in-the-ear style is possible but behind-the-ear instrument is preferred; supplemented in school with FM system
55–69	Moderately severe	60	Difficulty even with loud speech	Full-time hearing aid use; patient acceptance related to word discrimination ability; behind-the-ear styles most appropriate to yield best performance; direct audio input may be considered	Minimum choice is behind-the-ear units; may require special class and speech/language therapy; use of ALD system is essential

continues

TABLE 2–1. *continued*

ANSI (1989) Levels in Decibels	Classification	Approximate Discrimination (%)	Typical Speech Understanding (Unaided)	Typical Adult Amplification Considerations	Typical Child Amplification Considerations
70–89	Severe	36	Severe difficulty; loud or amplified speech might be understood	Full-time binaural hearing aid use; behind-the-ear aid is appropriate style; assistive devices considered, such as closed caption TV decoder	Minimum choice is behind-the-ear instruments; may consider body hearing aid; ALD system use is mandatory
90+	Profound	20	Understanding of speech severely limited even with amplification; use of amplification provides mostly environmental and speech clues	Minimum choice is power behind-the-ear instruments; may require body instrument; cochlear implant may be recommended in post-lingually deafened	Powerful behind-the-ear units may be possible; cochlear implant or vibrotactile aids may be considered; often requires special education program

Note. It should be pointed out that this table refers to limitations and needs related to cochlear hearing losses. Conductive, retrocochlear, and central disorders may follow a different pattern of handicap and needs. The three frequency speech average refers to the average dB value for pure tones 500 Hz, 1000 Hz, and 2000 Hz in the better ear. When appropriate, binaural amplification is preferred to monaural.

verbally demanding (e.g., truck drivers, farmers, industrial workers). Individuals who tend to socialize more (those who go to parties and the theater) will notice hearing losses sooner than people who tend to stay home and read, watch television, and relate only to close family members.

The influence of the degree of hearing loss is even more critical in the case of young children in the first few years of life, especially when the problem occurs before the development of language. In cases of profound hearing loss, voice, speech, and language are likely to be substantially influenced. Abnormal breathing patterns and improper use of the vocal folds will influence intonation and stress patterns (Whitehead & Barefoot, 1983). Also, the fundamental frequency of the voice is generally higher than normal (Gilbert & Campbell, 1980). Vocal onset confusions, which result from not knowing how to produce the sounds, affect both a child's understanding and production of voiced and voiceless consonants (Mashie, 1980). Vowels often are substituted for one another and final consonants frequently are omitted (Levitt & Stromberg, 1983).

Less severe hearing losses have correspondingly fewer communicative consequences; however, in any given group there will be notable exceptions. Often, because of unknown reasons, an individual with relatively little hearing will perform especially well. This is most obvious in classrooms for those with hearing impairment in which students with the poorer hearing may perform better in dealing with verbal information than those who possess milder hearing losses. Further, predicting a hearing handicap based on pure-tone thresholds in people who have cochlear implants can be quite perplexing. Even gross generalities do not hold, because of the great dissimilarity between normal or aided hearing versus the electrical stimulation through a cochlear implant.

Configuration of Loss

The shape of an audiogram helps to determine the frequency characteristics of the auditory information an individual receives. When both the audiometric configuration of a patient's hearing and the energy distribution of the incoming auditory signals are known, the audiologist can better understand the speech sounds the patient is generally able to hear. An audiologist often looks at the patient's binaural hearing to determine the sounds that she will hear best. This is done by noting the better threshold at each frequency for the two ears. Although this approach is likely a valid one, it is limited in a number of ways. Although it does consider hearing level, it does not consider the locus of lesion, the unilateral/bilateral nature of the loss, and the clarity of the incoming information.

The configuration of hearing loss is considered in the following text as if it were produced by acoustic filtering. Using this approach, the audiologist can obtain important information to better understand a patient's communicative abilities and deficits. Other variables that influence performance are discussed later.

Flat Configuration

A flat configuration is seen in a pure-tone audiogram in which there are relatively small differences in thresholds across the audiometric frequencies. However, this does not imply the same exact dB hearing level throughout the audiogram. In fact, slightly sloping and jagged patterns are frequently considered flat because they are not extreme enough to be classified as high- or low-frequency curves. Figure 2–3 is an example of an audiogram with a flat configuration.

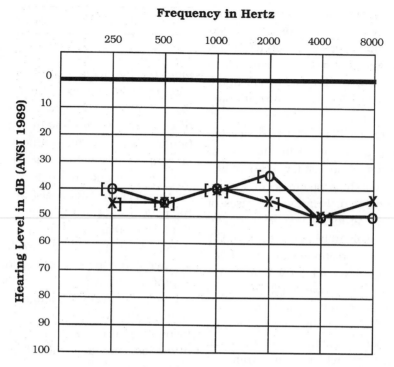

Figure 2–3. Example of a hearing loss with a flat configuration.

The audiologist can assume that a flat loss will limit the input evenly across the frequencies. The major energy component of speech is in the low frequencies (250 to 500 Hz). Despite the power of those frequencies, they contain relatively little information for identifying words. There is little speech energy in the high frequencies. In the normal listener, essentially complete and accurate intelligibility comes from the frequencies 300 to 3000 Hz. The frequencies of speech that contribute most to intelligibility are between 1000 and 3000 Hz (Hodgson, 1978). This information can help clinicians to understand hearing loss as a "filter effect." Because speech contains little high-frequency energy, a flat loss is likely to affect the high-frequency information most severely and the low-frequency information least of all.

High-Frequency Configuration

Although a flat configuration tends to impact heavily on the high-frequency portion of speech signals, a high-frequency loss has an even greater effect. This type of loss is analogous to a filter with a sharply sloping reduction for the high frequencies. In other words, the low frequencies are passed on to the listener, with the high frequencies impeded and not heard or heard less well. Figure 2–4 is an example of an audiogram that depicts a high-frequency hearing loss.

A person with a predominantly high-frequency hearing loss is keenly aware of speech and environmental sounds that contain a preponderance of low-frequency energy. Thus, she is able to hear such life-saving sounds as a car horn or a verbal warning, but misses nuances, confuses words,

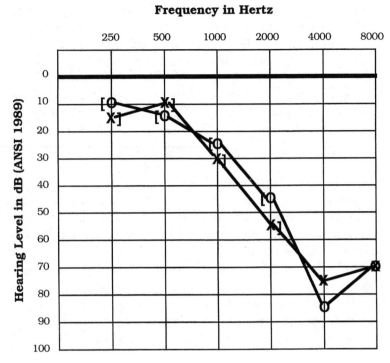

Figure 2–4. Example of a hearing loss with a high-frequency configuration.

and may not understand the punch lines of jokes. These individuals also have difficulty in locating the source of a sound, understanding speech from another room, and blocking out background sounds.

When there is a major difference between a person's hearing in the low and middle frequencies versus those in the upper frequency range, this difference may create a problem for the audiologist in planning appropriate amplification. The specific frequency at which a loss drops off is most important, especially if it is within the speech frequencies.

Individuals with high-frequency losses are often accused of hearing just what they want to hear or simply of not paying attention. For example, they may easily recognize their names and familiar phrases from

the low-frequency components, but fail to understand when the language or concepts become complex or abstract. Furthermore, their level of understanding can be expected to fall sharply when the listening environment is noisy or otherwise distracting.

Low-Frequency Configuration

Bilateral low-frequency audiometric configurations are less common and have the fewest disadvantages than most other configurations. Low-frequency information is the most powerful and the most expendable portion of the speech signal. Thus, from a simple filter effect, the patient retains the most important part of the frequency range and should have good discrimination for speech. The one exception to this rule is when the low-frequency loss is associated with brainstem pathology, which may result in reduced speech discrimination. Even in those instances, the patient's voice is generally unaffected and articulation usually remains normal. Figure 2–5 is an example of an audiogram that shows a low-frequency hearing loss.

Saucer-Shaped Configuration

Occasionally, a saucer-shaped audiometric curve is observed. This pattern is characterized by better thresholds for the high and low frequencies than for those in the midrange. Thus, the sounds that are most important for speech recognition are diminished the most. Although this configuration of loss would appear to be extremely hand-

icapping, we often find good speech thresholds and very good speech recognition scores. This may be because saucer-shaped losses are frequently congenital in nature. Therefore it is likely that, over the years, affected individuals refine their ability to derive phonemic cues from the higher and lower frequency information. Figure 2–6 is an example of an audiogram that depicts a saucer-shaped hearing loss.

Speech Thresholds and Word Recognition Scores

Standard speech threshold and discrimination/recognition tests are administered to understand a person's hearing ability under optimum conditions (such as those found

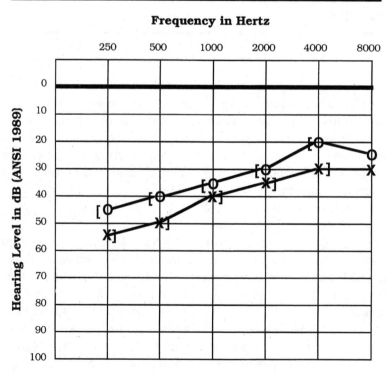

Figure 2–5. Example of a hearing loss with a low-frequency configuration.

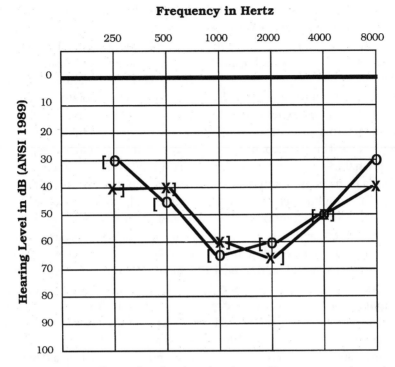

Figure 2–6. Example of a hearing loss with a saucer-shaped configuration.

in a sound-treated environment and spoken by an excellent speaker). The expected relationship between pure-tone thresholds and word recognition scores can be estimated by way of the percentage scores obtained to help identify those who have excessive difficulty with speech clarity (Dubno, Lee, Klein, Matthews, & Lam, 1995). Suprathreshold measures such as most comfortable loudness (MCL) and uncomfortable loudness (UCL) tests can be administered to help predict how comfortably an individual will handle amplified speech (e.g., a hearing aid).

Good speech recognition, along with a moderate speech threshold and a wide dynamic range of comfortable listening, encourages audiologists to think that an individual will obtain good results with properly fitted amplification. However, poor word discrimination with very poor pure-tone thresholds may complicate achieving excellent aided results. The hypersensitivity to moderate levels of speech may call for complex solutions to enable the individual to fully benefit from amplification.

Because standard speech threshold and discrimination measures generally employ single word tasks, they are not representative of normal conversation, not to mention the absence of background noise and use of professional speakers. The measures do not take into account the context of conversations, inflections, and visual cues. Thus, a variety of speech measures is needed to accurately represent a person's performance under normal listening conditions. The Central Institute for the Deaf's Everyday Speech Sentence lists (Davis & Silverman,

1978) and the Harvard Psycho-Acoustic Laboratory (PAL) question-and-answer type materials are often used for testing longer speech strings (Hudgins, Hawkins, Karlin, & Stevens, 1947).

Early tests of speech recognition failed to address the difficulties experienced by people with losses that primarily involved the high frequencies. This problem has been resolved somewhat by the use of tests such as the California Consonant Test (Owens & Schubert, 1977), a multiple-choice procedure that requires careful attention to high-frequency consonant sounds.

The evaluation of young children poses additional challenges to an audiologist. Speech threshold and recognition measures generally require modification, if they can be used at all. If time tested materials such as the Haskins Phonetically Balanced Kindergarten Word Lists (PBKs; Haskins, 1949) or the Word Intelligibility by Picture Identification test (WIPI; Ross & Lerman, 1970) are not successful, informal procedures can be employed.

Other Audiometric Tests

Other audiometric tests, many of which were more recently developed, enable the audiologist to obtain a better understanding of the patient. Acoustic immittance measurements are of great value in determining the need and type of rehabilitative services for an individual. Tympanometry, which measures the mobility of the tympanic membrane, permits an evaluation of middle ear status. If a middle ear problem, such as otitis media, is present, then medical referral is warranted. Determining the presence or absence of acoustic reflex thresholds may differentiate middle ear from inner ear deafness.

Another important procedure that is useful for young children and the difficult-to-test is the auditory brainstem response (ABR). Although hearing aid evaluations with those who can communicate effectively do not need such elaborate procedures to verify the benefit of a hearing aid, this might be necessary for young children and others who may not provide reliable responses to other test stimuli. ABR audiometry utilizes minute electrical potentials that can be measured on the scalp to monitor the activity of the acoustic nerve and central auditory system when auditory signals are presented to the ears. The audiologist can assess the levels at which the auditory system produces acceptable electrical responses from the CN VIII and brainstem. This will help an audiologist to ascertain if there is a functional auditory system when the child is too young to respond accurately, if an aid might be of benefit, and at what level the aid should be set.

A number of behavioral tests also can be of importance when assessing a patient for rehabilitation. Tests of central function may explain why a particular individual does not fully benefit from amplification (Stach, 1989). When central tests show that one ear is especially deficient (regardless of the peripheral test performance), then the other ear might be considered more strongly for amplification.

Tests that provide speech signals embedded in competing noises may be used as a more realistic measure of performance in real-life situations. Specially developed tests such as the Speech in Noise Test (SIN; Killion & Villichur, 1993) and the HINT (Hearing in Noise Test; Nilsson, Soli, & Sullivan, 1994) have been used to quantify the effect of background noise on speech understanding. In addition, the Speech Perception in Noise (SPIN; Kalikow, Stevens, & Elliot, 1977) test has been used for this purpose for many years.

Limitations of Audiometric Information

Audiometric data can accurately describe a person's hearing status, but cannot reveal with any precision how well an individual gets along in her personal and professional communication environments. The specifics and complexities of real-life situations are too idiosyncratic for audiologists to make accurate predictions about how each complex individual will perform or react (Hargus & Gordon-Salants, 1995). Thus, audiologists can make assumptions and generalizations, but they should try to validate them through interviews and informal testing. Certain information may never be known. The following examples illustrate these uncertainties.

Case 1

A college student inadvertently pushed a cotton swab through his tympanic membrane. He was tested audiometrically over time until his hearing improved to a level of about 10 dB poorer than his normal ear. At this point, both ears were within normal audiometric limits. After 5 years, the patient continues to feel that the hearing deviation has affected him greatly. He is annoyed because the two ears hear differently and he is highly distracted by background noise.

Case 2

At the other end of the continuum is a child who has severe-to-profound hearing impairment but who performs better than other individuals with normal hearing could be expected to perform. He excels in foreign languages, plays a musical instrument, and communicates without obvious handicap when facing the speaker at a distance of not greater than 15 feet. We believe that this is due, in large measure, to early binaural amplification and a mother who had been determined that her child would develop normal speech and language.

Educational and Vocational Considerations

Educational

The child or young adult who has hearing impairment will be faced with limitations in a mainstreamed classroom perhaps more than any other setting. Despite the numerous potential advantages of integrating a child with a hearing impairment into a typical class, the challenge may be considerable. By definition, school is a setting in which new information and unfamiliar concepts are presented. Unlike the rest of the class, the child or adult who has auditory impairment must attempt to determine what was said and then deal with it at the cognitive level that the teacher intended.

In recent years, many forms of assistive listening devices have become available to help people who are limited in their auditory function to pursue their education along with normally hearing individuals (Crandell & Smaldino, 1995). These devices and approaches are discussed in greater length elsewhere in this textbook.

Vocational

As in the classroom, the workplace provides many challenges to a person who has hearing impairment. People choose careers that are suited to their abilities but which may be affected by their limitations. Hearing-impaired individuals generally avoid jobs that require intensive communication. However, in recent years we have seen a growing number of students who are disabled enter fields that were in earlier years considered out of their reach. For example, individuals who are partially sighted or have hearing impairment now become physicians and lawyers. New vocational opportunities make the need for efficient and innovative management strategies even greater than in the earlier times when a person's options were more severely limited by her hearing impairment.

Summary

In this chapter we have discussed the implications of audiometric findings on the needs of individuals who have hearing impairment. Much information can be obtained from basic audiometric procedures that shed light on the auditory status and auditory capabilities of these people. This, in turn, helps in developing a rehabilitative plan that can address their communicative needs.

Although audiometric data provide crucial information in understanding a patient's problems, the audiologist must also be aware of the test limitations. It is often difficult to generalize from formal tests to a person's day-to-day life. To fill those gaps, audiologists must seek information from interviews, questionnaires, and other sources.

References

American National Standards Institute. (2004). Specifications for Audiometers. ANSI S3.6. New York: American National Standards Institute.

Bardon, J. I. (1986). Unilateral sensorineural hearing loss: From the inside out, a patient's perspective. *The Hearing Journal, 39*, 13–17.

Bess, F. (Ed.). (1986). The unilaterally hearing-impaired child. [Special issue]. *Ear and Hearing, 7*(1), 1–54.

Costello, M. R., & McGee, T. M. (1967). Language impairment associated with bilateral abnormal auditory information. In A. B. Graham (Ed.), *Sensory processes and disorders* (pp. 86–97). Boston: Little Brown.

Crandell, C., & Smaldino, J. (1995). An update of classroom acoustics for children with hearing loss. *The Volta Review, 1*, 4–12.

Dalzell, J., & Orwid, H. L. (1976). Children with conductive deafness: A follow-up study. *British Journal of Audiology, 10*, 87–90.

Davis, H., & Silverman, S. R. (1978). *Hearing and deafness.* New York: Holt, Rinehart & Winston.

Dubno, J., Lee, F., Klein, A., Matthews, L., & Lam, C. (1995). Confidence limits for maximum word-recognition scores. *Journal of Speech and Hearing Research, 38*, 490–502.

Gilbert, H. R., & Campbell, M. I. (1980). Speaking fundamental frequency in three groups of hearing-impaired individuals. *Journal of Communicative Disorders, 13*, 195–205.

Goetzinger, C. P. (1978). Word discrimination testing. In J. Katz (Ed.), *Handbook of clinical audiology* (pp.149–158). Baltimore: Williams & Wilkins.

Green, D. (1978). Pure tone testing. In J. Katz (Ed.), *Handbook of clinical audiology* (pp. 98–109). Baltimore: Williams & Wilkins.

Hargus, S., & Gordon-Salants, S. (1995). Accuracy of speech intelligibility index predictions for noise masked young listeners with normal hearing and for elderly listeners with hearing impairment. *Journal of Speech and Hearing Research, 38*, 234–243.

Haskins, H. (1949). *A phonetically balanced test of speech discrimination for children.* Unpublished master's thesis, Northwestern University, Evanston, IL.

Hodgson, W. R. (1978). Disorders of hearing. In P. Skinner & R. Shelton (Eds.), *Speech, language and hearing* (pp. 457–470). Reading, MA: Addison-Wesley.

Holm, V. A., & Kunze, L. H. (1969). Effect of chronic otitis media on language and development. *Pediatrics, 43*, 833–839.

Hudgins, C. V., Hawkins, J. E., Karlin, J. E., & Stevens, S. S. (1947). The development of recorded auditory tests for measuring hearing loss for speech. *Laryngoscope, 47*, 57-89.

Jerger, J., Silman, S., Lew, H., & Chmiel, R. (1993). Case studies in binaural interference: Converging evidence from behavioral and electrophysiologic measures. *Journal of American Academy of Audiology, 4*, 122-131.

Kalikow, D. N., Stevens, K. N., & Elliott, L. L. (1977). Development of a test of speech intelligibility in noise using sentence materials with controlled word predictability. *Journal of Acoustical Society of America, 61*, 1337-1351.

Kaplan, H., Bally, S. J., & Brandt, F. (1990). Communication Self-Assessment Scale Inventory for Deaf Adults. *Journal of the American Academy of Audiology, 2*, 164-182.

Katz, J. (1998). Central auditory processing and cochlear implant therapy. In M. G. Masters, N. Stecker, & J. Katz (Eds.), *Central auditory processing disorders: Mostly management* (pp. 215-232). Needham, MA: Allyn & Bacon.

Keith, R. (1979). An acoustic reflex technique of establishing hearing aid settings. *Journal of the American Auditory Society, 5*, 71-75.

Killion, M. C., & Villichur, E. (1993). Kessler was right—Partly. But SIN test shows some aids improve hearing in noise. *Hearing Journal, 48*, 31-35.

Lamb, S., Owens, E., & Schubert, E. (1983). The revised form of the Hearing Performance Inventory. *Ear and Hearing, 4*, 152-157.

Levitt, H., & Stromberg, H. (1983). Segmental characteristics of speech of hearing-impaired children—Factors affecting intelligibility. In I. Hochberg, H. Levitt, & M. J. Osberger (Eds.), *Speech of the hearing-impaired: Research, training, and personnel preparation* (pp. 32-41). Baltimore: University Park Press.

Mashie, J. J. (1980). *Laryngeal behavior of hearing-impaired speakers.* Unpublished doctoral dissertation, Syracuse University, Syracuse, NY.

Mongelli, C. (1978). *Central auditory involvement in two geriatric populations measured with the staggered spondaic word test.* Unpublished manuscript, University of California, Santa Barbara.

Nilsson, M., Soli, S. D. & Sullivan, J. (1994). Development of the hearing in noise test for measurement of speech reception thresholds in quiet and in noise. *Journal of the Acoustical Society of America, 95*, 1085-1099.

Owens, E., & Schubert, E. (1977). Development of California Consonant Test. *Journal of Speech and Hearing Research, 20*, 463-474.

Ross, M., & Lerman, J. (1970). A picture identification test for hearing impaired children. *Journal of Speech and Hearing Research, 13*, 44-53.

Secord, G. J., Erickson, M. T., & Bush, J. P. (1988). Neuropsychological sequelae of otitis media in children and adolescents with learning disabilities. *Journal of Pediatric Psychology, 13*, 531-542.

Speaks, C., & Jerger, J. (1965). Method of measurement of speech identification. *Journal of Speech and Hearing Research, 8*, 185-194.

Stach, B. (1989). Hearing aid amplification and central processing disorders. In R. E. Sandlin (Ed.), *Handbook of hearing aid amplification: Vol. II. Clinical considerations* (pp. 87-111). Boston: College Hill Press.

Stredler-Brown, A. (2009). Intervention, education and therapy for children who are deaf or hard of hearing (pp. 934-954). In J. Katz, L. Medwetsky, R. Burkard, & L. Hood (Eds.), *Handbook of Clinical Audiology* (6th ed.). Baltimore: Lippincott Williams & Wilkins.

Thompson, G., & Hoel, R. (1962). Flat sensorineural hearing loss and PB scores. *Journal of Speech and Hearing Disorders, 27*, 284-287.

Weinstein, B., Richards, A., & Montano, J. (1995). Handicap versus impairment: An important distinction. *Journal of the American Academy of Audiology, 6*, 250-255.

Whitehead, R. L., & Barefoot, S. (1983). *Air flow characteristics of fricative consonants produced by normally hearing and hearing impaired speakers.* Unpublished manuscript, National Technical Institute for the Deaf, Rochester, NY.

End of Chapter Examination Questions

Chapter 2

1. Audiologists make use of standard speech threshold and speech recognition tests to _____.

2. A person who possesses a conductive hearing loss may achieve very good speech recognition simply by _____.

3. As with other diagnostic information, audiometric data have inherent informational limitations. Describe three:
   a.
   b.
   c.

4. Severe congenital or prelingual hearing losses have a great impact on _____, _____, and _____ because an individual does not develop these skills without usable hearing.

5. According to the authors, although a flat frequency configuration hearing loss tends to impact heavily on the high-frequency portion of speech, a high-frequency hearing loss has an even greater adverse effect. Why?

6. The handicap resulting from a unilateral hearing loss is due not only to the loss of sensitivity, but also to the _____.

7. Both the classroom and the workplace provide many challenges to persons who have hearing impairment. From the information obtained in this chapter, describe four of those challenges.
   a.
   b.
   c.
   d.

End of Chapter Answer Sheet

Name _____ Date _____

Chapter 2

1. _____

2. _____

3. a. _____

   b. _____

   c. _____

4. _____, _____, and

   _____.

5. _____

6. _____

7. a. _____

   b. _____

   c. _____

   d. _____

3

The Psychosocial, Educational, and Occupational Impact of Impaired Hearing and the Vocational Rehabilitation Counseling Process

R. STEVEN ACKLEY with Information on Vocational
Rehabilitation Counseling by KAREN DILKA

Introduction

The incidence of hearing loss in the general population is variable and highly age-dependent. The often quoted incidence in newborns of "1 in 1000" births pertains primarily to those infants born with "significant bilateral permanent hearing loss" and does not take into account children born with mild hearing loss, unilateral hearing loss, or temporary conditions including otitis media (middle ear infection). In addition, it should be noted that consistent and systematic national statistics on incidence of hearing loss in newborns and young children are also lacking. State Early Hearing Detection and Identification (EHDI) programs provide this data on a state-by-state basis. On the basis of this contributed data, national projections can be derived, and the National Institutes of Health (NIH) have estimated national hearing loss prevalence for various age groups including the 0 to 5 year old population through the Epidemiology and Biostatistics Program of National Institute on Disabilities and Communication Disorders (NIDCD).

Prevalence of Significant Hearing Loss in Children (Ages 0–5)

NIDCD determined that the U.S. population consisted of 25 million 0 to 5 year old children. Based on mean data provided by the majority of states, an incidence rate of 1.11/1000 live birth newborns were identified with significant hearing loss, which translates to about 4385 newborns in this hearing loss category. Because the incidence rate has not varied substantially over the past decade or so, this number was multiplied by 6 to cover this age group, yielding 26,310 children under 6 years of age with hearing loss since birth. When accounting for delayed-onset congenital hearing losses, viral- or bacterial-induced hearing losses in this age range (CMV, meningitis, etc.), trauma, and other injuries, NIDCD predicted an overall prevalence of significant hearing loss of 30,000 children. As noted, this constitutes the population of children 0 to 5 years old with primarily moderate-to-profound hearing losses and does not include mild and/or unilateral hearing losses.

Prevalence of Significant Hearing Loss (Ages 0–19)

Perhaps somewhat less reliable than the data calculated on the 0 to 5 year old population is that reported on the 0 to 19 year old childhood population. Much of this data is derived via survey instruments developed and conducted primarily by the Centers for Disease Control (CDC) as part of their National Health Interview Survey (NHIS), which is conducted annually on 12,000 to 15,000 subjects. These data identify an incidence rate of 0.81/1000 children who are reported as deaf, yielding a total number of deaf children at 67,000. This would indicate that 3000 to 3500 children at any year of age are deaf in the United States. The estimate would be lower for newborns and higher for older children as more time has enabled more risk of deafness to be acquired. In other words, these data suggest that the incidence rate of deafness among 1-year-old children in the United States is near 3000 individuals and the rate for 18-year-olds would be around 3500 children. If the NIDCD 0 to 5 year old data are extrapolated out to 0 to 19 years of age, the prevalence would be closer to 90,000 to 100,000 children who have moderate-to-profound hearing loss. These data agree. The subset of deaf children in the population of those with moderate, severe, and profound hearing losses is significantly less than the total. Another measure of hearing loss incidence among school-age children is the number served under the Individuals with Disabilities Education Act (IDEA). Data for the 2000–2001 school year report more than 70,700 children receiving services for hearing impairment (U.S. Department of Education, 2002), which are primarily those 6 to 21 year old children with moderate-profound hearing loss and who do not report another

primary disability. Those children with multiple disabilities add to this number. Another study that is consistent with these reports is that done by Blanchfield et al (2001) who found that 738,000 people in the United States have severe-to-profound hearing loss and about 70,000 of them are under the age of 18 years. This also agrees with statistic that 3000 to 3500 children at any year of age are deaf (Figure 3–1).

Prevalence of Mild and Unilateral Hearing Loss

The CDC has been gathering data on the population of school-age children who have mild or unilateral hearing losses for several years. As expected, incidence rates for children with this condition are significantly higher than for the moderate-to-profound category. The incidence of school-age children with mild bilateral hearing loss is 10 to 15 in 1000, and for unilateral hearing losses in this group is 30 to 56 in 1000 (Ross, Gaffney, Green, & Holstrum, 2008). Applying the NIDCD 0 to 5 year old number of children in the United States (25 million) to this rate yields approximately 300,000 to 450,000 children in the 0 to 5 year old range with mild hearing losses and an additional 900,000 to 1,500,000 children in the 0 to 5 year old group with unilateral hearing losses in the United States. Taking the conservative estimates given here, the incidence rate of children with mild or unilateral hearing loss is 1 in 25 in the United States. However, the rate could be as high as 1 in 13 based on these calculated prevalence ranges. This constitutes a significant impact on classroom instruction in the United States, as these children perform poorly in conditions of moderate background noise levels, generally score more poorly on standardized

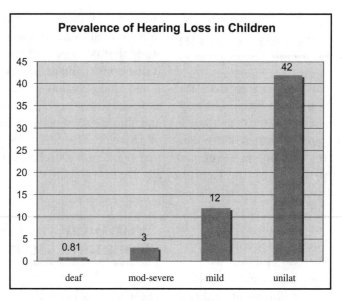

Figure 3–1. This graph shows the incidence rate of hearing loss among school-age children according to severity of hearing loss. *Note.* These data reflect statistics from Centers for Disease Control, 2008, EDHI Update, retrieved July, 2008 from http://www.cdc.gov/ncbddd/ehdi/FAQ/ questionsgeneralHL.htm; National Institute on Deafness and Other Communication Disorders, 2008, Statistics on Hearing Loss, retrieved July, 2008 from http://www.nidcd .nih.gov/health/statistics/hearing.asp; "Prevalence and Effects," by D. S. Ross, M. Gaffney, D. Green, & W. J. Holstrum, 2008, *Seminars in Hearing, 29*(2), pp. 141–148.

tests, develop speech and vocabulary later than peers with normal hearing, and often exhibit behavior problems, higher levels of frustration, and difficulty with overall socialization. They may be diagnosed with ADD or ADHD based on their behavior profile, when in reality they have behaviors consistent with auditory processing disorder (APD), which in these cases would be secondary to actual hearing loss. Again, these data are based on relatively conservative calculations provided by NIDCD and CDC. Another report, the NHANES study, gives an incidence rate of 73/1000 children with hearing loss in the 6 to 19 year old age range, of whom 96% had either unilateral loss (78%) or mild bilateral hearing loss (19%). These various reports corroborate a significant health-related issue that is profoundly impacting public and private education of school-age children in the United States.

Prevalence of Hearing Loss in Adults (Ages 20–69)

A comprehensive study was conducted by Agrawal, Platz, and Niparko at Johns Hopkins Medical Center. They evaluated national survey data on adults (ages 20–69) between 1999 and 2004 (Agrawal, Platz, & Niparko, 2008). They reported on hearing levels for 500 to 6000 Hz frequencies for this age group and found a prevalence of 31% of this population (55 million subjects) had hearing loss (12% unilateral and 19% bilateral). In addition, they found that males were 5.5 times more likely to have hearing loss than females, whereas African American individuals were 70% less likely to have hearing loss than either Caucasian or Mexican American subjects. If some of the behaviors listed for children with hearing loss can be applied to adults as well (higher levels of frustration, poor performance in background noise situations), most Caucasian and Mexican American men are affected, which signals an epidemic of hearing loss and resultant behaviors that may run the range from "mildly inconvenienced" to

"sociopath." NIDCD reports that 17% of the adult population, or 36 million individuals, have some noticeable complaint of hearing loss. This is much lower than the Johns Hopkins study because most people with mild high-frequency hearing loss are unaware of the damage, although they may still have unexplained symptoms such as poor understanding of speech in background noise situations. In addition, NIDCD reports a strong relationship between age and reported hearing loss: 18% of American adults 45 to 64 years old, 30% of adults 65 to 74 years old, and 47% of adults 75 years old or older have a hearing impairment (Figure 3–2a, Figure 3–2b, and Figure 3–2c).

In a 2008 report based on National Center for Health Statistics (NCHS) data obtained by CDC conducted annually from 2000 to 2006, Schoenborn and Heyman (2008) reported that 3.3% of U.S. adults aged 18 years and over were deaf or had a

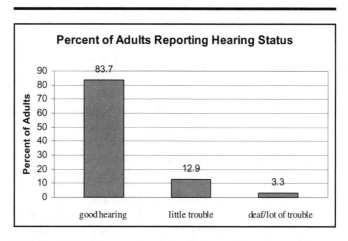

Figure 3–2a. The percent of adults and hearing status as reported to CDC on the NCHS survey 2000–2006. *Note.* From Centers for Disease Control, 2008, EDHI Update, retrieved July, 2008 from http://www.cdc.gov/ncbddd/ehdi/FAQ/questionsgeneralHL.htm; and by C. A. Schoenborn and K. Heyman, 2008, retrieved July, 2008 from http://www.cdc.gov/nchs/products/pubs/pubd/hestats/hearing00-06/hearing00-06

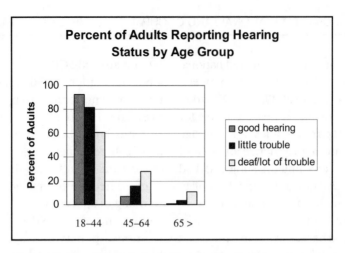

Figure 3–2b. Percent of adults reporting hearing status by age group. *Note.* From Centers for Disease Control, 2008, EDHI Update, retrieved July, 2008 from http://www.cdc.gov/ncbddd/ehdi/FAQ/questionsgeneralHL.htm; and by C. A. Schoenborn and K. Heyman, 2008, retrieved July, 2008 from http://www.cdc.gov/nchs/products/pubs/pubd/hestats/hearing00-06/hearing00-06

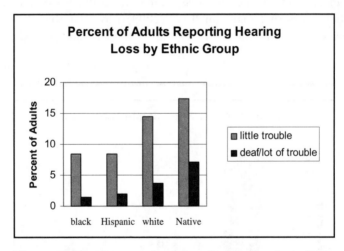

Figure 3–2c. Percent of adults with hearing loss ("little trouble" or "deaf/lot of trouble") according to ethnicity. The Native category includes Native Americans and Native Alaskans and represents the ethnic group in the United States reporting the highest incidence of hearing loss *Note.* From Centers for Disease Control, 2008, EDHI Update, retrieved July, 2008 from http://www.cdc.gov/ncbddd/ehdi/FAQ/questionsgeneralHL.htm; and by C. A. Schoenborn and K. Heyman, 2008, retrieved July, 2008 from http://www.cdc.gov/nchs/products/pubs/pubd/hestats/hearing00-06/hearing00-06.

lot of trouble hearing without the use of a hearing aid. Men (4.3%) were more likely than women (2.4%) to be deaf or have a lot of trouble hearing. Deafness or a lot of trouble hearing increased dramatically with age, rising from 0.9% among adults under age 45 to 3.1% among adults aged 45 to 64 and 11.1% among adults aged 65 and over. These age-related increases in deafness or a lot of trouble hearing were similar for men and women. Rates of a lesser degree of hearing trouble (i.e., a little trouble) also rose with age, increasing more than fourfold between ages 18 and 44 (6.7%) and ages 65 and over (27.8%). Non-Hispanic white adults and non-Hispanic American Indian or Alaska Native (AIAN) adults had the highest rates of any hearing trouble of the race/ethnicity groups studied. Adults with the most education (a bachelor's degree or higher) and those with the highest incomes were somewhat less likely than other adults to have any trouble hearing, although the differences were not large.

Cochlear Implants as Cure for Deafness

There is much debate about the effectiveness of cochlear implants among profoundly deaf users and their ability to understand speech and use a telephone. In many cases, this most desirable outcome is reported. However, in the majority of cochlear implant recipients, this level of improvement is not achieved. Still, the number of cochlear implant recipients in the Unites States is a small fraction of the hundreds of thousands of deaf individuals who could potentially benefit from this device. NIDCD reports that about 23,000 adults and approximately 15,500 children have received cochlear implants to date.

Quality of Life and Hearing Loss

In a survey of more than 40,000 households utilizing the National Family Opinion panel, hearing loss was shown to negatively impact household income on average up to $12,000 per year depending on the degree of hearing loss. However, the use of hearing instruments was shown to mitigate the effects of hearing loss by 50%. For America's 24 million hearing-impaired who do not use hearing instruments, the impact of untreated hearing loss is quantified to be in excess of $100 billion annually. At a 15% tax bracket, the cost to society could be well in excess of $18 billion due to unrealized taxes (Better Health Institute [BHI], 2007; Figure 3–3).

Comparing current data to what has been reported in the recent past, according to the NCHS in 1971 there were 69 persons per 1000 of the population with hearing impairment, and in 1991, the incidence was 86.1 per 1000. These data do not vary appreciably from currently reported hearing loss statistics. An NHIS report in 1994 stressed the relationship between aging and hearing loss (NCHS, 1994a), indicating that as the population ages, the incidence of hearing loss within the total population will likewise increase because hearing loss generally accompanies the process of aging.

Influences of Hearing Loss

Family Income

The 1994 report by NCHS found that persons with severe hearing loss were more frequently found in families with an annual

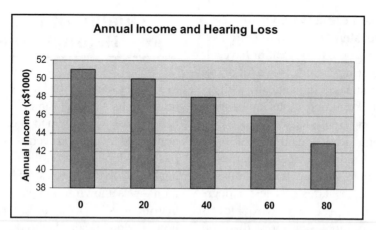

Figure 3–3. Impact of hearing loss severity on annual income. Values along the x-axis (0–80) represent percentage of hearing loss ranging from normal hearing (0% loss) to severe hearing loss (80% loss). Annual income is ranged from approximately $53,000 (normal hearing) to $43,000 (severe hearing loss). *Note.* From "S. Kochkin Report on Annual Income and Hearing Loss," Better Health Institute, 2007, retrieved July, 2008 from http://www.better hearing.org/pdfs/marketrak_income.pdf

income of less than $10,000, and less frequently found in families with incomes of $50,000 and more. According to that survey, 24.9% of persons with no hearing impairment were found in families earning $50,000 or more, and only 16% of those with hearing impairment were in that income group (NCHS, 1994a).

Employment Status and Type of Occupation

The 1994 NCHS report found that more persons with impaired hearing were unemployed than those with average hearing (NCHS, 1994a; Reis, 1993), ranging from 77.6% of persons with a severe hearing impairment, to 29% among those without hearing impairment. Utilizing the Bureau of Census categories of occupations, persons with moderate-to-severe hearing loss are sig-

nificantly underrepresented in occupations related to sales, service, and administrative support. Only around 37% of persons with hearing impairment were found in those types of occupations.

The economic problems of adults with severe hearing impairment have historically involved both unemployment and underemployment. A large part of the problem may be attributed to the myths concerning deafness and hearing impairment and ignorance by many employers about the capabilities of those with hearing impairment. It is not unheard of for companies that depend heavily on telephone communication, for example, to avoid hiring deaf employees. Studies cited by Meadow-Orlans (1985) present some interesting information on employment and employability of deaf workers in Europe, the Netherlands, and Scandinavia. Beuzart (1982) found that in one inquiry in France, 50% of workers lost their jobs upon onset of deafness. Others remained, but earned lower salaries. A survey by Thomas and Herbst (1980) found 236 respondents were significantly "less happy at work" than matched hearing controls. Breed, van den Horst, and Mous (1981) found members of a Dutch hard-of-hearing organization were most likely to do "lonely" work, away from their hearing counterparts.

Meadow-Orlans (1985) cites two studies in detail that elaborate on the impact of hearing loss on a person's economic future. Those include a study by Kyle and Wood (1983) that consisted of an interview with 105 persons ages 25 through 55 years with onset of hearing loss in the previous 10 years. According to Meadow-Orlans (1985), 91% of those persons could, with their hearing aid(s), "hear normal speech across a room." Despite their usable hearing, 35% "felt that promotion at work was relatively impossible (p. 43)." Sixty-three percent of persons who were prelingually deafened felt the same, compared with only 16% of those who possessed normal hearing. Kyle and Wood (1983) state that acquired hearing loss affects the quality of working life more than the level of earnings. In this study, it was found that when the workers discovered their hearing losses, only 39% informed their employers.

Another study described in detail by Meadow-Orlans (1985) involved adults in greater London who had hearing impairment. The study was conducted by Thomas, Lamont, and Harris (1982). All subjects were of employment age and had hearing loss greater than 60 dB. The study involved interviews with the workers and surveys. Representative responses by the workers related to the impact of their hearing loss on their ability to work included (a) difficulty coping with the public, (b) difficulty with the telephone, (c) difficulty doing their job, (d) difficulty with colleagues, (e) being

given less responsibility, and (f) altered job assignments.

Education

For persons 18 years and older, the number of persons with less than 12 years of education increases proportionately with the degree of hearing loss (NCHS, 1994b). The discrepancy between those who attend college and those who do not widens proportionately with degree of hearing loss. That is, as hearing loss increases, the number of persons attending college proportionately decreases (Adams & Benson, 1994).

Marital Status and Living Arrangements

Among persons with severe hearing loss, comparatively few have never been married as compared to persons with normal hearing, that is, only 8.2% (Adams & Benson, 1994). However, when comparing persons more than age 18 years who have severe hearing loss with those who have normal hearing, more in the hearing loss category are found to have been divorced, widowed, separated, or married but not living with a spouse (NCHS, 1994a), that is, 27.8% as compared to 20.3% among persons with normal hearing. Further, more persons with hearing loss that interferes with hearing and understanding speech in the age 18 years and above range live alone (23.4%) as compared to those with normal hearing (12.4%; Adams & Benson, 1994).

Births

Fewer children are born to women who are deaf than to normal hearing women. The reason for this is not clear, but it may perhaps be related to the marital status that the survey by the NCHS (1994b) listed as most prevalent among those with severe hearing loss. Those with severe loss tended to be divorced, widowed, separated, or never married. Among those who become parents, children born into families in which at least one parent is prevocationally deaf have normal hearing 88% of the time (Reis, 1993).

Vocational Impact of Hearing Impairment and Deafness and Vocational Rehabilitation Counseling

The purpose of rehabilitation is to provide comprehensive services to individuals with mental, physical, sensory, or emotional handicaps with the intent that they will "attain usefulness and satisfaction in life" (Wright, 1980, p. 3). This broad definition asserts that determination of a recipient's goals and objectives will vary along a continuum from those who have achieved independent living skills to those who have achieved gainful employment. The rehabilitation process encompasses a series of prioritized steps tailored to the unique needs and circumstances of each individual patient. Therefore, the associated time limit for successful completion of the rehabilitation process will depend on the extent and diversity of designated services. The expectation for accomplishment of a patient's initial goal(s) is correlated with his stamina, capabilities, motivation, and support base, which includes his family and significant others.

Unfortunately, the deaf/hard-of-hearing population does not have equivalent sociological, educational, and linguistic advantages that are inherent in the hearing society.

Undoubtedly, this is because a hearing loss, regardless of the type of remedial treatment proposed, significantly restricts the acquisition and comprehension of information that is readily accessible to the hearing majority. Divisional gaps deepen with demographic data indicating inferior educational and socioeconomic status of persons with hearing loss compared to their hearing counterparts (Phillipe & Auvenshine, 1985; Schein & Delk, 1974; Wooton & Mowry, 1986). To complicate the situation further, members of this minority group do not necessarily have homogeneous characteristics. For example, school environments, parental acceptance and leadership, exposure to cultural experiences, onset and degree of loss, and most importantly self-esteem are all variables that affect individual growth and development. Hence, the accumulation of the listed factors compounds any career dynamics associated with occupational choice, mobility, adjustment, and work-related functions.

The literature regarding technological advancements in business and industry is replete with references that detail the rapid changes and breakthroughs in industrial mechanization. The forecast of career profiles reflects this shift, with a move from manual labor toward administrative and executive positions. Concurrently, a concentrated effort must be made by all professionals serving individuals who are deaf or hard of hearing to empower and prepare them to take advantage of these trends.

Vocational Rehabilitation Process

The structural framework of vocational rehabilitation is mandated by public law (PL 93-112, Rehabilitation Act of 1973; PL 93-516,

Vocational Rehabilitation Act of 1973) and consists of specific phases of implementation.

Preliminary Phase

The preliminary phase combines (a) patient referral, (b) an intake interview, and (c) evaluations to determine the patient's eligibility or potential for employment. Two critical components are (a) the interview in which valuable personal, educational, vocational, and financial information is collected; and (b) an aggregate of evaluations (medical, audiological, visual, vocational, and psychological) to assess a patient's physical, mental, and work-related abilities and limitations. Consideration of appropriate testing instruments and administration procedures with persons who are deaf/hard of hearing predominates in this phase of the rehabilitation process. A wide range of communication possibilities and cultural experiences collectively influences the sequential movement of preparation toward vocational achievement. Emphasis is placed on individual assets and liabilities. However, regardless of a patient's circumstances, the following requirements must be met to receive further specialized assistance through the government program.

1. The individual is mentally, physically, or sensorily impaired or disabled.
2. The disability creates a barrier or handicap to attainable employment.
3. The individual will obtain and sustain employment on completion of services provided by vocational rehabilitation.

Development of Individualized Rehabilitation Plan

The next phase entails the development of an individualized written rehabilitation plan (IWRP) to focus on pertinent occupational goals and establish a course of action. Vocational guidance, under the direction of a vocational rehabilitation (VR) counselor, is imperative at this stage to develop a realistic perspective regarding preparation, duration of the task, extent of provisions, and financing. At this juncture, the patient and counselor jointly decide on career aspirations, orientation, timeliness, and procedures.

The data gathered on job placement for persons with hearing loss consistently indicate that they tend to be underemployed rather than unemployed (Schroedel, 1987; Steffanic, 1982; Williams & Sussman, 1976). Job stereotyping and employer discrimination have contributed to this situation (Phillips, 1975). Individuals who are deaf/hard of hearing are predominantly hired in the operative and clerical areas (El-Khiami, 1986). Therefore, there is a severe underrepresentation of persons who are deaf/hard of hearing in what are considered to be high-status professions (Schroedel, 1987).

Restoration Phase

Although all phases of the vocational rehabilitation program compose essential elements, the categories of restoration and training are exclusively oriented to the needs of the patient and, therefore, considered the core of the process. Auditory devices such as hearing aids, telephone accessories, and other assistive equipment/appliances for communication or personal management are necessary. Additionally, medical, surgical, or prosthetic intervention may be necessary, as well as the correction of visual problems to enhance patients' communicative effectiveness via sign language and/or lipreading. Another option might be classes to improve the communication techniques of auditory training and speechreading, manual communication systems, and/or American Sign Language (ASL) when they will assist the patient.

Training Phase

As the patient progresses, formal training begins. Training activities will vary for the person who is deaf/hard of hearing, depending on the results of previous evaluations and his occupational interests. Support services are interwoven throughout the rehabilitation process. However, access to information provided during training is crucial to the application of new skills. Individuals who are deaf/hard of hearing may derive benefit from the availability of interpreters, oral or manual. Other auxiliary resources may be requested for full participation in community or educational settings. Note takers and tutors also facilitate instruction and learning for a person with hearing loss.

Employment Phase

For a patient who has more severe hearing impairment or deafness, the final phase of vocational rehabilitation solidifies the original plan by the formulation of a tangible conclusion—employment or independence. Job opportunities will have, at this point, been solicited and placement of the patient proceeds. Continual observation provides the counselor with insight into the success or failure of the arrangement. Patients' freedom to express themselves and be understood by management contributes to their performance level. Both patient and employer satisfaction determine which procedures a counselor will select for follow-up sessions. If the situation is unfavorable, then an attempt to gain employment elsewhere is investigated. It must be noted that provisions need to be made in each phase to disqualify a patient from services and from receiving further assistance through vocational rehabilitation, if extenuating circumstances arise.

Role of the Rehabilitation Counselor

The vocational rehabilitation (VR) process is designed to offer counseling and personal or career consultation at all phases of a patient's program. At times, the counselor's role involves intensive therapeutic interaction with the patient to resolve personal issues that interfere with the ultimate goal of employment. Therefore, demonstrated proficiency in the preferred language of the individual who is deaf/hard of hearing, irrespective of the mode or method, creates an atmosphere of trust and respect vital for a positive patient-counselor rapport. Rehabilitation counselors provide direction, supervision, and advocacy for a patient while arranging, organizing, and monitoring the delivery of an array of services. These responsibilities cover a gamut of vocational, educational, and professional transactions (operations).

Case Studies

The following vignettes are presented to illustrate the diversity of service alternatives within the realm of VR and the individualization embedded in the system. The three patients described represent a spectrum of the deaf/hard-of-hearing population whose needs are interwoven into the IWRP. The ability of the rehabilitation counselor to tailor the IWRP is one of the unique strengths of the rehabilitation process.

Acquired Hearing Loss Rehabilitation

Wendy was a skilled home economics teacher. She had enjoyed teaching high school students for 12 years. Her goal was to continue teaching for 13 more years and then retire with her husband. As Wendy was driving to work one morning she had a serious car accident and was hospitalized for several weeks. Although she recovered from her physical injuries, Wendy was left with a severe bilateral sensorineural hearing loss. This traumatic experience left Wendy angry and frustrated. Her acquired hearing loss created obstacles that were extremely difficult to cope with both emotionally and physically. Wendy tried to return to work only to discover she no longer had control of her classes and could not communicate with her students or colleagues. Subsequently, Wendy chose to give up her teaching position.

Wendy's home life was also affected by her postlingual loss of hearing; family relationships were strained because of the lack of spontaneous communication or compensatory techniques. Misunderstandings frequently arose and she began to remove herself from social gatherings with family and friends. Feeling isolated and seeking alternatives, Wendy decided to contact a local organization for those with hearing impairment. She was eventually referred to a VR counselor, from whom she gained information about her hearing loss and opportunities for revised career development.

After the initial interview and application procedure, Wendy was sent to an otologist for a thorough examination of the hearing mechanism and to her family physician for a medical update. The next step entailed an audiological evaluation to assess the extent of the hearing loss sustained in the accident and an ophthalmological evaluation to ascertain the integrity of her visual system. With relevant information obtained from the audiologist, Wendy became aware of a wide range of assistive devices, hearing aids, and communication strategies to enhance adjustment to her hearing loss.

Wendy met all the necessary requirements for eligibility for VR and proceeded to develop, in conjunction with the counselor, an IWRP. Wendy identified an aspect of home economics she wanted to pursue (fashion editor) and the IWRP document detailed her new career direction, including training, resources, essential materials, a proposed schedule of activities, and anticipated outcomes. It was recommended that Wendy return to the audiologist to purchase bilateral hearing aids. She also inquired about the purchase of a telephone device for the deaf (TDD) and a lighting system for her house, so she would know when the doorbell or telephone rang. VR approved and paid for these items on Wendy's behalf. Concurrently, arrangements were made for Wendy to enroll in an auditory training and lipreading class sponsored by a local speech and hearing clinic. Wendy's preference was to continue to use an oral method of communication, and the instruction was designed to maintain speech production and diminish the frustration of adjustment to auditory stimuli. VR contributed financial support to Wendy's endeavors; however, the amount was based on her income and economic status reports.

The relationship between Wendy and her counselor developed into a warm, respectful exchange of thoughts, ideas, and information. Communication became less of a challenging task and more of a relaxed acquisition of messages. Personal and career counseling were an integral part of Wendy's IWRP.

The onset of a sudden hearing loss can evoke emotional turmoil that an individual is not psychologically prepared to manage without the help of a professional trained in the area of hearing loss. Gradually, Wendy began to acknowledge and ultimately accept her disability. She gained confidence in her communication abilities, focusing on the positive aspects of change. This significant progress was due, in part, to the effective guidance and monitoring techniques employed by her VR counselor.

Through specialized courses, Wendy studied interior design. She assumed responsibility for payment of all supplies and materials for the courses; however, she was reimbursed for tuition by her local office of VR. Wendy finished the program within 1 year and later found employment at a woman's publishing company. The VR counselor proceeded to conduct an in-service for the manager of the publishing company on practical communication strategies and disseminated similar information to departmental employees. Wendy's goals were consequently achieved in a 2-year time frame, resulting in an occupational shift and successful rehabilitation closure.

Congenital Hearing Loss Rehabilitation

Scott was deaf from birth because of autosomal recessive genetic hearing loss (connexin 26). Although "culturally Deaf," he decided at the end of his high school term to look into the cochlear implant option. He was accepted into Gallaudet University and performed in that environment with ease because of his fluency in ASL. However, after cochlear implant surgery and subsequent training with his new device, he found that he was understanding speech much more effectively than he anticipated

and his speechreading ability was vastly superior to his pre-implant condition. In most conversational situations Scott was able to understand 95% or more of the conversation when he could maintain face-to-face eye contact. In the auditory-only mode, he would still pick up between 50 and 65% of the conversational speech. In addition, his speech improved dramatically and he found that it was not necessary for him to repeat himself as was common before his implant.

Scott's VR counselor had him set up to attend Gallaudet in the fall with tuition covered. Scott was now in a situation where he felt that he might be able to function in the primarily auditory environment of his state university, assuming support services including classroom interpreters. He felt that he might be able to function in certain classroom situations without an interpreter— such as where the instructor lectures from a podium without turning to the blackboard or away from the audience. Even then, he would always need to position himself directly in front of the instructor and rely heavily on an effective note taker. He had a month or so during the summer to decide if his progress post-implant would be adequate in his mind to give him the confidence to take on the new challenge of the state university.

It was Scott's decision to give the state university a try. The VR counselor contacted Gallaudet and then verified that all support services were in place at the state university, including interpreters and note takers in all of Scott's classes. Scott was a golfer and planned to join the university golf team, which was in part his motivation to attend the state university rather than Gallaudet, which did not have a golf team. Everything was in place and he started classes that fall semester. As the semester progressed he found that being in huge lecture hall-type classes was distracting, and despite interpreters and note takers his grades were not quite what they had been in high school. His cochlear implant was less effective in lecture halls than in one-on-one situations, and so he found that he was relying on his implant less and less in the classroom environment. As a diversion he was able to meet the golf coach, who arranged for him to practice with some of the varsity golfers. Interestingly, he wore his implant consistently to play golf because he found that the auditory feedback he received from the contact the club made with the ball helped improve his shots. Still, he was not performing as well as he hoped and he decided he would not try out for the golf team after all.

By the end of the fall semester, Scott had decided to look into transferring to Gallaudet. His grades at the state university were average and his dream of becoming a star golfer were somewhat dashed, and he thought the classroom size of 20 or so students at Gallaudet, where ASL would be used by all, might be a better fit for him. His VR counselor was able to make all the transfer arrangements including helping with transfer of courses so that he lost no time or credit in his spring semester entry into Gallaudet.

The move to Gallaudet turned out to be a very positive experience for Scott, because he excelled academically, became involved with student government and various clubs on campus, and even started a golf team that played unofficially as a club sport with other small colleges in the DC region. Ironically, Scott used his cochlear implant more frequently in the classroom situation at Gallaudet than he had while attending the state university. The smaller class size enabled him to better approximate the one-on-one situation that was optimal for him to realize implant success. In addition, he found that the audiologists working in the on-campus clinic at Gallaudet were knowledgeable and experienced in dealing with his implant programming needs and other assistive technology requests he had. And because the entire campus, including the audiologists, communicated in his native ASL he found no communication barriers.

Genetically-Based Conductive Hearing Loss Rehabilitation— Apert's Syndrome

Stanley was born with an autosomal dominant disease diagnosed as Apert's syndrome. He had multiple handicapping conditions, including a moderate hearing loss (SRT of 50 dB HL), skull and facial malformations, decreased cognitive capacity, fusion of the hand and toe digits (syndactyly), and spina bifida. Stanley's extremely high forehead and facial anomalies were primary indicators of the genetic syndrome at birth. Therefore, Stanley received early medical, otological, and audiological intervention.

Throughout the developmental years, Stanley underwent numerous surgeries to correct the cranial and facial anomalies. The multidisciplinary management team also performed several operations on Stanley's hands and feet to separate the digits. However, only the thumb and smallest finger could be detached from the solid mass. This allowed Stanley to manipulate objects, even though he did not have optimal functioning of his hands. Otological intervention was necessary to improve his hearing acuity for the acquisition of speech and language. The stapes footplate was removed and a prosthesis put in place; however, further reconstructive surgery to remediate his hearing loss was not possible. After treatment, Stanley had an audiological evaluation that signified an increase in his hearing ability to within the mild range. Simultaneously, Stanley was fitted with a bone conduction hearing aid.

Education for Stanley was difficult. His mobility was restricted because of his spina bifida and, therefore, he used a wheelchair. During his school years, he was assigned to a self-contained classroom for the trainable mentally handicapped and later transferred to the district's vocational setting. Stanley enjoyed the hands-on work that was expected of him in this new environment. The precision with which he assembled products was recognized by his teachers. The quality of his workmanship was consistently above average. Prior to graduation, Stanley's instructor contacted the VR counselor, starting the VR process. Stanley was 21 years old.

Diagnostic data were collected regarding Stanley's medical, audiological, educational, and vocational history. Fortunately, current information was available in all these specialty areas, expediting the determination of eligibility. The years of training and work experience gained at the vocational school were noted for consideration when Stanley's future placement was discussed. Using that and scores from a battery of work sample evaluations to measure Stanley's occupational aptitudes and input from the immediate family, an IWRP was developed. This document focused on independent living skills and extended employment at a sheltered workshop.

It was decided that a combination of community resources would benefit Stanley in his pursuit of independence. An occupational therapist taught Stanley functional self-care tasks. This helped him attain a higher level of autonomy within the family unit. The services of a physical therapist were contracted to administer a therapeutic exercise program aimed at strengthening body parts, enhancing circulation, and reducing the possibility of muscular atrophy. Of course, it was apparent to Stanley's family that he would always need additional support, as he had multiple disabilities affecting his mental, physical, and emotional health. Restorative devices allowing freedom of movement were purchased, including an automatic wheelchair and a contemporary bone conduction hearing aid. These items were deemed essential for Stanley to cope constructively with the barriers in the environment. This significant expenditure of money was shared by VR and Stanley's parents.

Job placement at a local sheltered workshop for rehabilitation patients complied with Stanley's IWRP objectives. He was tentatively accepted at the facility and a conference was scheduled for the VR counselor and appointed supervisor to exchange relevant competency-based information. A brief transitional period from school to work was allotted before actual training sessions were set up. Stanley's performance was assessed for several weeks. It was eventually established that he met the criteria for extended employment. The counselor remained in contact with the center until closing Stanley's file. Follow-up conferences were positive and his supervisor reported he was an asset to the facility.

Discussion of the Case Studies

As indicated in the case studies, a distinction is evident between the terms, *rehabilitation* and *habilitation*. The first implies that an individual becomes disabled because of a medical condition or an injury, after possessing work-related skills. In contrast, the latter term signifies that the individual has a congenital disability and must be introduced to the complexities of employment. Although these terms are used synonymously throughout the literature, the difference is considerable when selecting appropriate facilitative methodology.

Wendy, Scott, and Stanley obviously have very different needs, idiosyncratic qualities, and lifestyles. Optimally, a VR counselor will develop a plan for the delivery of services that accentuates each recipient's aptitudes and talents. Often, this will require unlimited resources and a longer period of training than is usually allocated for completion of the VR process. Consequently, the enormous challenge facing both patient and counselor necessitates a creative and flexible program to derive maximum benefits that will lead to a profitable future.

Combining Vocational Rehabilitation and Audiology

Networking between professionals, their sponsoring agencies, and organizations affiliated with hearing loss is a powerful tool for the collection and dissemination of information. Most VR counselors recognize networking as the key to a smooth vocational transition for the patient who is deaf or hard of hearing. It expands patient opportunities and negates bias factors that have, in the past, prohibited the participation of those with hearing loss. Networking breaks down the barriers involved in professional "turf guarding" and allows for positive interaction and valuable input into the rehabilitation process (Woodrick, 1984). Without this cooperative working relationship among service providers, the patient will have delayed progress due, in part, to external matters beyond his control. Additionally, the lack of communication and/or miscommunication between professionals interrupts the continuity and flow of services. In return, this affects a patient's personal motivation and has a profound impact on

the patient's perspective toward specialized personnel. Confidence in the system and associated professionals begins to deteriorate. Therefore, prompt and accurate information, exchanged in an efficient and timely manner, eliminates conflict and unnecessary obstacles. Through the avenue of networking, many of these intrusive problems can be avoided or resolved.

Given the continuum of audiological needs exhibited by persons with hearing loss, the role of the audiologist is significant in all phases of the VR process. Considering the proliferation of new developments in technology, the audiologist's knowledge and expertise is vital to programming success. Contemporary hearing aids and devices are capable of refining a patient's auditory skills and enabling each individual to develop strategies for the enhancement of overall communication.

A VR counselor cannot possibly keep abreast of the latest improvements in hearing aids and devices and, for this reason, must regularly consult with the audiologist. This is especially true for adult patients who have recently acquired a hearing loss. Most often the VR counselor is the patient's first contact, so most likely the counselor has not been introduced to these sophisticated instruments. The patient, therefore, may require in-depth counseling by the audiologist. It becomes apparent in these particular situations that the charge for both professionals is interrelated, with counseling and supervision as shared responsibilities. However, the VR counselor and audiologist's complementary roles come from distinctive knowledge bases from which each can solicit useful information. The VR counselor is accountable for the patient's vocational habilitation/ rehabilitation program, whereas the audiologist's focus is primarily on the auditory/ communicative aspects of rehabilitation.

Summary

The placement and retention of individuals who are deaf/hard of hearing in quality work environments is the ultimate goal of VR. Counselors are trained in the area of deafness to diligently seek out new frontiers for employment, to liaise with other professionals, and to provide assistance to patients in their efforts to obtain personal and occupational independence. The underlying commonality that VR counselors share is the advancement of people who have hearing impairment into the labor market.

Acknowledgment. Portions of the content of this chapter were originally prepared by Karen Dilka for the fourth edition of *Aural Rehabilitation* (2001). This author wishes to acknowledge her contributions to the information prepared for the previous edition, particularly as it pertains to the role and function of the VR counselor.

References

Adams, P. F., & Benson, V. (1994). Current estimates from the National Health Interview Survey, 1993. *National Center for Health Statistics, 13,* 181.

Agrawal, Y., Platz, E. A., & Niparko, J. N. (2008). Prevalence of hearing loss and differences by demographic characteristics among US adults. *Archives of Internal Medicine, 168*(14), 1522–1530.

Better Health Institute. (2007). S. Kochkin Report on Annual Income and Hearing Loss. Available at http://www.betterhearing.org/pdfs/marketrak_income.pdf

Beuzart, J. G. (1982, November). *Deafened workers in France: Characteristics and conditions.* Paper presented at the International Congress of Audiophonology, Besançon, France.

Blanchfield, B., Feldman, J., Dunbar, J., & Gardner, E. (2001). The severely to profoundly hearing-impaired population in the United States: Prevalence estimates and demographics. *Journal of the American Academy of Audiology, 12,* 183–189.

Breed, P. C., van den Horst, A. P., & Mous, T. J. M. (1981). Psychosocial problems in suddenly deafened adolescents and adults. In T. Hartmann (Ed.), *Congress report* (pp. 1023–1054). Hamburg, Germany: First International Congress of the Hard of Hearing.

Centers for Disease Control. (2008). EDHI update. Available at http://www.cdc.gov/ncbddd/ehdi/FAQ/questionsgeneralHL.htm

Dilka, K. (2001). A psychosocial, educational, and economic profile, and vocational rehabilitation counseling for the hearing impaired and deaf. In R. Hull (Ed.), *Aural Rehabilitation: Serving Children and Adults* (pp. 41–58). San Diego, CA: Singular.

El-Khiami, A. (1986). Selected characteristics of hearing-impaired rehabilitants of general VR agencies: A socio-demographic profile. In D. Watson, G. Anderson, & M. Taff-Watson (Eds.), *Integrating human resources, technology and systems in deafness: Proceedings of the Tenth Biennial Conference of the American Deafness and Rehabilitation Association* (pp. 136–144). Silver Spring, MD: American Deafness and Rehabilitation Association.

Fellendorf, G., Atelsek, F., & Macklin, E. (1971). *Diversifying job opportunities for the adult deaf.* Washington, DC: Alexander Graham Bell Association for the Deaf.

Kyle, J. G., & Wood, P. L. (1983). *Social and vocational aspects of acquired hearing loss. Final report to the Ministry of Social Concern.* Bristol, UK: School of Educational Research Unit, University of Bristol.

Meadow-Orlans, K. P. (1985). Social and psychological effects of hearing loss in adulthood: A literature review. In H. Orlans (Ed.), *Adjustment to adult hearing loss* (pp. 35–58). San Diego, CA: Singular.

National Center for Health Statistics. (1975). Persons with impaired hearing: United States. *Vital and Health Statistics, 10,* 101.

National Center for Health Statistics. (1994). Current estimates from the National Health Interview Survey, 1990. *Vital and Health Statistics, 10*(1991), 181.

National Center for Health Statistics. (1994). Prevalence and characteristics of persons with hearing trouble. (Series 10. No. 188. Data from the National Health Survey, pp. 5–10). Washington, DC: Department of Health and Human Services.

National Health Interview Survey. (1994). Prevalence and characteristics of persons with hearing trouble: United States, 1990–1991. *Vital and Health Statistics, 10*(188), 1–8.

National Institute on Deafness and Other Communication Disorders. (2008). Statistics on hearing loss. Available at http://www.nidcd.nih.gov/health/statistics/hearing.asp

Phillipe, T., & Auvenshine, D. (1985). Career development among deaf persons. *Journal of Rehabilitation of the Deaf, 19,* 9–17.

Phillips, G. B. (1975). Specific jobs for deaf workers. *Journal of Rehabilitation of the Deaf, 9,* 10–23.

PL 93-112. (1973). Rehabilitation Act of 1973.

PL 93-516. (1973). Vocational Rehabilitation Act of 1973.

Reis, P. (1993). Hearing ability of persons by sociodemographic and health characteristics: United States, 1993. *National Center for Health Statistics, 10,* 140.

Ross, D. S., Gaffney, M., Green, D., & Holstrum, W. J. (2008): Prevalence and effects. *Seminars in Hearing, 29*(2), 141–148.

Schein, J. D., & Delk, M. T., Jr. (1974). The deaf population of the United States. Silver Springs, MD: National Association of the Deaf.

Schoenborn, C. A., & Heyman, K. (2008). Information on Hearing Products. http://www.cdc.gov/nchs/products/pubs/pubd/hestats/hearing00-06/hearing00-06

Schroedel, J. G. (1987). The educational and occupational aspirations and attainments of deaf students and alumni of postsecondary programs. In G. B. Anderson & D. Watson (Eds.), *Innovations in the habilitation and rehabilitation of deaf adolescents: Selected proceedings of the Second National Conference on Habilitation and Rehabilitation of Deaf Adolescents* (pp. 117–139). Afton, OK: American Deaf Adolescent Conference.

Steffanic, D. J. (1982). *Reasonable accommodation for deaf employees in white collar jobs* (Monograph 10). Washington, DC: United States Office of Personnel Management, Office of Research and Development.

Thomas, A., & Herbst, K. (1980). Social and psychological implications of acquired deafness for adults of employment age. *British Journal of Audiology, 14,* 76–85.

Thomas, A., Lamont, M., & Harris, M. (1982). Problems encountered at work by people with severe acquired hearing loss. *British Journal of Audiology, 16,* 39–43.

U.S. Department of Education. (2002). To assure the free appropriate public education of all Americans: Twenty-fourth annual report to Congress on the implementation of the Individuals with Disabilities Education Act. Washington, DC: Author.

White, K. R., & Munoz, K. (2008). Screening. *Seminars in Hearing, 29*(2), 149–158.

Williams, W., & Sussman, A. E. (1976). Social and psychological problems of deaf people. In A. E. Sussman & L. G. Stewart (Eds.), *Counseling with deaf people* (pp. 13–29). New York: Deafness Research and Training Center.

Woodrick, W. E. (1984). Utilization of existing potential programs and facilities for serving multihandicapped deaf persons in Region IV. *Journal of Rehabilitation of the Deaf, 18,* 17–20.

Wooton, S. C., & Mowry, R. L. (1986). A follow-up study of hearing-impaired vocational rehabilitation clients closed successfully by a state VR agency. In D. Watson, G. Anderson, & M. Taff-Watson (Eds.), *Integrating human resources, technology and systems in deafness: Proceedings of the Tenth Biennial Conference of the American Deafness and Rehabilitation Association* (pp. 410–419). Silver Spring, MD: American Deafness and Rehabilitation Association.

Wright, G. N. (1980). *Total rehabilitation.* Boston: Little Brown.

Yoshinaga-Itano, C., Johnson, C. D., Carpenter, K., & Brown, A. S. (2008). Outcomes of children with mild bilateral hearing loss and unilateral hearing loss. *Seminars in Hearing, 29*(2), 196–211.

End of Chapter Examination Questions

Chapter 3

1. **Unilateral hearing loss occurs in children at a rate of**
   a. 250 per 1000
   b. 1 per 250
   c. 2.7 per 1,000
   d. 42 per 1,000

2. **People with a hearing loss may miss out on which of the following?**
   a. group interaction
   b. social knowledge
   c. career development
   d. all of the above

3. **(True or False) Cochlear implants restore hearing to normal understanding of conversational speech in 90% of cases.**

4. **(True or False) A hearing impairment affects all aspects of the individual's life.**

5. **(True or False) Loss of hearing is the most common physical impairment experienced by people in the United States.**

6. **Describe four areas in your own life that would be changed if you had hearing loss.**
   a.
   b.
   c.
   d.

7. **After reading the reasons given for the increase in the incidence of hearing loss given in this chapter, give another reason why you believe there has been such a large increase.**

8. **List three job situations where it would be impossible to work if you had a severe hearing loss, and tell why.**
   a.
   b.
   c.

9. **Choose an area of life in which a person might have difficulty (school, work, home, shopping, etc.) and describe what changes could be made to accommodate his hearing impairment.**

End of Chapter Answer Sheet

Name _____ Date _____

Chapter 3

1. Which one(s)?   a   b   c   d

2. Which one(s)?   a   b   c   d

3. Which one(s)?   a   b   c   d

4. Circle one: True   False

5. Circle one: True   False

6. a. _____

   b. _____

   c. _____

   d. _____

7. _____

_____

_____

8. a. _____

   b. _____

   c. _____

9. _____

_____

_____

4

Introduction to Hearing Aids and Amplification Systems

JOSEPH J. SMALDINO

Chapter Outline

Introduction

Hearing aid selection and assessment are important components of the process of hearing habilitation/rehabilitation. An impaired auditory system typically involves reduced function in the perception of intensity, differentiation of frequency, and/or analysis of the temporal components of incoming sound. When that incoming sound is speech, the impaired system can affect the development of normal speech and language or significantly reduce ability to accurately perceive speech (Boothroyd, 2008; Sanders, 1993; Smaldino & Crandell, 2005). Primarily, these impairments are produced by loss of receptor cells in the cochlea and/or reduction in the number of neurons in the auditory nerve and are permanent. The function that remains is residual hearing, and it is the goal of hearing aid selection procedures to enable the hearing-impaired individual to have access to all of the residual hearing potential that remains.

This discussion of hearing aids includes (a) basic components, (b) electroacoustic properties, (c) styles of aids, (d) implantable aids, (e) earmold acoustics, and (f) programmability/digital signal processing. Consideration of hearing aid selection, assessment philosophies, and procedures in regard to children are covered in Chapter 6. Hearing aid orientation guidelines for adults are discussed in Chapter 13 and other hearing aid considerations in older adults are found in Chapter 20. A thorough discussion of other assistive listening devices can be found in Chapter 14.

Hearing Aid Components

Modern hearing aids are very complex signal processing devices. However, there are basic components that compose all hearing aids. A basic hearing aid circuit block diagram is pictured in Figure 4–1. The actual components of a hearing aid are shown in Figure 4–2. Each component modifies the incoming signal in prescribed ways. All of the components working together result in the frequency, intensity, and overall response characteristics of a given hearing aid.

All hearing aids amplify sound for the listener. Acoustic waves entering at the hearing aid microphone are converted into electrical signals that mimic the pressure variations of the sound waves. The electrical signal from the microphone is amplified by the amplifier section of the hearing aid and delivered to the receiver of the aid, which converts the electrical signal back into its

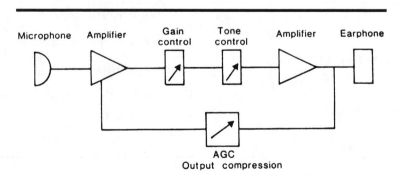

Figure 4–1. Basic hearing aid circuitry.

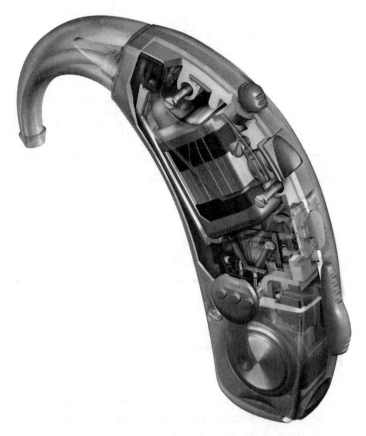

Figure 4–2. Image of a typical hearing aid (Photo courtesy of Phonak).

acoustic form to be heard by the listener. Along the way, adjustments can be made to various aspects of the amplification process; the person fitting the aid sets some aspects, and some are automatically adjusted by the hearing aid circuitry. The overall goal of a hearing aid fitting is to make sound audible and clear, without exceeding a person's level of comfortable listening.

The Microphone

Sound energy is transduced (changed) to electrical energy by the microphone. The electret microphone is the most versatile and is used in virtually all modern hearing aids. According to Killion and Carlson (1974), the electret microphone offers (a) an excellent response to a wide range of frequencies, even at low intensities, (b) low sensitivity to mechanical vibration, and (c) low noise. Figure 4–3 is a diagram of an electret microphone.

An electret microphone is made from a permanent electrically charged element (the electret). A very thin metallically-coated diaphragm is suspended just above the electret material. As sound waves strike the diaphragm, the vibration causes a fluctuating

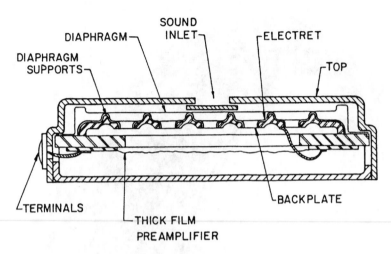

Figure 4–3. Diagram of an electret microphone.

charge to be generated, which is amplified by a transistor in the microphone housing and is delivered to the next hearing aid component.

Microphones can be classified as omnidirectional and directional. Directional microphones are typically more responsive to sound from the front and help the hearing aid user hear better in noise by allowing the user to point the microphone toward the wanted signal and away from the unwanted noise.

Some hearing aids are equipped with a telecoil (T-coil) for telephone use. The telecoil bypasses the microphone by picking up electromagnetic energy produced by a telephone or induction loop and directing it to the hearing aid amplifier. Many hearing aids are also equipped with a direct audio input (DAI), which permits other technology (such as an FM receiver) to be plugged into the hearing aid and become a part of the hearing aid processing. Recently, Bluetooth connectivity has been added to some hearing aids that permits other Bluetooth enabled devices, such as a cell phone, to directly provide input to the aid.

The Amplifier

The electrical signal from the microphone is small and in analog form (the electrical signal mimics the acoustic signal picked up by the microphone) and must be strengthened to be useful to a hearing aid user. Before development of the integrated circuit (IC), the amplifier was the largest hearing aid component. The integrated circuit amplifier increases the signal intensity by combining transistors and other components on a very small silicon chip. In virtually all modern hearing aids, the signal from the microphone is converted to digital form (digitized) before amplification and processing occurs. The amplified signal is then converted back to analog form and delivered to the hearing aid speaker or receiver.

The components are interconnected, which permits a wide variety of electroacoustic characteristics to be specified for a particular hearing-impaired user. For instance, differing amounts of amplification (gain) can be prescribed, or certain frequencies can be amplified, which specifies the frequency response of the amplifier, or the maximum amplification permitted by the amplifier can be set to accommodate various degrees of loudness discomfort.

In modern hearing aids, several IC amplifiers can be combined on a silicon chip to provide even greater ability to modify the electroacoustic characteristics. Some of these circuits permit programming of characteristics to suit the needs of a user in a variety of listening situations. Also, automatic features are included that permit the hearing aid response to vary depending on the acoustic environment without manual user controls. The most sophisticated amplifiers incorporate digital signal processing, which allows a broader range of signal modification to better match a patient's needs. Figure 4–4 is an example of a hearing aid amplifier.

Basic amplifier electroacoustic performance can be adjusted using specific controls (in digital hearing aids the adjustments are performed in a software program designed for the particular aid). Typically, there is a control to regulate the volume and others to change the frequency response and maximum output of an aid. Advanced amplifier circuits have additional controls for sophisticated signal processing, including circuits specifically designed to automatically prevent squealing (feedback).

The Receiver

The receiver works like a microphone in reverse and converts an electrical signal to an acoustic signal to be received by the ear. Most modern hearing aids incorporate

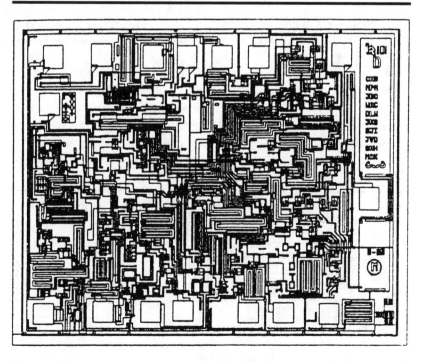

Figure 4–4. Example of a hearing aid amplifier.

an internal air conduction receiver that is connected by tubing to the outside of the hearing aid case or to the earmold. Some receivers, like those found in body-style aids, are coupled directly to the earmold. Air conduction receivers are generally of the balanced-armature magnetic type, because these can faithfully reproduce an amplified wide-band signal and can be constructed in an extremely small package (Staab & Lybarger, 1994). Figure 4–5 is a diagram of a receiver.

The alternating electrical signal from the amplifier causes the electromagnetic field around the armature to change strength and be more or less attracted to the permanent magnets. As the armature is attracted to the diaphragm, the movement of the armature causes the diaphragm to vibrate and produce sound. Bone conduction receivers are used when factors contraindicate the use of air conduction receivers. These receivers are designed to directly vibrate the skull and may have less desirable electroacoustic performance than air conduction receivers.

Batteries

The power source for the increased signal strength and output produced by the amplifier is the battery. Modern hearing aids are typically powered by zinc-air or mercury batteries. Long shelf life and less environmental impact make the zinc-air batteries more desirable. These batteries are basically containers of stored power, and the rate at which the hearing aid drains the stored power will determine how long a battery lasts. The storage capacity of a battery is rated as *milliampere-hours* (mAh), and each hearing aid circuit consumes at a certain mAh rate. Usually the greater the gain, signal processing, and output demands placed on the hearing aid circuit, the greater its current consumption and the shorter the battery life. To extend battery life in this type of aid, a larger battery is needed for increased storage capacity. Hearing aids with lower current drain requirements can use smaller batteries with less storage capacity.

Electroacoustic Properties of Hearing Aids

To select a set of hearing aid components that will meet the needs of a specific hearing-impaired person, knowledge of how the hearing aid components will affect a signal is crucial. As the hearing aid selection process

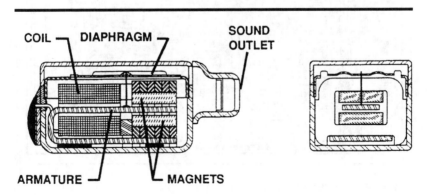

Figure 4–5. Diagram of a hearing aid receiver.

often involves a comparison of hearing aid performance, a standard method of comparing key amplification properties allows comparison across circuits and manufacturers. Currently, the American National Standards Institute (ANSI S3.22, 2003), Specification of Hearing Aid Characteristics, provides the standard measuring techniques for linear hearing aids, with ANSI S3.42-1992 (R2007) (2007), Testing Hearing Aids with a Broad Band Noise Signal, specifying the techniques for nonlinear aids. The standards are revised periodically as hearing aid technology changes. Additional tests are also performed in the actual patient's ear (real-ear measurements) using actual use settings to verify the adequacy of the fitting. Although these measurement standards are not reviewed in detail here, important electroacoustic properties of hearing aids are briefly discussed.

Saturation Sound Pressure Level

Saturation sound pressure level (SSPL) is the maximum sound pressure level that can be produced by a hearing aid when the input signal to the hearing aid is at a high level. The SSPL is usually set below the point at which a user considers the sound to be uncomfortably loud.

Acoustic Gain

The gain of a hearing aid is determined by measuring its output across the frequency spectrum when compared to the level of the sound input to the hearing aid. Gain is a measure of how much the sound is amplified by a hearing aid. Hearing aid gain is determined by the capabilities of the amplifier and the degree to which the user adjusts the volume control, among other things. For example, persons with severe-to-profound

hearing losses will require more acoustic gain than persons with a mild hearing loss.

Frequency Response

The frequency response of a hearing aid is a measure of the range of frequencies amplified by the aid. The frequency response is usually presented as a graph showing the output of the aid as a function of frequency, under conditions specified in a measurement standard. Figure 4–6 depicts the frequency/intensity response curves of a typical hearing aid using the methods specified in ANSI S3.22 (2003).

Distortion

If the signal delivered by the hearing aid to the ear of the user contains sounds that were not present at the hearing aid microphone, the hearing aid system is said to

Standard Frequency Response 007 HX-RPC-1

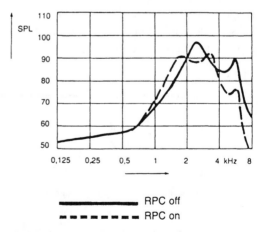

RPC off
RPC on

Figure 4–6. Frequency/intensity response curves of a typical hearing aid.

have added distortion to the input signal. It is generally agreed that distortion reduces the clarity and perhaps the intelligibility of speech and should be minimized in an amplification system. One characteristic of hearing aid component malfunction is high levels of distortion. ANSI S3.22 (2003) specifies ways to measure a type of distortion referred to as harmonic distortion. Other types of distortion, including intermodulation and temporal, may prove to be important in the future.

Styles of Hearing Aids

Early electrical hearing aids were bulky and required large batteries to furnish the power needed to run them. By 1955, the invention of the transistor allowed engineers to design aids that were dramatically smaller. Subsequent miniaturization in the size of microphones, receivers, and batteries plus the development of integrated circuits has permitted the production of ever-smaller hearing aids. This trend toward miniaturization has been driven by the public's desire for the "invisible hearing aid."

Modern hearing aids come in a wide range of styles. The suitability of a particular style depends on the shape of the user's outer ear, circuitry requirements, and age,

among other things. Hearing aids can be classified as body-worn, eyeglass, behind-the-ear, in-the-ear, in-the-canal, completely-in-the-canal, and implantable. Figure 4–7 shows examples of hearing aid styles.

Body-Worn

Body-worn and eyeglass hearing aids together make up less than 2% of hearing aid sales (Kirkwood, 2006). Body-worn aids have a receiver that is separated from the rest of the hearing aid by a lengthy cord. The separation enables the aid to provide sufficient gain without feedback to persons with extreme hearing loss. Because of the size of body-worn aids, circuitry compromises are usually not necessary; therefore, the aids typically allow for many features and adjustments. Batteries can be larger to accommodate the larger current drain required of a high-gain hearing aid.

Eyeglass

Typically the microphone, amplifier, and receiver are built into the eyeglass temple or sidepieces. A major drawback of the style is that the wearer is forced to wear her glasses when the hearing aid is to be used.

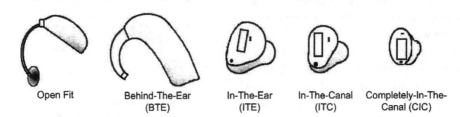

| Open Fit | Behind-The-Ear (BTE) | In-The-Ear (ITE) | In-The-Canal (ITC) | Completely-In-The-Canal (CIC) |

Figure 4–7. Examples of hearing aid styles.

Behind-the-Ear

Behind-the-ear (BTE) hearing aids are designed to fit behind the pinna. The size requires little circuit compromise, and larger capacity batteries can be utilized. They are available in many sizes and configurations for hearing loss from the mild to profound categories. They can easily be adapted for use with classroom amplification and so are frequently used for children.

Recently the so-called mini-BTE open fit has become very popular. These ultra-small BTE instruments channel sound to the ear through very thin tubing or by placing the receiver in the ear canal (called receiver-in-the-ear or RITE hearing aids). The tubing or receiver is held in place with a fitting dome, and by so doing the ear canal is left largely open instead of closed off, as is the case in traditional custom hearing aid products. The open fit was intended for individuals with primarily high-frequency hearing losses and as a means to avoid the unpleasant sound of the patient's own voice produced by the occlusion effect.

In-the-ear (ITE) hearing aids are self-contained packages that fit within the concha and ear canal, with all of the components located in the concha section of the pinna. This positioning of the hearing aid takes advantage of the natural sound enhancements produced by the pinna and possibly the ear canal (Staab & Lybarger, 1994). The ITE hearing aid was made possible by the development of smaller electret microphones, smaller receivers, and smaller yet longer-lasting batteries. The cosmetic appeal of the all-in-the-ear concept has led to wide acceptance of this design. Although the ITE is compact, it is large enough to include such connectivity options as a telecoil or DAI, and a large capacity battery can be used.

In-the-Canal

In-the-canal (ITC) hearing aids were conceived with further miniaturization of the microphone, receiver, and battery. They are self-contained and fit into a small section of the concha and the ear canal. Most of the hearing aid components fit into the concha section, but some reside in the ear canal section. This position in the ear takes advantage of the natural high-frequency resonance of the pinna, unblocked concha, and deep ear canal insertion. The smaller receivers used in the ITC provide more high-frequency response than the larger receivers found in the ITE (Staab & Lybarger, 1994). Although less visible than the ITE, the small size also makes them inappropriate for older patients and persons with disabilities who have dexterity or visual problems, which would make handling of the small aids and small batteries difficult.

Completely-in-the-Canal

Completely-in-the-canal (CIC) hearing aids are self-contained and fit completely within the external auditory canal. Because they are inserted deeply in the ear canal they terminate very close to the tympanic membrane. An example of a CIC hearing aid is shown in Figure 4–8.

Deep CIC insertion in the ear canal provides a number of acoustic benefits to the user. The aids are more cosmetically pleasing, because they are nearly invisible; termination close to the eardrum permits less gain and output to be needed for a given loss, and gain availability is enhanced; and the deep insertion reduces the "head in a barrel" effect (occlusion), provides a secure fit, allows normal use of the telephone, reduces

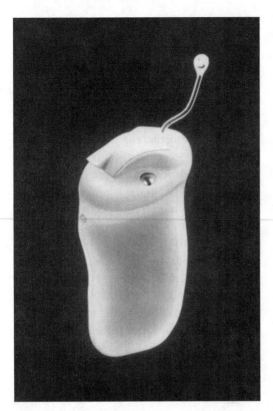

Figure 4–8. Example of a CIC hearing aid.

wind noise, makes feedback less likely, and reduces the amount of cerumen that can clog hearing aid receivers (Staab, 1992).

The small size of the CIC hearing aid and its deep location in the ear canal limit the connectivity options available for this style, and so they may not be appropriate when assistive technologies are recommended for use with the hearing aid. Because the aid fits completely in the ear canal, some persons with small canals are not able to use these small devices.

Implantable Hearing Aids

As the name implies, this category of hearing aid requires a surgical implantation of part of the aid into the auditory pathway. Typically, the electronics, battery, and microphone are not implanted and require a connection to the implanted transducer.

Cochlear Implants

This type of aid converts sound into electrical impulses that are delivered through an electrode that has been surgically placed within the cochlea. The electronics process the acoustic signal and encode it into electrical patterns that can be used to directly stimulate the auditory nerve. The implanted individual must undergo a learning process to efficiently interpret patterns of sound.

Historically, only patients with profound postlingual hearing loss who did not benefit from standard hearing aids were considered cochlear implant candidates. As implant technology has improved, patients will less severe hearing loss have been receiving implants.

According to Schow and Nerbonne (2007), not everyone is a candidate for a cochlear implant. Typical candidacy criteria for cochlear implant referral for adults include (a) a 70 dB HL or greater hearing loss in the mid- to high frequencies; (b) aided word recognition scores of poorer that 50% in the ear to be implanted (60% in the unimplanted ear); and (c) high motivation and realistic expectations. For children to be candidates for cochlear implantation, the child must (a) possess a hearing loss of 90 dB HL or greater in the mid- to high frequencies; (b) demonstrate failure to progress in speech-language-listening development or have a best aided word score of less than 30%; (c) have high parent motivation and realistic expectations, among other requirements. Additional information on the use of cochlear implants can be found in Chapter 9 and Chapter 10 in this text. Figure 4–9 is an illustration of a cochlear implant.

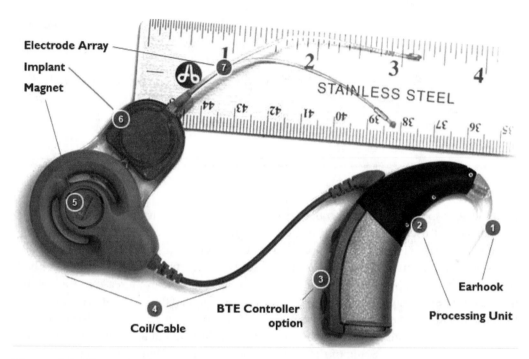

Figure 4–9. Example of a cochlear implant.

Middle Ear Implants

These aids use a magnet, piezoelectric crystal, or other driving device to physically vibrate the tympanic membrane or one of the middle ear ossicles. According to *The Hearing Review* (Tech reports, 1999), middle ear implants are designed for persons with a moderate-to-severe hearing loss and who for whatever reason do not or cannot benefit from air conduction hearing aids.

Bone-Anchored Hearing Aids

These aids use a vibrator that is surgically affixed into the skull. Sound causes the skull to vibrate and the individual hears by bone conduction. The so-called bone-anchored hearing aid (BAHA) uses a sound processor attached to a small titanium implant that is placed in the temporal bone. The temporal bone, then, provides a pathway for sound to the cochlea by passing the ear canal and middle ear (Tech reports, 1999). The manufacturer of the BAHA is Cochlear Corporation (see http://www.cochlearamericas.com).

Earmold Acoustics

Careful ear impressions are necessary to accurately reproduce the geometry of the ear canal, prevent acoustic feedback, and ensure user comfort. Earmolds can be fabricated from ear impressions into many different types and can be made of hard to very soft plastic. Figure 4–10 shows examples of earmold types.

Earmold acoustics are important to understand, because they can be used to

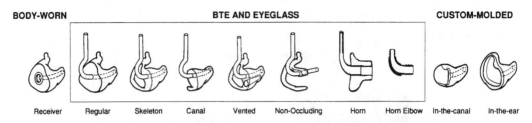

Figure 4–10. Examples of earmold types.

modify the response of the aid to better fit the needs of a user. However, the marketplace shift to ITE, ITC, and CIC hearing aid styles limits the acoustic modifications that were once possible. Nonetheless, BTE hearing aids still require an explicit earmold and tubing coupling to the ear, which can be modified to change the sound delivered through the aid to the ear canal. Some of the modifications can also be applied to hearing aid styles for aids that reside in the concha or ear canal.

As can be seen in Figure 4-11, the frequency response of a hearing aid can be dramatically modified using different earmold acoustic modification techniques (Killion, 1980). These changes in hearing aid response are often necessary to fine tune a hearing aid response to a user's residual hearing. The techniques in common use can be categorized as the following. (a) Venting (primarily affecting the low frequencies) is the making of an opening through the hearing aid from the outside to the ear canal, usually parallel with the receiver tubing of the hearing aid. The diameter of the hole may range from 0.065 mm to simply release pressure against the eardrum when inserting the earmold, up to a 3 mm diameter, where maximum acoustic effects are expected. (b) Damping (influencing mostly the mid-frequencies) works by inserting occluding devices that restrict the flow of acoustic energy at specific frequencies, depending on the resistance and the location of the damping device in the tubing or earmold. These devices are frequently used to reduce the gain when peaks occur in the frequency response. (c) Horn effects (affecting primarily the high frequencies) are an increase in the volume of the ear canal end of an earmold. This increase in volume acts much like a "horned" musical instrument to emphasize certain frequencies, depending on the size and shape of the horn (Killion, 1976; Libby, 1981).

The diameter and length of the tubing used in the earmold type can also produce major changes in the frequency response. Although the acoustic effects of earmold modifications are somewhat predictable, obtaining a desired result is often done by trial and error and can be a lengthy process.

Programmability and Digital Signal Processing

Hearing aids used to have relatively fixed electroacoustic characteristics selected to generally meet the residual hearing needs of the user. Fine tuning of these devices was sometimes difficult, and so an approximate fitting to the user's needs was often considered acceptable. Modern digital hearing aids are designed to have a wide variety of electroacoustic characteristics built into them, along with a programming function, which allows the aid to be finely tuned to the needs of a user. Electronic control of the electro-

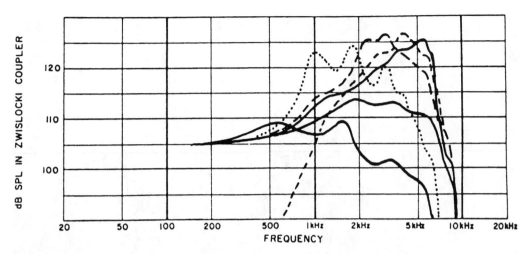

Figure 4–11. Examples of frequency response modifications using different earmold modification techniques.

acoustic modifications is more predictable than purely acoustic modification through earmold changes. Until recently, most programmable hearing aids were programmed using a computer (programming was digital), but the actual functioning of the aid did not convert the acoustic signal into digital form (so the amplification remained analog). The latest digital aids employ both digital programming and digital signal processing during amplification. These offer an increasing selection of processing options to more precisely meet the amplification needs of each patient.

A diagram of a programmable hearing aid is shown in Figure 4-12. Typically, the user's audiometric data is input into a computer program that makes calculations for desirable electroacoustic characteristics based on established predictive equations. The hearing aid dispenser selects additional features that are required by the dynamics of the hearing loss and user needs. Given the different combinations of gain, output, frequency response, output limiting, and number of channel combinations possible, the dispenser has literally thousands of aids

to choose from to meet user needs. In the most sophisticated aids, multiple programmable memories are built in, which allows the user to switch from one set of electroacoustic characteristics to another to maximize the characteristics for particular listening situations. Of course, if the user's hearing and listening needs change, the programmable aid can be reprogrammed without the purchase of an entirely new aid.

Summary

Designing and fitting hearing aids to enable the hearing-impaired individual to use all of the residual hearing potential has been and continues to be a challenge. Advances in hearing aid technology have allowed us to come closer than ever to meet the challenge, but our understanding of how to repair a broken auditory system is still incomplete. As more is learned about the function and dysfunction of human hearing, it is a certainty that hearing aids will be designed to utilize that knowledge.

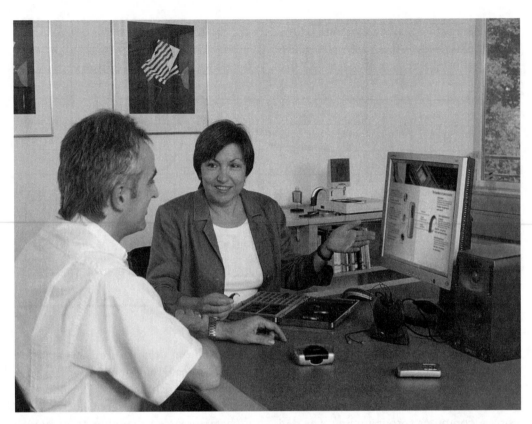

Figure 4–12. Modern digital hearing aids are programmed through a computer using specific fitting software. Here a typical fitting session is shown (Photo courtesy of Phonak).

References

American National Standards Institute. (2003). *Specification of hearing aid characteristics.* ANSI S3.22-2003. New York: Author.

American National Standards Institute. (2007). *Testing hearing aids with a broad-band noise signal.* ANSI S3.42-1992 (R2007). New York: Author.

Berger, K. (1984). *The hearing aid: Its operation and development.* Livonia, MI: The National Hearing Aid Society.

Boothroyd, A. (2008). The acoustic speech signal. In J. Madell & C. Flexer (Eds.), *Pediatric audiology* (pp. 159–167). New York: Thieme.

Hearing Industries Association. (1992). *Statistical report for the quarter ending December. New units sold by type and origin.* Washington, DC: Author.

Holmes, A., & Rodriguez, G. (2007). Cochlear implants and vestibular/tinnitus rehabilitation. In R. Schow & M. Nerbonne (Eds.), *Introduction to audiologic rehabilitation* (pp. 77–112). New York: Pearson.

Killion, M. (1976). Experimental wide band hearing aid. *Journal of the Acoustical Society of America, 59*(Suppl. 1), S62.

Killion, M. (1980). Problems in the amplification of broadband hearing aid earphones. In G. Studebaker & I. Hochberg (Eds.), *Acoustical factors affecting hearing aid performance* (pp. 121–132). Baltimore: University Park Press.

Killion, M., & Carlson, E. (1974). A sub-miniature electret microphone of new design. *Journal of the Auditory Engineering Society, 22,* 237–243.

Kirkwood, D. (2006). Led by BTE, sales rise for fourth straight year to surpass 2.3 million. *The Hearing Journal, 59*(12), 11–20.

Libby, E. (1981). Achieving a transparent, smooth, wideband hearing aid response. *Hearing Instruments, 32,* 9–12.

Sanders, D. (1993). *Management of hearing handicap.* Englewood Cliffs, NJ: Prentice Hall.

Schow, R. & Nerbonne, M. (2007). *Introduction to Audiologic Rehabilitation* (5th ed.). New York: Allyn and Bacon.

Smaldino, J., & Crandell, C. (2005). Speech perception in the classroom. In C. Crandell, J. Smaldino, & C. Flexer (Eds.), *Sound-field amplification: Applications to speech perception and classroom acoustics* (pp. 49–56). Clifton Park, NY: Thomson Delmar Learning.

Staab, W. (1992). The peritympanic instrument: Fitting, rationale and test results. *The Hearing Journal, 45,* 21–26.

Staab, W., & Lybarger, S. (1994). Characteristics and use of hearing aids. In J. Katz (Ed.), *Handbook of clinical audiology* (pp. 657–722). Baltimore: Williams & Wilkins.

Tech reports. (1999). Update on implant technology: Part 2. Implantable hearing aids. *The Hearing Review, 6,* 12, 13, 33, 34.

End of Chapter Examination Questions

Chapter 4

1. What is the overall goal of a hearing aid fitting? Briefly describe that goal.

2. Some hearing aids utilize an earmold. In general acoustical terms, what does an earmold do?

3. The author describe six basic styles of hearing aids in this chapter. What are they? What are their benefits and limitations?

4. Define the following terms, and describe how they contribute to the overall function of a hearing aid:
   a. Saturation sound pressure level
   b. Acoustic gain
   c. Frequency response
   d. Distortion

5. In regard to styles of hearing aids, which recent style has been developed specifically to amplify high frequencies and eliminate the occlusion effect?

6. Define the following terms as they relate to earmold acoustics:
   a. Venting
   b. Damping
   c. Horn effects

End of Chapter Answer Sheet

Name _____ Date _____

Chapter 4

1. _____

_____

_____

2. _____

_____

_____

3. _____

_____

_____

4. a. _____

b. _____

c. _____

d. _____

5. _____

6. a. _____

b. _____

c. _____

Part II

Introduction To Aural Rehabilitation: Children With Impaired Hearing

5

Family Involvement and Counseling in Serving Children Who Possess Impaired Hearing

DALE V. ATKINS

Chapter Outline

Introduction

Acknowledging that one's child has impaired hearing is a long and often challenging emotional process that no one, aside from another parent of a child whose hearing is impaired, can fully understand. It is the first and most important fact that each professional needs to accept before, during, and after provision of service to any family with a child who possesses a disability. This chapter presents information on the families of children who have impaired hearing, the role of the family in the support of the children, and the role of the professional involved with their families.

Preliminaries for the Professional

There is much that professionals can do to help in the navigation of an unfamiliar and confusing road. Whether trained as teachers, doctors, speech and language pathologists, audiologists, or counselors, professionals must always be mindful of who they are and what their role is in the process of working with parents and children. Professionals may wish to make their patient's pain go away; they may wish to fix everything and see themselves as saviors, miracle workers, or persons on whom parents rely to cope better with their situation. They may, intentionally or not, raise parents' expectations based on their own desire to have everyone feel better.

Certainly, it is well within a professional's realm to be encouraging, hopeful, and positive in spirit. It is not within a professional's realm to promise what cannot be delivered. Early in this author's career of working with families of children who have

hearing impairments, a mother of a happy, popular, highly communicative 12-year-old girl who used total communication (i.e., a combination of sign language, voice, and audition) kept insisting that her daughter mostly use her voice instead of signing when talking with me. Afterward, in my private conversation with the mother, she said she felt like a failure whenever her daughter chose not to speak. When asked why, she replied, "I'll never forget the first professional I met in the field of deafness. She was a therapist who told me that if I worked hard enough, my daughter would speak as well as any 'normal' child. You know, I devoted my entire life to trying to teach her to speak well. Since she doesn't speak well, I feel as if I didn't do enough."

Another family has been waiting for life to return to the way it was before their son lost his hearing at age 26 months. The father, upon reflection of the doctor's words, recalled him saying, "Things will be as good as new; even better because you all have survived such a terrible trauma." Contrary to what the doctor predicted, things were far from better. The household was in chaos and the older, 6-year-old brother felt confused, abandoned, and neglected because of his parents' involvement with his younger brother. They were waiting for things to go back to "the way it was." It was already more than 4 years and the family was still trying to sort out their lives. Things were hardly "as good as new."

When we experience loss, our lives change. Things do not return to the way they were because *we* have changed and our family dynamic has also changed. This does not mean life will not be better. Often it is. But it will not be the way it was. The *challenge* is to discover the meaning of this experience, notice how we are transformed, integrate the experience into our lives, and move forward. This is a process and for each of us it takes a different form and period of time. Life events do matter. Richard Lucas, a psychologist at Michigan State University, in studying happiness and the effect of major changes in life circumstances found that they can indeed have long-term impact on happiness levels.

Individual differences play an important role as well as what people experience during the adaptation process. People who are more positive emotionally and have good social relationships may be more likely to integrate these changes better than those who are and do not. It is important to understand the various ways people react to life factors they anticipate having difficulty dealing with (Lucas, 2007).

Professionals must be mindful that each person's experience is unique, and that discovering that one's child has a disability changes each person in some way. In all families, parental actions are heavily influenced by various factors, among which are the child's responses. Also vital are the parents' family backgrounds and interpersonal stories, how they were raised, marital harmony or discord, finances, chronic or acute stresses and means of dealing with them, strengths and support of friendships, expectations for themselves and their children, knowledge about and attitudes toward disability, maturity, and attitude toward life's challenges. Further, there are cultural differences in how persons with disabilities and their families are perceived (Yacobacci-Tam, 1987).

In a reflection on his long and important career in the field of deafness, David Luterman, an audiologist by training and one of the pioneers in parent counseling in the field of deafness, said,

> My own view, based on 40 years of observing children who are deaf, is that a variety of approaches are needed and that the child will tell us which is the best way for him or her to be taught. Ongoing research needs to be conducted so that we can match the child to the methodology sooner. At the present time it is more trial and error. (Luterman, 2004)

How professionals see themselves and interpret their roles will greatly affect the course of treatment for a family as a whole and a child individually. Helping people to approach their lives from a perspective of strength and expediting their discovery and utilization of their own inner resources, while sorting out the maze in which they find themselves, is within the professional's domain. The rate at which a family's progress occurs is outside the professional's domain and is determined by the persons themselves and their response and interaction with the long process of healing, coping, and living. Specialists need to be unintimidating, cooperative teammates who have chosen a field of study and have developed considerable experience and training in specific areas, but who are open to learning from the people who have come for guidance. They must present themselves as human beings first, people who have selected a particular profession and, as a result, have accumulated some knowledge. They cannot be all-knowing, superior, or condescending. Rather, professionals must embark eager to learn in a partnership with people whom they view positively and respectfully.

Preliminaries for the Family

The family is a primary, powerful emotional system that shapes and influences the lives of its members. In systems theory, the family is conceptualized as a dynamic unit. The theory posits that family relationships are interdependent and mutually interactive; change in one part of the system stimulates compensatory change in other parts. Erikson (1964) found that the stability of a family hinges on the complicated and sensitive pattern of emotional balance and interchange. The behavior of each member affects and is affected by the behavior of other members. Families are the greatest potential resource for personal well-being, as well as for psychological distress.

Luterman (1979) states that in families with children who possess a disability, the family as a whole may initially attempt to adjust to the disability without changing the existing family structure. However, members may eventually reach a point where they cannot continue to meet previous social, economic, and personal roles and expectations, and where they may become dissatisfied with their relationships with each other. A role organization crisis may occur that is associated with elevated tension, in which delicately balanced family priorities may shift. Siblings may be expected to take over adult responsibilities and the quality and frequency of recreational activities may change; grandparents may shy away from sharing child care responsibilities or may offer help and be rejected. Previously earmarked finances may need to be budgeted for the funding of hearing aids, tactile stimulators, private therapy, or attendance at conferences. Longstanding friendships may be critically scrutinized and personal time and energy all but disappear. When family disequilibrium persists and parents feel particularly stressed, there is a risk of severe personal or relational problems developing.

All too often, the actual issues that are troubling a family are not addressed and symptoms rather than causes are confronted. In a rather typical example, a father in one family became increasingly more involved in his work after the diagnosis of his son's hearing impairment. He attended evening work meetings, traveled more, and accepted business-related phone calls at home. Whenever he was scheduled to attend a clinic appointment, invariably someone from his office would call. This put a severe strain on his relationship with his wife. She felt she was alone and they argued frequently. The symptoms appeared to indicate marital distress, but, in truth, the man needed to become totally absorbed in his work to get his mind away from the pain he was experiencing about his child who was hearing impaired and to reassure himself of his importance. The father needed to believe that he could still control much of his world even though he felt helpless over not being able to change his son's hearing impairment.

The Role of the Professional

Interactions with the Family

In the beginning of a professional association, the professional does not know the people seeking help (parents or children), and they (the parents and children) do not know the professional. Professionals are viewed as "the experts." The danger of this for professionals is that they may maintain the parents' expectation of them and forget that they, too, are involved in a learning process. This "halo effect" is a dangerous illusion for a professional who does not understand the lengthy process in which the parents are immersed. Parents desperately need to know they are not lost, that their family, particularly their child, will be okay. They desire reassurance about the decisions confronting them. Parents are thrown into a new world (with its own language and conflicts in the field) and are required to make serious decisions for and about their child, based on recommendations of various professionals.

Even before a child's hearing aids arrive, the parents need to select one of many early intervention programs representing different philosophies. If cochlear implantation is an option, how is it presented? "What should we do? What would you do if you were in my shoes?" asks the overwhelmed parent. The professional is often, during these moments, viewed as much more than human and asked to make decisions for the parents about their family's future. The professional's job is not to make decisions for the family, but rather to help the parents become sufficiently informed and comfortable so that they can make their own decisions. It is a difficult position to be in because of the nature of the counseling required.

Counseling

As speech and language pathologists, teachers and audiologists are not trained to be professional counselors, social workers, or psychologists; thus they sometimes feel inadequate to deal with the range of emotional responses they encounter while performing the service for which they were trained. Many of these professionals feel competent working with children, but find themselves interacting at arm's length with the child's parents as well as siblings, grandparents, and caregivers. Frequently, an entire family (extended and nuclear) will show up for an appointment and the professional feels unprepared to handle the different people and the various emotions expressed.

It is essential that a clinician understand that his role is not to become a counselor. However, to be more proficient, the profes-

sional does need to be sensitive to and unafraid of the multifaceted nature of his work, which is simultaneously content- and emotion-based. Both aspects are equally important to the success of the interaction. At times, content may come more to the fore, but that does not mean that emotional underpinnings are absent.

The Professional as Counselor

To enable professionals to feel prepared for these encounters, it is useful for them to learn basic counseling theories, with the understanding that they will, for the most part, be dealing with a "well patient" model. Unlike in psychotherapy, where the main goal is to help reorganize and reinterpret a patient's intrapersonal conflicts, which may be characterized by anxieties, depression, guilt, confusions, or ambivalence, counseling in this context is done with psychologically normal individuals who are presently trying to confront and cope with a major disruption or series of major disruptions in their lives (Clark, 1990, p. 5).

Counseling is supportive and builds on renewed insights into the persons, their family, goals, and specific aspects of their lives. For a more intense examination of the various models and their use with a population that has hearing impairment, the reader is referred to the works of Harvey (1989), Luterman (1979), and Rollin (1987). One can attempt to be familiar with a variety of theories and then blend them, depending on the need of a patient and the situation.

Whatever a professional's orientation, no response will compensate for the loss that the family is going through. The gaping hole cannot be filled by words. The hurt may be soothed over time—usually years.

Professionals must be active and involved listeners, committed to the process: active in that they encourage parents to express their emotions and the circumstances underlying those emotional states; involved in that they recognize when questions need a direct, informal response. It is essential to be straightforward yet compassionate and empathetic, confident yet neither pompous nor omniscient, respectful of the family and sensitive to their plight and concerns, so that the family will be able to perceive and accept the professional as a viable and trustworthy partner.

Trust has more chance of developing if a professional learns the parents' personal hopes and their goals for themselves and their children. These people have a lot to teach. Refraining from making assumptions is vital for a professional. The extent to which the news of a hearing impairment affects a family can only be discovered by listening to and observing each particular family. Yet the professional can view them against a backdrop of knowledge that has been garnered from other families.

Emotional Responses of Families

From research and observation of families of children who have impaired hearing, professionals find that in the area of emotional response, these families experience reactions similar to those of children who have other disabilities. The response cycle is not unlike that experienced by any person involved in grieving a major loss. For years, this process was likened to that described by Kübler-Ross (1969) in her classic treatise entitled, *On Death and Dying*. Predictable stages were described as shock, recognition, denial, acknowledgment, and constructive action. Because parents lost the child they had envisioned, their task at hand is to adapt to the thought and reality of life with this different child. What was previously normal suddenly undergoes reassessment. Somehow, a new "normalcy" needs to be established. There is an ending to the relationship with the child who was believed to have normal hearing and a beginning of a new relationship with a child who has impaired hearing. With neither warning nor preparation, the parents are thrust into an unfamiliar world filled with information and people they would have otherwise gone a lifetime without confronting. To add to the predicament, there really is no choice. They enter this world reluctantly and apprehensively. The professional's function at this point is to serve as a supportive guide through the maze.

This process of parental grieving is different from that of losing a child completely. It is also unlike the discovery that one's child has a more visible disability that may have been obvious at birth. Deafness is referred to as "the invisible handicap" and, thus, the extent of the disability is not known to most people. Additionally, as deafness is rarely discovered at birth, parents initially bond with the child whom they believe is 100% as expected. They sing, talk, and in general relate to the baby as if there were normal function. When the suspicion that the child may have a hearing problem is confirmed, there is, understandably, shock, sadness, guilt, anger, resentment, vulnerability, overprotection, confusion, denial, depression, and remorse on the part of the parents and other family members (Luterman, 1987). These feelings frequently appear and reappear over the years, although the families rebuild their lives and deal with their loss constructively. It is essential that parents go through, rather than avoid, the mourning process. "It enhances their parental capacity for satisfaction in childrearing" (Leigh, 1987). Nancy Miller, in her book, *Nobody's Perfect* (1994), describes four stages of adaptation experienced by parents of children who have disabilities. These stages are familiar to parents of children with hearing impairments. They are dynamic, nonlinear, and often overlap. They are: surviving, searching, settling in, and separating. Each stage has its own set of experiences and reactions that go along with them for each person.

Hearing the News

Often, on hearing the news, parents question their ability to parent a child, feel unprepared, and don't know what to do. They question everything they do know about their child and wonder if they will ever relate to this different child from whom they feel estranged and with whom they imagine they will be unable to communicate. Previously held feelings of competency about their own parenting skills are called into question as they begin to worry about what will happen to their children, their relationship, and their family. One mother mused:

> I knew that music was my whole life and I had spent so much time thinking about how great it would be to have a child to sing with. I played soothing classical music during my pregnancy, sang all the time while he was an infant, and brought him every musical toy that I could find. I truly do not know what I'm supposed to do. I'm just so utterly sad.

On the recent discovery of his fourth child's hearing impairment, one father lamented,

> I don't think I can rely on anything I did with my other kids to be right. I don't know how to deal with Mickey since he cannot hear me. How will I discipline him? How will I find out what he wants? I'm questioning everything I ever knew about children, because I see how much I don't know.

The overwhelming sense that they will not know what to do or that there is too much to learn and they are not equipped to handle all that will be required can cause some parents to question everything they know about children.

To help parents realize their full potential, their initial perceptions of weakness and helplessness must be gradually and consistently replaced by confidence and competence. The clinician's role is to enable parents to work effectively with a child, while providing objective, individualized support, guidance, and critique. The professional's role changes over time. At first, their words are the only words of guidance and instruction that are available to the family. Later, they serve as a sounding board.

It is at this point that the message "child first and foremost" needs to be conveyed to parents gently and consistently. Usually, parents focus on the aspect of their child that is impaired rather than focusing on the whole child. This is a natural response. It is up to the professional to relate to the child as a child first, considering the hearing impairment second. Even though the family sees the professional for issues regarding the hearing impairment, the nature of the professional's interaction, questions, and manner should be that of a person interested in the functioning of a whole child within a whole family. A mother of a newly diagnosed 20-month-old daughter insisted that, whenever her husband interacted with their daughter, he wear the microphone for her FM unit. At times he resisted, especially when he wanted to "roughhouse" with his daughter. This incited tension between the couple. She felt she was the only one working with Angela, while he was just there for the fun. The mother felt they did not have time to "fool around." Without realizing it, the mother sent disapproving messages to her husband, so that he felt his way of relating to his daughter was not valuable. Much of his time was not engaged in "teaching language"; therefore, it was deemed unimportant. She felt he was not giving his daughter anything that she needed. He claimed, "I don't do as well as my wife does in the structured setting. At least I can still develop a relationship with my daughter. Isn't that worth something?" Intuitively he knew that he was doing well with Angela, but the pressure of needing every waking hour to be involved in a structured language experience had taken over and dictated their lives. The valuable, delicate balance had not yet been struck.

Feelings, Doubts, and Questions

Feelings are complex and confusing. Doubts abound. Questions are asked. Some are unanswerable, thus adding to the frustration and the sense of feeling unfamiliar and incompetent. Parents of newly diagnosed children frequently report feeling numb. They are overwhelmed with a horrible sense of disbelief and shock and unable to process information they are given about hearing loss, audiograms, cochlear implants, hearing aids, educational options, and state support services, while attempting to look attentive with tears welling up or running down, fighting enormous lumps in throats, resisting nausea and a generalized feeling of being in another place or time zone, with people who are unfamiliar (Buscalia, 1975; Featherstone, 1980; Moses, 1985).

Maria Forecki (1985) recounted her experiences with her son, Charlie, who has impaired hearing, in Speak to Me. She recalled her initial experience this way:

> Mourning manifested itself in not wanting to speak to Charlie, or anyone else. I unplugged my radio and refused to watch television. I surrounded myself with the absence of sound so as to make sound not exist. It was impossible to live with the fact that Charlie could not experience sound. (p. 29)

One father described hearing the news this way:

> It was as if I was knifed in my stomach; my insides were threatened to come out and the more I tried to hold them in, the more I lost control. The audiologist just kept staring at me with a shocked expression on his face. I must have looked like something had snapped inside of me . . . in fact, it did.

Delivering difficult news is something most of us are not comfortable with. At various stages in the families' journey they will meet many professionals who will be in the position of delivering, if not bad, then difficult news. The first person to confirm the parents' suspicion of hearing impairment is usually a pediatrician, otologist, or audiologist. Although the news may be delivered gently and tactfully, it may not be received in that way.

Many professionals perceive their role as being one of delivering news and then asking the parents for questions. When the parents do not ask any, the professional assumes all is understood as it was presented and continues to talk. It is useless to deliver news and information if you do not validate that it is actually received and understood.

Yet when the news is difficult, professionals often avoid the very probing that is necessary, not wanting to "upset" the parents more. The professional must make a serious and consistent effort to listen to what is and what is not being said. Whenever professionals are in the position of delivering news, they must be conscious of several factors, among which are environment, participants, timing and sequencing, language or symbols, strength ability, and resources (Kroth, 1987). Because the sorrow of having a child who has impaired hearing is often chronic, professionals need to be supportive and mindful of these factors throughout the years of their interactions with parents. One mother thought aloud:

> Sometimes, today, 15 years later, I still feel like I did at that first meeting with the audiologist. When I hear important information about Jackie, my emotions get in the way of my being able to listen attentively, and I have a hard time hearing what is being said. I guess because we have been through so much, people expect me to have an unfeeling filter through which I hear all of the facts. It just isn't so.

If a professional is furnishing information, it is imperative that attempts be made to assist the parents in feeling less overwhelmed by making enough time to give information and to answer questions. Language needs to be carefully chosen and words that may be unfamiliar should be explained. Few situations are more intimidating to parents than listening to professionals talk about their child, using words that are unfamiliar. In the area of hearing impairment, where there are unfamiliar terms and symbols (e.g., interpreting an audiogram), handouts should be provided with terminology, phrases, and definitions, with resource sheets and pamphlets

readily available in their own language. Parents need time to ingest what is discussed. They need to be assured that a follow-up meeting or phone call is scheduled to ensure clarification of points made.

Enhancing Communication between Professionals and Parents

Because much of the information that is presented may or may not be heard or processed, it is essential to frequently review what has been previously discussed. One mother tape recorded every session she had with the otologist and audiologist so that she could review the tape with her husband who was unable to attend many of the appointments with her. As her child grew up, tape recording became a useful habit. She taped teachers' meetings and individualized educational plan (IEP) sessions. Some professionals she encountered were uneasy, but she countered by saying that she wanted to concentrate on what was being said, wanted to feel free to ask questions, and wanted to have time to review all of the answers when she was in the privacy of her own home. Professionals who feel comfortable with this idea can expand it by providing prerecorded tapes of the information to be covered or by taping their sessions and giving the parents the audiotape. In this age of CDs, hearing an old fashioned audiotape recorder is often helpful. Additionally, it is helpful to appreciate how much families benefit from receiving a packet of information sheets, booklets, lists of national and local organizations and resources, and books for themselves and to share with family members. The information packet should be available in as many languages as the community served. This practice is especially helpful when parents travel a great distance and the likelihood of frequent follow-up meetings or immediate contact with other parents is slim or if their extended family lives in another town or country.

Realizing that only a portion of a message is going to be received is an important lesson for all professionals. Messages, particularly those that are not entirely welcome, are frequently distorted as they are filtered through our thoughts and feelings. Whenever professionals are in the position of giving news to parents, they must be aware that parents also need to hear what the possibilities are for their children and for their families. One father remembers:

> The therapist seemed so upbeat, hopeful, and positive. It helped us because, like us, our friends and family were all so down and grief-stricken. Every conversation we had was about Joey and his hearing. Heaven knows what was happening in other aspects of our lives since it seems now that we didn't deal with anything else. We were sad, but we also wanted to do something constructive.

Referring to his own participation he said:

> I realized that I began to enjoy the sessions because I was learning while I was getting to know Joey in a different way. Instead of focusing on the fact that he could not hear, I began to think of ways I could broaden his ability to hear. It became exciting. That is when I began to feel hopeful.

Families seem to do better when they are confident that a professional is familiar and current with different educational programs. Visiting area schools and keeping up professional associations with those in the same and related fields is helpful for the clinician's personal and professional growth. It is invaluable when sharing knowledge with families. Professionals who attend conferences and participate in workshops designed for parents can develop sensitivity to the situation faced by those parents. Teachers who visit local hearing aid dispensers and hearing and speech centers at local hospitals and clinics where families receive services have a better chance of connecting with families and understanding the complex network with which the families interact. Too often, parents are the link in a large network of services. When they discover that professionals are unacquainted or unfamiliar with one another, their confidence in the professionals and the system can wane. If they perceive that there is a larger, interconnected structure of which they are a part, they feel less isolated.

Exchanging Roles

A strategy at seminars and workshops is to encourage parents and professionals to assume the role of the other when involved in a particular problem-solving exercise or sensitivity-training role play. By reversing roles, empathy is likely to develop, and the process of working together can be accomplished more smoothly. In one such exercise, a speech-language pathologist expressed anger over a parent's tardiness for her son's sessions. The clinician interpreted this chronic lateness as the mother's resistance to having her son in therapy. When the speech-language pathologist took the role of the mother, she discovered that the mother needed to travel 2 hours on public transportation to attend therapy. After discovering this, the pathologist became more alert to such situations in her patients' lives. In this case, there was an effort to address the problem directly, enlisting a community ride service, which helped to ease the transportation problem.

Professionals are well advised to develop sensitive communication skills that consider a family's needs and comfort. Professionals who work with children who have hearing loss and their families are closely involved with them in exploring solutions to their challenges The overriding message the professional can convey is that the family will be able to cope, and the professionals the parents encounter will assist them and be a part of their journey, making their task easier. Parents' existing coping skills may enable them to deal with their situation better than professionals expect. Some people are more resilient than others. Conversely, developing coping skills may be what is needed to facilitate better adjustment and adaptation, and therefore, the professional's role may be expanded to include helping parents discover how to efficiently negotiate the maze of people, places, and things related to and about hearing loss. Professionals can help their patients incorporate family and friends into their lives in ways that can be beneficial to all involved. Finally, professionals are in the privileged position of providing a safe place where families can recognize and explore their fears and develop the courage to deal with them. This transition and transformation happens when there is, at the core of the relationship, a fundamental trust.

Parent Support Groups

Most professionals know the value of connecting families with other families who are in similar situations. At times, there may be initial reluctance by patients to meet other parents. Perhaps talking to one professional is all a family can handle at the moment. Perhaps meeting with other parents is too

threatening, too definite an acknowledgment that they have a child who has impaired hearing. But the eventual sharing that occurs among families is potentially the most therapeutic and healing remedy that any family can undertake. Bonds of friendship, understanding, empathy, and humor form among families who, under other circumstances would not have met. They give one another strength as well as hope. Helen Keller wrote:

> We bereaved are not alone. We belong to the largest company in all the world—the company of those who have known suffering. When it seems that our sorrow is too great to be borne, let us think of the great family of the heavy-hearted into which our grief has given us entrance, and, inevitably, we feel about us their arms, their sympathy, their understanding. (Keller, 1954, p. 56)

It is the parents who grow together, leaving behind feelings of helplessness and despair, as they try jointly to make sense out of the new world into which they have reluctantly been thrust.

Professionals must encourage attendance at parent support groups, and if none exist, commit to starting such a program with one or two interested families. These discussion groups augment parent-to-parent phone connections, membership in organizations, attendance at panel discussions featuring parents of teenagers and young adults who have hearing loss, older children who have hearing loss, grandparents, and siblings, and interaction with adults and professionals who have hearing loss. All are of inestimable value in the adaptation of families with children who have hearing losses.

It is other parents who can offer solace when a grandparent appears to favor one child over another and the parents do not know how to address this with their own parents. It is other parents who understand what it is like when a child who has hearing impairment is not asked for "playdates" by the neighborhood kids. It is other parents who can talk openly about their feelings of neglecting their other children in favor of the child who has a hearing loss, because the "need" is greater. Other parents can truly understand the difficulty of not having the time or energy for their spouses or their children. They can notice other parents placing expectations on the siblings who have normal hearing to behave maturely and accept responsibilities beyond their ages.

Parents in a parent group can organize a sibling day, arrange to have all of the families meet at a picnic site, and emphasize the normalcy of their families so that the siblings can see other families with children who wear hearing aids (Atkins, 1987). These events help families and siblings, in particular, feel less isolated. It is in a parent group that parents can let their hair down and not have to be "supermom" or "superdad." It is in a parent group that parents can discuss what it is like to have one's personal and familial identity quickly transformed into the "father of" or "family with the deaf kid," recognizing that wherever they go people look at them and make assumptions, sometimes asking questions, sometimes not, sometimes offering suggestions, sometimes not. One mother received nods of recognition from group members when she said, "Running to the market used to be so easy. Now when I take Alex, everyone in the check-out line stares at his hearing aids. One woman asked if he was listening to a Walkman. I'm embarrassed to tell you that I said, 'Yes'!"

Only other parents can identify with the sinking feeling when every eye in the store is on you when your child has a tantrum. Upon reflections on his daughter's tantrum in a toy store, one father admitted:

It is worse when your kid is deaf, because when she closes her eyes and pulls her hearing aids out of her ears there really is no way to reach her. While I am waiting for her to calm down, it seems like everyone in the store has passed me and I'm convinced they think I am the most incompetent father in the world.

It is also parents who are going through a similar process who can encourage other parents to be patient while witnessing the progress of their friends' children and not seeing any discernible change in their own children:

Sometimes when we see my sister's kids, I can't help feeling envious of her. She has it all so easy! We were pregnant at the same time, planned it so that the cousins would be close and play together, and now I wonder how they will ever get along. I don't want my nephew to feel that Billy is a drag to be around.

Another mother commented:

Years ago when I saw other mothers playing with their children in the park I would feel intensely jealous. Now I know that many of my friends envy my relationship with my daughter because we really are close. Maybe that has to do with how hard we have worked at communicating. I needed a lot of patience.

Other Family Members

Another means of assisting parents adapt to life with a child with impaired hearing is acknowledgment by professionals that there are other important influences in their lives. Attending to the needs of their child who is hearing impaired is often dominant, but it is not the only important aspect in their lives. Relationships with other children in the family, spouses or significant others, grandparents, friends, and one's self need to be addressed.

Parents and Siblings

Other children in the family fare better when their needs are also recognized, when they are included in family decisions, and when they are spoken to openly and honestly about what has transpired and what is happening in their family. Explanations take time and need to be repeated and broadened as children grow and develop. Books written for and about sibling issues are available, and most professionals welcome brothers and sisters attending an occasional session so that they can become informed, participate if they care to, and listen through hearing aids. Siblings can help in very specific ways, thus alleviating some of the pressure felt by the parents. It is imperative to remember at all times, however, that the responsibility for the child who has impaired hearing, whether lessons or care, does not lie with a sibling. In addition to making brothers and sisters feel welcome and important, professionals can offer correct, easy explanations embellished by pictures, CDs andIinternet video, and the actual apparatus that is used for testing, while providing answers to questions that help siblings respond when their friends ask them questions about hearing loss.

Professionals and parents can organize the sibling days devoted to the education and involvement of brothers and sisters. Age-appropriate information can be shared about facts and myths about hearing impairment, family adjustment issues, and coping techniques for specific situations. Children of all ages need to know that they are not responsible for their brother's or sister's hearing impairment. They need to be reassured that their school performance, for example, is unrelated to their brother's or sister's. A 44-year-old teacher of children who have hearing impairment remembered her own household:

> Everyone made such a fuss when Kristen did well in school. If she got a "B" it was cause for celebration. I was happy for her too, but sometimes I would have liked some recognition for my hard work. Granted, things came easier for me because I had my hearing, but school was still hard. I had a straight "A" report card throughout high school and it was as if it was expected. I was the model kid. I know my folks had enough on their minds. I didn't want to add to their heartache, so I never brought them my problems.

To help siblings face their own feelings, parents need to be encouraged to provide full, age-appropriate explanations, with emphasis on the feelings the family and siblings are experiencing. This is particularly beneficial when helping siblings deal with feelings of sadness, guilt, disappointment, confusion, anger, jealousy, overprotection, fear, embarrassment, responsibility, pride, love, comfort, interest, concern, tolerance, patience, and sympathy. Encouraging siblings to express their feelings is difficult for some parents, if they themselves have been avoiding their emotions. Allowing children to express their feelings is a gift.

It is also worthwhile to know the parents' perception of their normally hearing child's role in relation to the sibling who has impaired hearing. Is the parental perception communicated to the sibling? If so, by what means? If not, is this a problem for the sibling? Most children need to know that the feelings they are having are okay. Parents do not need to do anything except listen in a nonjudgmental and loving way.

When parents attempt to deal openly with their own feelings related to having a child with a hearing loss, they are more likely to be able to address the issue with their other children. Some are unable to do this. One mother who was deep in grief interpreted her normal hearing daughter's "needy requests at bedtime" for "another glass of water and just one more story and please straighten out the dolls" as the daughter's willful attempt to be uncooperative and a pest. The daughter, however, realized that this was the only time during the entire day that her mother spent any time alone with her. She was determined to extend those moments as long as she could, even if her mother became impatient with her. It was better than nothing.

One father observed that his only chance to be with his children occurred when he returned from work in the evening and on weekends. He tried to divide his time so that he could have separate time with each of the children while still maintaining family time:

> I try to make everyone feel important, emphasizing not only what they do for themselves, but what they do for each other. I try to have them develop pride in how they help one another. Everyone gives to everyone else in this household. Dana teaches us things and we teach her things. That's just the way it is. I expect the same behavior out of all the kids. It is just harder to get Dana to understand what I expect. What's funny is that frequently, the older kids understand Dana better than I do, and they are the ones who help me understand what she is trying to say. I have to be careful though, that they are not always used as her interpreter. I don't want her

to become too dependent on them. They really do look out for her though.

This father noticed many aspects of sibling interaction within his own family. Siblings in all families serve many roles—friends, playmates, caregivers, teachers, models, interpreters, socializers, and confidants. The challenge in families with children who have hearing impairment is to try to accentuate the positive aspects of sibling relationships, promote healthy bonding, while encouraging each child to develop his individuality and to feel good about himself as a valuable, contributing member of the family. Their role in the family is as important as any other child's. Their needs are as significant. When parents are unable to be totally available to all of their children, they can enlist the help of friends or family members who may be eager to help but may not otherwise know what they can do.

Grandparents

Grandparents are often a source of support for families of children who have hearing impairment. Sometimes the diagnosis facilitates the healing of old family wounds because of the need. Like parents, grandparents also have expectations for their grandchildren. They, too, have dreams about their relationship and how it will develop. One woman said:

> When my daughter was pregnant I fantasized about how I would tell my grandchild stories about our life before we came to America. My English isn't very good, so I thought I would teach her Spanish and she would become bilingual and travel with me to Mexico and meet her relatives. Now I worry that she will not understand me. How will I talk to her?

This grandmother needed reassurance that she was not inadequate. The love and caring that she wanted to give her granddaughter could still be transmitted effectively. She continued to talk to her granddaughter. Instead of withdrawing, she helped to encourage attendance at meetings of Spanish-speaking grandparents. Her involvement with her granddaughter was invaluable and a close relationship developed.

If grandparents live nearby, they can play a more consistent role in the lives of their grandchildren, especially in the case of single-parent households. Their support of their children and their "extra pair of hands" can, in some families, enable parents to cope successfully with their situation. It behooves the professional to understand the role that grandparents have undertaken and interact with them respectfully and in accordance with their position. When a grandparent cares for a child all day while the parent is at work, it is advisable that both the parent and the grandparent be involved in lessons and any informational sessions that may be scheduled. This important relationship between parents of the child who has hearing impairment and their own parents is one that is a potential source of support or a potential source of stress. Without a doubt, it comes under scrutiny when a child is diagnosed as hearing impaired.

When grandparents live a distance from their children and grandchildren, one of the best investments the family can make is in a camera that attaches to a computer. Frequent and consistent viewing using the computer helps both the grandparents and the child not only recognize each other but develop a strong connection where the foundation for conversation will develop. Being a part of a grandchild's life despite the miles helps everyone feel connected and a part of everyone else's life.

Having said this, there are often expectations on the part of the parents as well as the grandparents regarding what is an appropriate role and what are appropriate boundaries regarding the care and involvement of the grandchildren. Disappointment can occur on both sides. Grandparents may have "their own lives" and just may not be available for caregiving or help in the way their children want and expect them to be, thus contributing to friction among the adults.

Parent Self-Care

Encouraging parents of children who have impaired hearing, particularly mothers, to take care of themselves physically, mentally, emotionally, and spiritually is of utmost importance. For women who work outside of their homes, the conflict surrounding caring for their children and caring for themselves is profound. Arranging time off from work to attend professional meetings and appointments is frequently difficult and can cause distress, even with the most understanding employers and coworkers. One mother stated, "My performance on the job diminishes, and taking care of my own needs doesn't even make the list of 'things to do.'" Another mother reflected:

My boss was wonderful to me when I discovered Hillary's hearing loss, but now I feel I have to make up the time. People assume that once you get hearing aids, and your child is enrolled in a program, your involvement is virtually over, and you can return to your 9 to 5 job. I feel apologetic when I ask for time off to visit school programs, audiologists, and to attend a mothers' group. The mothers' group is really for me and me alone, but I can't attend regularly because it meets in the daytime. Almost all of the things that I have to do for Jenny take place during working hours. Believe me, as much as I love my job, if I did not have to work I would not.

Single mothers are not the only ones who have difficulty with inflexible work schedules that clearly add to the stress in their lives. Every parent who works outside of the home needs to take into account the time it takes to travel between appointments. Professionals need to be as flexible as possible when scheduling sessions, if the goal is to have parents participate.

The Long Process

Professional versus Parental Expectations

Professionals are sometimes unaware of the time it takes for parents to see results and believe that a particular method will work for their child. Because auditory technology has come so far in the last several years, professionals in the field of hearing impairment have tremendous confidence in the value of cochlear implants, hearing aids, and auditory stimulation. This confidence is frequently conveyed to parents, but the context of an appropriate time frame is not. It is helpful to communicate a variety of examples illustrating the kinds of responses that have been observed with other children, so that the family has a framework within which to work. Many parents have no way of knowing that learning to attend auditorily is a process that takes years. As assurances cannot be given, parents are asked to proceed on faith. Professionals implore them to be patient.

It is not only parents who become impatient for their children to begin show-ing progress. Professionals, at times, have a specific time frame in which a parent's acceptance of the hearing loss is supposed to fit. At a meeting of several professionals who had contact with one family, one commented: "This mother has been denying her son's deafness long enough." Another added, in a particularly frustrated way, "I can't handle this father's anger any longer. He really should be moving on; he's known about his son's hearing loss for two years already!" Their frustration demonstrates that sometimes professionals have their own internal requirements for the "rate of recovery." But what about a mother who was doing fine with her daughter's deafness, in fact was the mother most often found comforting and helping other parents in a parent group? She was thrown into a tailspin when her mother died and she began mourning the loss of her daughter's hearing all over again. The knowledge that she was now on her own, without her own mother to take care of her (even though the mother had lived 2,000 miles away), was enough to stimulate her bereavement again. Subsequent losses are felt more severely; previous losses may be reexperienced more intensely.

Integrating and Moving Forward

It is imperative that both professionals and parents are mindful of the emotional seesaw of frustration, fear, anger, denial, recognition, and adaptation. Families who overly identify with their children may attribute to them aspects of life that may be inappropriate. "Deaf people are so isolated; Annie will never be able to make friends." This mother's comment reflects her own pain and does not take into consideration Annie's personality and ability to socialize, communicate, or interact. Coming to terms with one's own feelings as separate from those of one's child and the child's situation takes time, experience, and exposure to other children and adults who have hearing loss. Accepting one's feelings, no matter what they are, is imperative to establishing a healthy relationship with self and loved ones, especially children. Acceptance of one's feelings is a positive precursor to acceptance of one's situation.

> With help, the feelings associated with a communication disorder can be transmuted into productive behavior. The confusion becomes a spur to learning; the recognition of vulnerability leads to a re-ordering of priorities; anger becomes the energy to make changes; and guilt transforms into commitment. The grief becomes compassion for all suffering, but in particular for people and families dealing with disabilities. (Luterman, 2006, p. 124)

Adapting to life with a child who has impaired hearing means accepting change. By nature, some of us do this better than others, but all of us have the ability to learn how to do it. What helps many people is paying attention to what I refer to as the five basic elements of sanity saving:

- *Self*—Maintaining a healthy body, mind, and spiritual connection
- *Support*—Being with people in your life who you care about and who care about you . . . with whom you can be your true self and who understand the journey you are on at this time and the challenges you are facing
- *Surroundings*—Connect with nature and create a peaceful place for yourself so you can go there and reflect on the changes in your life and take stock of how you are doing

- *Stimulation*—Live a life with purpose, curiosity, and passion as you learn so many new things
- *Savor*—Take time to "be," have fun, laugh, and appreciate the gifts in your life (Atkins, 2007).

Summary

There are numerous and varied aspects to the adjustment to life with a child who has a hearing impairment. Parents and professionals need to work together to help families find a balance that suits them. Whole families can learn much about themselves as individuals and as a family unit. Among the many challenges they face is that of discovering and tapping their inner resources. This is a long process requiring courage, strength, and patience.

References

Atkins, D. (1987). Siblings of the hearing-impaired: Perspectives for parents. In D. Atkins (Ed.), *Families and their hearing impaired children* (pp. 32–45). Washington, DC: Volta Bureau.

Atkins, D. (2005). *I'm OK you're my parents.* New York: Random House.

Atkins, D. (2007). *Sanity savers: Tips for women to live a balanced life.* New York: Harper-Collins.

Bevan, R. (1988). *Hearing-impaired children: A guide for concerned parents and professionals.* Springfield, IL: Charles C. Thomas.

Buscalia, L. (1975). *The disabled and their parents: A counseling challenge.* Thorofare, NJ: C. B. Slack.

Clark, J. (1990). Counseling in communicative disorders: A responsibility to be met. *Hearsay, 12,* 4–7.

Clark, J., & Martin, F. (1994). *Effective counseling in audiology: Perspectives and practice.* Englewood Cliffs, NJ: Prentice Hall.

Erikson, E. (1964). *Childhood and society.* New York: W. W. Norton.

Featherstone, H. (1980). *A difference in the family: Life with a disabled child.* New York: Basic Books.

Forecki, M. (1985). *Speak to me.* Washington, DC: Gallaudet College Press.

Harvey, M. (1989). *Psychotherapy with deaf and hard-of-hearing persons.* Hillsdale, NJ: Lawrence Erlbaum.

Keller, H. (1954). *The story of my life.* Garden City, NY: Doubleday. [Originally published 1903].

Kroth, R. (1987). Mixed or missed messages between parents and professionals. In D. Atkins (Ed.), *Families and their hearing impaired children* (pp. 1-10). Washington, DC: Volta Bureau.

Kübler-Ross, E. (1969). *On death and dying.* New York: Macmillan.

Leigh, I. (1987). Parenting and the hearing impaired: Attachment and coping. In D. Atkins (Ed.), *Families and their hearing impaired children* (pp. 11-21). Washington, DC: Volta Bureau.

Lucas, R. (2007). *The state of human happiness* (pp. 114-116). *Science Daily.* Ann Arbor: Michigan State University.

Luterman, D. (1979). *Counseling parents of hearing-impaired children.* Boston: Little, Brown.

Luterman, D. (1987). *Deafness in the family.* Boston: Little, Brown.

Luterman, D. (2004). Children with hearing loss: Reflections on the past 40 years. *The ASHA Leader, 11*(4), 6-21.

Luterman, D. (2006, March 21). The counseling relationship. *The ASHA Leader, 11*(4), 8-9, 33.

Miller, N. (1994). *Nobody's perfect.* Baltimore: Paul H. Brookes.

Moses, K. (1985). Infant deafness and parental grief: Psychosocial early intervention. In F. Powell, T. Finitzo-Hieber, S. Friel-Patti, & D. Henderson (Eds.), *Education of the hearing-impaired child* (pp. 115-127). San Diego, CA: College Hill Press.

Rollin, W. (1987). *The psychology of communication disorders in individuals and their families.* Englewood Cliffs, NJ: Prentice-Hall.

Yacobacci-Tam, P. (1987). Interacting with the culturally different child. In D. Atkins (Ed.), *Families and their hearing impaired children* (pp. 46-58). Washington, DC: Volta Bureau.

End of Chapter Examination Questions

Chapter 5

1. From the information in this chapter, describe what is and is not the role of the professional when navigating parents of a disabled child.

2. A professional should not _____.
   a. encourage
   b. be hopeful
   c. be positive in spirit
   d. promise outcomes of services

3. A "role organization crisis"
   a. causes family members to become dissatisfied with family relationships
   b. causes elevated tension
   c. causes siblings to take on additional responsibilities
   d. causes family members to adjust to a disability

4. What is the goal of the audiologist in counseling the family of a hearing-impaired individual?

5. Name the four stages of adaptation experienced by parents of children with disabilities.
   a.
   b.
   c.
   d.

6. A message the audiologist should stress to the parent of a hearing-impaired child is:
   a. child first and foremost
   b. focus mainly on the child's impairment
   c. a structured language setting is not necessary for language development
   d. both a and b

7. Briefly describe why parent support groups and family involvement are important when coping and dealing with a disabled child.

8. Professionals must be _____ when scheduling sessions if the goal is to have parent participation.

9. A way for parents to "come to terms" with their child's disability is to:
   a. identify with their child's disability
   b. accept their feelings as their own
   c. show patience only as needed
   d. not separate parent/child feelings

End of Chapter Answer Sheet

Name _____ Date _____

Chapter 5

1. _____

_____

_____

2. Which one? a b c d

3. Which one? a b c d

4. _____

_____

_____

5. a. _____

b. _____

c. _____

d. _____

6. Which one? a b c d

7. _____

_____

_____

8. _____

9. Which one? a b c d

6

Considerations and Strategies for Amplification for Children Who Are Hearing Impaired

WILLIAM R. HODGSON

Chapter Outline

Introduction

The American Speech-Language-Hearing Association (ASHA, 2006) has published guidelines for hearing aid selection and fitting for children. The guidelines stipulate that the process of audiologic (re)habilitation includes:

1. ongoing audiologic (re)habilitation to establish and verify hearing loss parameters,
2. counseling of parents regarding the nature of hearing loss and its effects on development of language and speech,
3. the use of amplification to minimize auditory deprivation,
4. counseling on optimum communication systems and educational opportunities,
5. attention to nonauditory factors such as consideration of stigmatic peer response to hearing loss and other factors associated with psychosocial development, and
6. counseling the child regarding acquisition of behavioral coping strategies.

Children who wear hearing aids are not a homogeneous group. There is a world of difference among the needs of a child with profound congenital hearing loss, an older child with acquired sensorineural loss, and a child with a small, fluctuating conductive loss. A child with profound congenital loss faces the almost insurmountable obstacle of learning to use minimal residual hearing and of acquiring speech and language through the use of partial auditory clues to supplement those available through vision. An older child with acquired sensorineural loss, although having the advantage of normal language and speech, faces social stigma associated with hearing loss and hearing aid use, and the task of learning in a noisy classroom with an impaired sensory system. The child with small hearing loss, perhaps a fluctuating conductive disorder, may have the handicap unrecognized, misunderstood, or underestimated, and there may be difficulty developing the discipline required for effective hearing aid use.

Because children with congenital losses comprise the most visible and perhaps the largest part of this disparate group, the majority of this chapter is devoted to them. However, attention is also given to the very different but also severe problems of children in the other two groups.

During the last 30 years, significant changes have occurred in the etiologies of hearing losses in children. Hearing losses from maternal rubella and problems associated with Rh-factor incompatibility have been substantially reduced. The prevalence of hearing losses from unknown causes remains at 40% of identified cases (Upfold, 1988). Increased availability of genetic counseling may have had some impact on the prevalence of hereditary disorders. These factors have led to a reduction in the number of severe and profound hearing losses and the proportional increase in the number of mild and moderate losses. The latter are not being identified and aided at an early enough age (Matkin, 1984).

Significant improvements have been made in miniaturization and flexibility of hearing aids. Digital and programmable hearing aids have improved accuracy and flexibility of fitting, but still amplify unwanted noise along with the desired speech signal. Better identification procedures for children with smaller hearing losses, better techniques for preventing hearing losses, and smarter hearing aids are goals to work for in the immediate future.

Early Identification and Adequate Evaluation

Amplification is the foundation on which the structure of aural habilitation for hearing-impaired children is built. If the structure is to be sound, the hearing loss must be detected early in life, so children can learn the meaning and utility of sound, can develop language and speech, and can acquire an education even though all auditory stimuli are filtered through an impaired sensory system. Therefore, the impact of an impairment must be minimized as early as possible through amplification, stimulation, and training in uses of residual hearing. Additionally, early identification is vital to provide time for parents to progress through a sequence of events commonly reported to occur in the parents of hearing-impaired children. Those include disbelief, grief, anger, and acceptance. Because of the crucial role parents must play in habilitation of a hearing-impaired child, they must also have time to acquire the knowledge that will make them an effective part of the aural habilitation team.

Importance of Early Amplification

The negative effects of sensory deprivation in children born with profound hearing loss may be both physiologic and behavioral. Evans, Webster, and Cullen (1983) reported incomplete maturation in the central auditory nervous system associated with auditory deprivation in animals. Kral et al. (2000) reported functional deficits in the auditory cortices of congenitally deaf animals, and suggested that similar deficits are likely to occur in congenitally deaf children. An *unaided ear effect* has been established in children with bilateral hearing losses who are fitted monaurally versus binaurally. Hurley (1999) reported significant reduction in word recognition ability in subjects' unaided ears relative to scores in the aided ears. The delay in language, speech, and educational development in children with congenital hearing losses is well documented (Northern & Downs, 1991). These findings corroborate the need for early amplification.

Children who acquire hearing loss may also experience problems in language, speech, and educational development dating from the onset of the loss. Delay between the onset of the hearing loss and the fitting of amplification may increase resistance to acceptance of amplification. Because of all these factors, decisions about the type of stimulation to be adopted and the fitting and use of amplification must begin as soon as possible. A prerequisite to the implementation of these decisions is detection and evaluation of the hearing loss.

Strategies for Identification and Evaluation

Physiologic measures, such as auditory brainstem response (ABR) testing and otoacoustic emissions (OAE) testing, provide the most accurate results in infants under 6 months of age. These measures add materially to the quantification of hearing loss in young children (Harrison & Norton, 1999; Jacobson, 1985). Beyond 6 months of age, behavioral methods for the identification and evaluation of hearing loss become increasingly useful and include conditioned orientation reflex audiometry (Suzuki & Ogiba, 1961), visual reinforcement audiometry (Liden & Kankkunen, 1969), and conditioned play audiometry. These techniques have the advantages of eliciting frequency-specific information and of being applicable to either unaided or aided testing. Therefore, in addition to quantification of the hearing loss, the amount of functional gain delivered by a hearing aid can be evaluated. Using behavioral assessment methods, Wilson and Thompson (1984) established that reliable estimates of hearing status can be established for children under 1 year of age.

Although skilled clinicians who are experienced in the evaluation of young children can obtain useful estimates of hearing sensitivity, evaluation is an ongoing process involving continued refinement of original findings (Figure 6-1). Final determination of the exact extent and fine details of an auditory impairment for each ear is usually not completed until a child is 2 or 3 years of age. This consideration calls for fitting of hearing aids that are flexible enough to be modified appropriately as more is learned about a child's hearing loss. Fortunately, hearing aids that can be substantially modified in gain, maximum output, and frequency response are available and should be used when fitting young children.

Immittance measures also help to identify the presence of conductive components, as well as giving information about the sensorineural system (Guidelines for Screening, 1989). In addition to usefulness in the initial diagnostic process, immittance measures should always be part of ongoing audiologic monitoring to detect development of conductive components that may require treatment and that can render an otherwise appropriate hearing aid fitting inadequate.

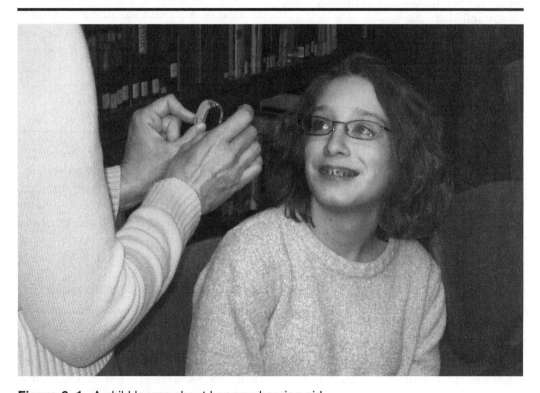

Figure 6–1. A child learns about her new hearing aid.

Language Considerations

When a hearing-impaired child is identified, language development should be evaluated. This information may be useful in estimating the degree of handicap associated with the hearing loss and in mild hearing loss may help to suggest whether or not a hearing aid is needed. Information regarding language development can be solicited from parents or teachers and receptive language level can be assessed by a scale such as the revised Peabody Picture Vocabulary Test (Dunn & Dunn, 1981).

The clinician should also be alert for the possibility of impairments in addition to hearing loss that may complicate the aural habilitation plan. Wolff and Harkins (1986) reported additional problems such as visual impairment, mental retardation, and learning disabilities in 30% of hearing-impaired children. A parent questionnaire, such as the Minnesota Child Development Inventory Profile (Ireton & Thwing, 1974), provides information about gross development, motor development, self-help ability, and personal-social development, in addition to receptive and expressive language development. Low profiles in areas outside language development indicate the need for additional evaluation to explore for the possibility of multiple handicaps.

Children with significant hearing losses must learn to use vision for clues that a defective auditory system cannot provide. For this reason, screening of a child's visual acuity is important and good visual health care must be maintained. This consideration is particularly important, as some causes of hearing loss are also associated with visual abnormalities.

It is important that preschoolers and children in regular classes from kindergarten onward enjoy a good hearing conservation program designed to prevent the development of hearing loss (through awareness of the hazard of noise exposure, for example). Screening audiometry is part of a good school hearing conservation program for identifying hearing losses that develop during the school years (Guidelines for identification audiometry, 1985). School hearing conservation programs are also still needed for another purpose: to detect unilateral as well as small, long-standing hearing losses that may be undetected until a child starts school.

Downs (2007) reminds us that children with unilateral losses tend to have delayed language, to fail grades in school, to have difficulty understanding speech in noise, and to have impaired sound localization ability. Strategies to reduce the effects of unilateral loss include preferential classroom seating, placing the child close to and with the impaired ear oriented towards the teacher. Monitoring of seating placement is important to assure that the assigned seating is maintained. Sound-field amplification systems may help the child with unilateral loss. A small amplifier/speaker is placed near the child's classroom seat, delivering the teacher's voice, usually by a microphone/FM system carried by the teacher. This arrangement in effect places the teacher's voice near the child, reduces the negative effect of reverberation, and improves signal-to-noise ratio. Alternatively, several arrangements of wearable hearing aids may be considered. If the impaired ear is aidable, a conventional aid might be placed on that ear. This arrangement may be especially helpful to the child with fluctuating conductive loss. The aid is worn only when the loss is present.

Careful monitoring to detect when the presence of the loss justifies using the hearing aid and medical conditions associated with occluding the ear canal must be considered. In cases where the impaired ear is unaidable, a very mild gain aid could be coupled to the normal ear via an open earmold, or a CROS-type arrangement can be explored, wherein a microphone placed on the side of the impaired ear carries the signal to the unoccluded normal ear. This arrangement gives the child hearing from both sides of the head, reducing the significant head-shadow effect, and possibly also helping with sound localization. Updike (1994) reported better understanding of speech in classroom conditions by children using FM systems compared to conventional or CROS hearing aids. These results are to be expected considering the improved signal-to-noise ratio obtainable with FM systems.

Unfortunately, it is not possible to predict which children with unilateral hearing loss will have academic difficulty, and it is also difficult to generalize about the efficacy of amplification. However, McKay (2002) reported that when children with unilateral hearing loss were fitted with hearing aids, parents generally but not universally reported that the children showed improved performance in social and academic situations. The American Academy of Audiology (2003) has recommended that decisions be made on a case-by-case basis.

Parent Counseling and Education

Without the understanding, acceptance, and commitment of parents or other primary caregivers, aural habilitation of a hearing-impaired child cannot be successful. Parents must understand the nature and implications of hearing loss. Hearing is generally taken for granted and the general public knows substantially nothing about how ears function. Parents must learn how the ear works and what can go wrong to understand their child's hearing problem. Carney and Moeller (1998) reviewed studies that found that family counseling enhanced realization of treatment goals for children with hearing impairment.

Early reactions of parents to the statement that their child has hearing impairment are likely to be emotionally driven and result in rejection of the statement, as well as feelings of doubt, anxiety, and guilt. A starting point for reducing these negative emotions is an explanation of auditory function, along with discussion of the potential of residual hearing to be realized through successful aural habilitation. The advantages and limitations of amplification must be thoroughly discussed, for parents will know nothing more of hearing aids than they know of the basic auditory processes.

Questions must be answered reducing groundless fears that parents may have. Parents should be reassured regarding their concern about a possible causal relationship between deafness and mental retardation. Research indicates a similar distribution of performance IQ scores in the hearing-impaired and hearing populations (Vernon, 1968). Audiologists should keep in mind, however, that hearing loss associated with some etiologies may be accompanied by brain damage or other organic disorders. For example, these conditions have been substantiated in meningitis and post-maternal viral syndromes (Mindel & Vernon, 1987). In addition, parents should be made aware of the genetic origin of some hearing disorders. Hopefully, those who carry these traits will learn about the probabilities of having hearing-impaired children. In this way, they can make an informed decision.

As cochlear implants continue to improve, parents are faced with an early decision to consider an implant versus conventional amplification. Issues include the greater cost of the implant, the long-term intensive training vital to an implant program, and the difficulty of preoperatively predicting the degree of success. On the positive side is the possibility of achieving better understanding of speech than would be likely with conventional hearing aids. It is important that a team of professionals evaluate each child and educate parents in the process of deciding which habilitation route to take.

Children with no residual hearing may nevertheless benefit from amplification that provides tactile clues to supplement visual communication. However, it should be anticipated that not all children with congenital hearing loss can learn to communicate by verbal language alone. A total communication approach, helping the child to learn verbal language, speech, and sign language, may be considered in some instances.

Two situations may apply: First, there are cultural factors to consider. Deaf parents who use sign language may well prefer that their deaf child learn manual communication. Second, the task of learning verbal language and speech is incredibly difficult for the child with complete congenital hearing loss and may be successful only if optimum conditions, including motivated parents and an excellent training program, are in place. If these factors do not obtain, learning manual language may give the child an intact communication system and may also expedite the task of learning verbal language.

Positive professional support and encouragement must accompany instruction as parents learn to accept a hearing problem and commit themselves to a long-term program of aural habilitation. Development of a goal-oriented program that includes the acquisition and successful use of hearing aids can reduce the anxiety, guilt, and feeling of helplessness as parents learn about hearing loss and what can be done.

Hearing Aid Evaluation and Fitting

After an evaluation has established hearing levels, the next step before hearing aid fitting is medical clearance. Federal regulations require medical clearance prior to fitting hearing aids on children (Food and Drug Administration, 1977). This regulation should be conscientiously followed to facilitate the general otologic health of each child, to look for correctable disorders, and to establish that there are no medical contraindications for hearing aid use. Following the initial medical examination and fitting of hearing aids, regular otologic examinations should be part of the aural habilitation plan. This practice will help to ensure good otologic health and reduce the probability of encroaching conductive disorders. For example, ear wax or middle ear problems can cause further damage to a child's hearing or render the selected amplification units inadequate.

Selecting Electroacoustic Characteristics for Children

Several prescriptive procedures designed to specify overall gain, gain-versus-frequency, and maximum output have been developed for use in fitting linear hearing aids. Most incorporate modification of the half-gain rule suggested by Lybarger (1963), who observed that adults with sensorineural loss preferred hearing aid gain that amounted to about one-half of their hearing loss. Subsequently, other individuals (Berger, Hagberg, & Rane, 1977; Byrne & Tonisson, 1976; McCandless & Lyregaard, 1983) modified the half-gain rule to reduce overamplification of low frequencies and to make other adjustments to maximize audibility of speech.

With the prevalence of digital technology and various kinds of compression amplification in today's hearing aids, newer procedures have been developed. For example, Cornelisse, Seewald, and Jamieson (1995) and Dillon (1999) reported strategies for fitting nonlinear hearing aids. Additionally, various computer software programs are available to facilitate hearing aid fitting. In general terms, all of the procedures aim to make as much as possible of the aided speech spectrum comfortably audible. This goal is clearly important for children learning new vocabulary on a daily basis.

Modification of Prescriptive Procedures for Children

Each prescriptive procedure used with adults can be adapted for use in hearing aid eval-uation and selection for children, although some call for loudness judgments that very young children cannot make. The following paragraphs suggest ways in which prescriptive procedures designed for adults can be modified to be appropriate for evaluation for children.

Probe-Tube Microphone Measurements

Of particular interest in evaluating the function of hearing aids on children is the use of probe-tube microphone measurements (Figure 6–2). Once a hearing loss is established and a hearing aid is selected, the probe-tube system can be used as an objective measurement to determine quickly and definitively the real-ear performance of the hearing aid. Desired changes in response can then be made and again measured, with the

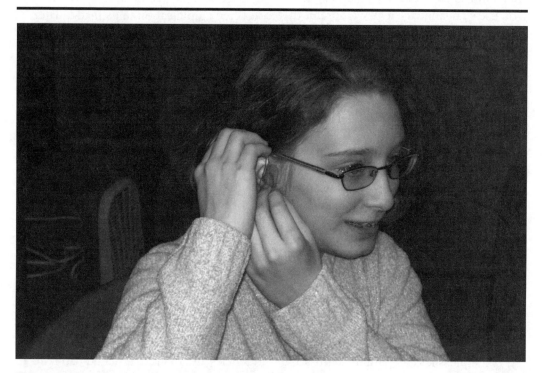

Figure 6–2. It is important that children learn to place the aid on their own ear successfully as a part of their aural habilitation program.

process continuing until the ideal response is realized. These measures are much faster than behavioral testing, during which a child may become restless and inattentive before the evaluation is completed. Hawkins, Morrison, Halligan, and Cooper (1989) presented a plan to use probe-tube microphone measurements to evaluate hearing aids in children. They reported success in their goal of amplifying and packaging the long-term speech spectrum into a child's residual hearing.

Electroacoustic Performance

The relationship between hearing aid electroacoustic performance as measured in the 2 cm^3 coupler and performance in the human ear is not very good even when adult ears are considered, because of coupler-real ear differences. This disparity may be increased in a child's ear (Seewald & Scollie, 1999). Because of the smaller size of a child's ear canal relative to the adult, greater sound pressure levels (SPLs) will be generated in a child's aided canal. Jirsa and Norris (1978) reported SPLs about 5 dB greater in the canals of preschool children relative to that of adults. Although these values may be accurate on average, they cannot account for the considerable variability in the volume of ear canals of different children. A decided advantage of probe-tube measures in hearing aid evaluations is the measure of the SPLs actually generated in ear canals under aided conditions.

Amplification-Induced Threshold Shift

There appears to be a remote possibility of further change in the hearing of children who wear hearing aids because of exposure to high sound levels. Sporadic accounts of individual cases appear in the literature. Rin-telmann and Bess (1977) in an early study surveyed the literature on this topic and conducted their own investigation. They concluded that sufficient evidence existed regarding isolated instances of amplification-induced threshold shift to justify careful limitation of maximum outputs according to the degree of loss and to emphasize the importance of careful audiologic monitoring. Subsequently, a federal regulation was enacted requiring a warning to accompany hearing aids whose maximum output exceeds 132 dB SPL, that the hearing aid may be hazardous to residual hearing (Food and Drug Administration, 1977).

Concerned about the possibility of damage to a hearing-impaired child's remaining hearing through amplification-induced threshold shift, Matkin (1986) recommended the following SPL limits for maximum output of hearing aids: with profound loss, 125 dB; moderate loss, 120 dB; and mild loss, 110 dB. He further recommended that 5 dB be subtracted from these values when fitting preschool children. More specifically, Skinner (1988) recommended that 6 dB be subtracted from the otherwise appropriate maximum output for infants to 2 years of age and that 3 dB be subtracted for children between the ages of 2 and 5. It should be noted that Kawell, Kopun, and Stelmachowicz (1988), in a study of loudness discomfort levels (LDLs) in children, did not find systematic differences between children older than 7 years and adults, and concluded that there may be no reason to reduce maximum output of the hearing aid for older children beyond the levels necessary for adults.

Maximum Comfort Levels

Maximum output values are usually selected when fitting hearing aids for adults by determining LDLs and selecting output levels below a patient's LDL. Young children cannot report LDLs reliably and it may be necessary to select output values based on those found to be uncomfortable on subjects with loss of hearing sensitivity comparable to that of the child in question. Estimated levels may be obtained by reference to the average LDLs obtained from subjects as a function of the magnitude of sensorineural loss.

Finally, it should be noted that appropriate procedures may permit assessment of LDLs in older children. Kawell et al. (1988) reported reasonably reliable LDL measures on children as young as 7 years. They used five loudness categories from "too soft" to "hurts." While listening to signals at various levels, children judged loudness by pointing to pictures of human faces whose expressions represented typical reactions to each of the five loudness levels.

Binaural Amplification

It is generally recognized that most adults who have bilateral hearing loss and aidable hearing in each ear perform better with two aids than with one. Advantages include (a) improved localization ability, (b) reduction of the head shadow effect that obtains with one hearing aid, (c) improved audibility of speech in noise (the squelch effect), (d) more natural "three-dimensional" sound quality, and (e) the ability to set the volume controls at a lower level because of binaural summation (about 5 dB, according to Byrne, 1981). However, some hearing-impaired individuals appear to function better with one hearing aid than with two, possibly because of defects in the central auditory system that prevent the interaction of signals coming from each ear as they ascend in the central pathways. Additionally, large differences between the impairment in the two ears may reduce the advantages of binaural amplification. These caveats call for careful evaluation and trial use in problem cases. Adults may be able to judge whether they function better with two aids, but small children cannot. Skinner (1988) suggests careful observation while a child is aided with one versus two aids to evaluate the ability to localize and to respond to speech with each aid alone, plus language and speech development during trial periods of monaural and binaural amplification.

As mentioned earlier, evidence is accruing that a hearing-impaired ear, left unaided, may be subject to deterioration in word recognition ability as a result of auditory deprivation. Silverman and Silman (1990) reported that in two adult cases there was a reduction over time in word recognition scores in the unaided ears relative to the performance of the aided ears. Moreover, on eventual binaural fitting, there was significant improvement in the performance of the previously unaided ears. Additionally, Gelfand and Silman (1993) reported a reduction in word recognition scores in the unaided ears of a group of monaurally fitted subjects, whereas they observed no such reduction in the ears of a similar group of binaurally fitted subjects.

Type of Hearing Aid

As is the case with adults, when fitting children, decisions must be made about the type or style of hearing aids. Concern about cosmetics plays a large role when adults are fitted. The same will be true for older children and for the parents of younger children. This concern must be considered, for aids considered stigmatic may not be worn. However, every attempt should be made to reduce these concerns on the part of a child and parents, so that appropriate amplification is the primary basis on which the decision of hearing aid type is made.

Conventional Hearing Aids

Beauchaine, Barlow, and Stelmachowicz (1990) point out that behind-the-ear (BTE) hearing aids are ideal to meet many of the special amplification needs of children, in that they (a) permit frequent earmold remakes, (b) simplify provision of loaner instruments, (c) provide strong telecoils and connections for direct audio input, and (d) are available with directional microphones. Today, BTE aids are available with sufficient power and flexibility to fit most hearing losses. They offer the advantage of ear-level hearing, which may be important in binaural functions, and reduce clothing noises and cord problems previously associated with body-type aids. However, for the very young child, it is easier for parents to see and manipulate controls of body aids. Body-type amplification is more feasible for an infant before the child sits and walks. For the child who requires extremely high gain, serious feedback problems may limit effective amplification if BTE aids are used. For example, Matkin (1984) reported that 8 of 11 preschoolers surveyed were receiving inadequate gain from ear-level aids, because the volume controls were turned down to avoid feedback problems.

To receive maximum gain without feedback, earmolds must be well designed and frequently replaced. Full-shell earmolds should be used and earmolds made of soft material are reported to reduce feedback problems (Seewald & Ross, 1988). Additionally, soft earmolds reduce the risk of injury if a child falls or is struck on the head. Especially with ear-level aids, frequent replacement of earmolds is necessary to maintain adequate gain without feedback. Constant monitoring of gain and earmold adequacy is necessary. Matkin (1984) suggests that children younger than 3 may need new earmolds at 3-month intervals to maintain an adequate seal. Technological advances in hearing aid performance now permit increased gain without feedback (Harris & Muller, 2003) and may facilitate the use of open earmolds to reduce undesirable ear canal occlusion effects in children with small hearing loss.

As children grow older, particularly as they approach adolescence and changes in size and shape of the external ear are reduced, cosmetic concerns may lead them to ask for in-the-ear (ITE) aids. Such a change is justifiable, if the hearing loss is appropriate for this type of aid, remembering that ITE aids generally do not provide as much overall gain or high-frequency amplification without feedback and that the cost of recasing ITE aids as a youngster's ear changes shape and size is greater than that of replacing earmolds.

Non-Hearing Aid Assistive Listening Devices for Children

Hearing-impaired children, especially those with more serious losses, should not be confined to conventional, wearable amplification. Systems used in the classroom, and others designed for personal use, are generally classified as *assistive listening devices*. They are designed to improve signal-to-noise ratio and reduce effects of reverberation by moving the system's microphone closer to the person who is speaking. Examples include the FM radio transmitting/receiving unit designed for either classroom or personal use (Figure 6–3). Behind-the-ear hearing aids are now available with built-in FM receivers so that the aid can be used as a conventional amplifier, as an FM receiver only, or with both input modes activated. In the latter case, a child can hear her own amplified voice while still maintaining a favorable signal-to-noise ratio for the primary signal. An older unit is the induction loop system, which sends an electromagnetic

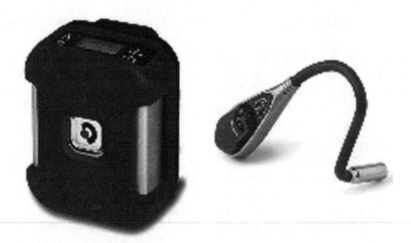

Figure 6–3. FM transmitter and receiver. With the addition of an external microphone, this system provides effective amplification for classroom or personal use. (Photo courtesy of Phonak.)

signal from a person speaking to a child's hearing aid.

It is necessary that the selected hearing aids be compatible with the classroom or personal units that are used. That is, if an induction loop system is to be used in the class or in the home, the child's hearing aids must have induction coils (*telephone switches*, or *T-coils*) that pick up the electromagnetic signals. These coils should be evaluated to ensure appropriate function, as hearing aids may operate quite differently with induction coil function than when the microphone is the input transducer.

The child's hearing aids should have input jacks for hardwired external microphones that can be located close to the mouth of the person speaking. An example of such an aid, with direct audio input via an external microphone, is shown in Figure 6–4. When use of the hardwired arrangement is feasible, the result will be vastly improved signal-to-noise ratio compared to a conventional hearing aid. However, hardwired units reduce classroom mobility. To summarize,

FM systems are the general choice of devices using remote microphone technology, because they provide greater flexibility and can be used either in or outside the classroom.

Consistent with a child's age and auditory needs, other assistive devices, such as telephone and television aids, should be introduced. The former may consist of telephone amplifiers or visible printouts of telephone messages (TTDs). In the latter case, various systems improve pickup of TV audio. The signal may be sent directly to a child's amplification system via hardwire, FM, infrared, or induction loop carriers. These arrangements reduce amplification of room noise. For more severely impaired children a close-captioned decoder will reveal on the TV screen the printed subtitles that are available on many TV programs. A complete amplification program should include these and the many other alerting, warning, and auditory devices that are available.

The American Speech-Language-Hearing Association (2002) issued guidelines for

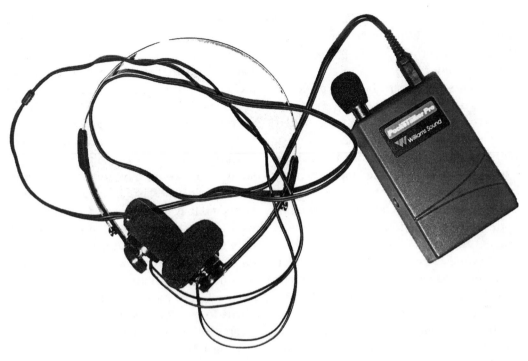

Figure 6–4. Hearing aid with hardwired external microphone. (Courtesy of Unitron Industries and Williams Sound.)

fitting and monitoring FM systems. The guidelines include criteria for selecting and monitoring the systems as well as training in their use. The guidelines conclude that these assistive devices have much to offer in terms of improved fidelity and signal-to-noise ratio, and that parent and child orientation, training, and counseling are critical to their successful use.

Learning Effective Hearing Aid Use

Three principles ensure effective hearing aid use by a child: (a) the parents must learn how to operate and care for hearing aids; (b) the child must learn and assume responsibility for hearing aid use and care, learn-ing as soon as possible optimum setting of controls and reporting of hearing aid problems; and (c) an effective monitoring system must be in place involving the audiologist, the parents, the child, and others such as teachers, who are a part of the aural habilitation team.

Duties of Parents and Children

Parents, and children as they are able, must become aware of the physical components and the functioning of a hearing aid. They must learn to operate the switches, rotate the volume control, and replace the battery. Prior to first hearing aid use, all concerned should be warned of the toxic nature of batteries and the danger of accidental ingestion. Parents should be instructed to call their doctor if a battery is accidentally swallowed and should be given the National Battery Hotline number, (202) 625-3333, which they can call for help.

Parents must learn how to place the earmold in the ear and remove it. They should be assisted in teaching their child to assume this responsibility as early as possible. Care and maintenance of the aid and troubleshooting of simple problems must be learned by the parents and assumed by the child in a graduated fashion, beginning with the concept of responsibility for the hearing aids.

Beyond learning the physical aspects of hearing aid manipulation and care, parents and the child must develop effective listening strategies. They must learn to survey the environment and assess factors that contribute to or detract from successful communication. They must learn to help the hearing aid by moving it closer to desired speech signals and further away from interfering noises. They must learn to reduce background noise levels when possible, and to adjust the hearing aid's volume control for maximum intelligibility in various noise levels. They must even learn the assertiveness necessary to inform those who talk to them of the presence of the hearing loss. Parents must remember to improve communication by getting the hearing-impaired child's attention before speaking, limiting conversation to line-of-sight situations when possible, and speaking more slowly. Parents and the child must acquire the ability to interpret signs that indicate if these strategies to improve communication are being successful or if additional effort is needed.

Of vital importance, a program of hearing aid monitoring must be developed involving the audiologist, the parents, the child, and others who are in frequent contact. With remarkable consistency, surveys taken over the years to determine how well hearing aids worn by children are functioning have shown that at any given time about half of them are defective or set inappropriately (Blair, Wright, & Pollard, 1981; Gaeth & Lounsbury, 1966; Porter, 1973). These surveys also suggest that parents have little knowledge about hearing aid function. For example, in the early Gaeth and Lounsbury study, when asked how long the batteries in the child's aid lasted, 9% of the parents answered longer than a year. Eleven percent were more honest and admitted that they didn't know. Although it is of great importance that parents learn to monitor the hearing aids and help to keep them operating well, it is most critical that the child learns to assume this responsibility, as the wearer is the only person who can monitor hearing aids full-time.

It is important to have a systematic program to document the goals and needs of the new hearing aid user and to establish a measure of improvements. Such a program for adults was developed by Dillon, James, and Ginis (1997), designated as the Client Oriented Scale of Improvement, and the scale was subsequently revised for use with children (COSI-C). There are separate sections for promoting hearing aid use with (a) infants, (b) toddlers, and (c) preschoolers and primary and secondary school children. When using the scale, the audiologist and parents establish goals and strategies to achieve the goals, and select a date by which the goals will be achieved. The scale provides a comprehensive and well-organized program for achieving successful hearing aid use. More information is available on-line (National Acoustic Laboratories).

The guide provided in Table 6–1 may be helpful to assist parents to detect problems via a daily check of the childs hearing aids. Initially, the audiologist should instruct

TABLE 6–1. The Hearing Aid Check

1. *Visual inspection of aid, tubing, and earmold.* Each should be clean and free of wax. All can be wiped clean with a dry tissue. The earmold and tubing can be removed from the earhook of the aid, washed in warm soapy water, rinsed, and dried completely. Afterwards, the earhook, not the hearing aid, should be held firmly while the tubing is replaced. If the tubing is discolored, cracked, dry and brittle, or loose where it fits into the earmold or onto the earhook, a trip to the dispenser is needed to replace the tubing.

2. *Battery check.* The battery should deliver its specified voltage, which can be learned from the dispenser, and discarded if this is not the case. It should be free of corrosion, as should be the battery case.

3. *Listening check on the parental ear.* Using the hearing aid stethoscope or a custom earmold, the parent should ascertain that speech is understandable through the aid, that speech quality has not deteriorated from its usual level, that there are no unexpected noises generated by the aid, and that the expected loudness is delivered when the volume control is rotated. While turning the volume control, the parent should ascertain that there are no scratchy noises or dead spots. Speech should smoothly grow louder as the volume control is rotated. The parent should tap the case of the aid and listen for intermittency, suggesting loose battery contacts. Additionally, with body aids, the cord where it inserts into the aid and into the earphone should be twisted gently, for the same purpose. Problems in any of these areas necessitate a visit to the dispenser.

4. *Listening check on the child's ear.* Separately, each aid should be inserted and the volume control rotated to the level recommended by the audiologist. Feedback (squealing) should not occur. Parents should learn that feedback results when too much sound leaks out of the aided ear canal and re-enters the hearing aid microphone. Causes of feedback at recommended volume control setting are: (a) wax in the ear canal that reflects too much sound back to the hearing aid; (b) an incompletely inserted earmold; (c) loose connections along the sound delivery route between hearing aid, earhook, tubing, and earmold; (d) an earmold that no longer fits well enough to create an adequate seal; and (e) internal feedback (squealing), which occurs when the acoustic isolation between the hearing aid microphone and earphone is destroyed. Additionally, feedback can occur momentarily when a hand is cupped over the hearing aid or the child stands close to a wall or other reflecting surface. The listening check on the child's ear should be completed by making sure the child can hear and understand speech in the usual fashion, consistent with the amount of hearing loss that is present.

parents and provide supervised practice in this hearing aid check. Parents then should assist the child to assume responsibility of those parts of the hearing aid check for which normal hearing is not a requisite.

Some equipment is needed for this hearing aid check. For listening to the hearing aid, the parent will need a hearing aid stethoscope or a custom earmold that fits the parental ear. These are shown in Figure 6-5.

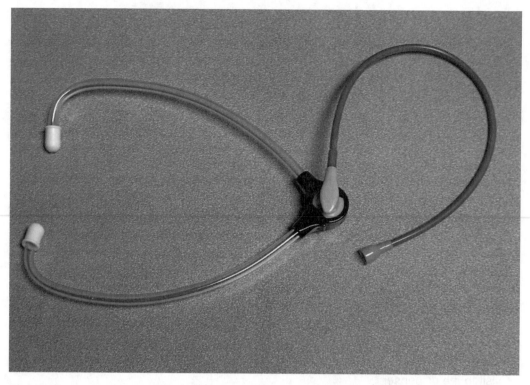

Figure 6–5. Hearing aid stethoscope for hearing aid checks. (Courtesy of Hal Hen.)

A voltmeter for testing the battery is useful. Batteries have been improved until they deliver almost their full voltage until near the end of their life and then die suddenly. Therefore, a battery that delivers anything less than its specified voltage should be discarded and spare batteries should always be carried, in case a battery dies between hearing aid checks. Figure 6-6 illustrates an inexpensive battery tester. As shown in Figure 6-7, a small brush and a wire loop may be helpful to remove accumulated wax from the sound channel of the earmold. Also illustrated is a hand syringe, which is useful to dry out tubing after the earmold has been removed and washed. Fluids other than water should not be used on the earmold and, of course, the hearing aid itself should never be exposed to fluids of any kind.

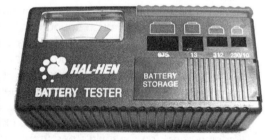

Figure 6–6. Inexpensive battery tester. (Courtesy of Activair and Hal-Hen.)

Parents must learn, and assist their child in learning, simple hearing aid troubleshooting procedures that may correct some problems and prevent a visit to the audiologist when problems arise. Some of these are presented in Table 6-2. Parents should not

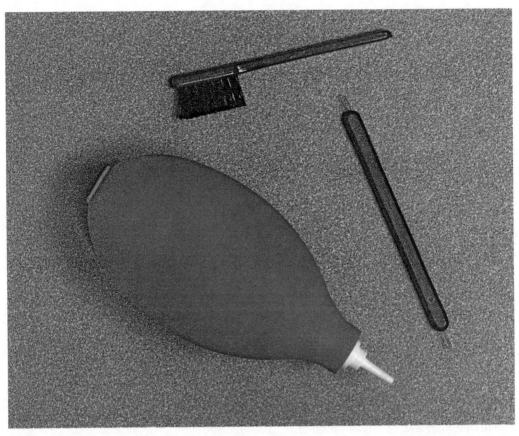

Figure 6–7. Hand syringe for cleaning water from hearing aids and a brush and wire loop for removing debris. (Courtesy of Hal-Hen.)

try to go beyond these simple procedures and should never attempt to open the case to repair the aid. Finally, as hearing aids are expensive and repairs and replacement are costly, parents and the child must learn certain fundamentals of care and maintenance. Some of these are detailed in Table 6–3.

Summary

For children born with hearing loss, early identification and amplification are crucial, because amplification is the foundation on which aural habilitation is built. Today, behavioral and electrophysiological test batteries can reliably establish the existence of hearing loss even in infants, and estimate magnitude and configuration. After fitting with hearing aids, a period of continuing evaluation and modification of amplification characteristics will follow. For this reason, it is important to prescribe flexible hearing aids with provision for considerable modification in electroacoustic characteristics. At the same time, parents must learn about hearing and hearing loss and the advantages and limitations of amplification and become dedicated to the long-term habilitation process.

TABLE 6–2. Hearing Aid Trouble Shooting

1. *Symptom:* No sound.
   Possible causes: Off-on switch may be set to off or the T (telephone) position. Battery may be the wrong kind, dead, or inserted backwards. Corrosion on the battery contacts may be responsible and may be cleaned gently. There may be a mechanical blockage of the sound route, such as perspiration in the tubing, which may be dried with a hand syringe after the tubing is removed from the earhook. Aids fitted with acoustic filters are particularly prone to this problem because the filter consists of a very small opening that is easily blocked. If the problem persists, a drying kit can be purchased, into which the aid can be placed each night. The earmold sound channel may be blocked by wax, which can be removed with the wire loop described in the text. It is possible, with the aid on the ear, that a kink or twist may close the tubing and block sound, necessitating correct placement or a new tube.

2. *Symptom:* Weak sound.
   Possible causes: Weak battery, sound channel partially blocked by moisture or wax, or the tubing may be bent partially closed. These problems can usually be corrected by the parents. If these causes are not evident there may be an internal problem that will require repair by the dispenser.

3. *Symptom:* Intermittent sound.
   Possible causes: Loose battery caused by bent contacts. With body aids, broken cords or loose connections may be the problem. Solutions are best left to the dispenser.

4. *Symptom:* Loudness does not change appropriately as volume control is rotated. Volume control rotation may be accompanied by noise, no change in loudness, or a sudden loudness at a given rotation.
   Probable causes: Dirty or broken volume control, requiring repair by the dispenser.

5. *Symptom:* Unnatural sound quality or noise.
   Possible causes: Remembering that all hearing aids sound different from unamplified speech and that some audible noise is present in normal function, the parents must learn to discern abnormalities that develop. Dirty controls can produce noise, and turning them back and forth may dislodge the dirt responsible for the problem. Unnatural sound quality may result from a nearly dead battery or from an inappropriately set tone control. Other noise and quality problems will require attention by the dispenser.

6. *Problem:* Feedback (squealing).
   Possible causes: Earmold incompletely inserted, volume control set above recommended level, loose connections between earhook, tubing, and earmold. These problems may be solvable by the parents. Other causes of feedback, for which parents must seek help, are wax in the ear canal and poorly fitting earmolds. Internal feedback can be diagnosed by removing the earhook and holding a finger over the sound outlet while rotating the volume control on. If the feedback is internal, the squealing will continue.

TABLE 6–3. Hearing Aid Care and Maintenance

1. Do not drop the aid. Hearing aids are more resistant to shock than previously but a long fall onto a hard surface may damage the case or contents. It is a good practice to sit on the bed or other soft surface when inserting or removing the aid.

2. Moisture, heat, and dirt are damaging to hearing aids. Therefore, the aid should be removed before showers or before applying hair spray. If the child forgets and takes a dip in the pool while wearing the aid, a trip to the dispenser is necessary. As mentioned elsewhere, a kit that contains a drying agent is available from the dispenser if moisture from perspiration is a problem. Opening the battery cases after removal of the aids each evening may permit some drying out, and will ensure that the aids are turned off. Batteries should be removed if the aids are to be unused for a period of time. The aid should never be left in a really hot place such as a windowsill or the dashboard of the car.

3. Earmolds and their tubing can be removed from the earhook of the aid and washed. A hand syringe is useful to blow water out of the tubing before replacing it. Brushes and wax picks should be used to keep the earmold sound channel and vents free of wax. Small pressure equalizing vents are especially liable to become occluded by wax, and a broom-straw may be helpful to clean them. A wire should not be used, especially with soft earmolds, because vents are not always straight and the material is easily damaged.

4. A safe place should be reserved to keep the aids when they are not in use. Audiologists who have been dispensing very long have witnessed the problem of temporarily or permanently lost hearing aids, or aids damaged or completely ingested by the family dog. As an additional safeguard, parents may want to consider insurance for the hearing aids.

5. Parents should institute a regular schedule of visits to the audiologist where, in addition to evaluation of the child's hearing, the performance of the aids and integrity of the earmolds can be evaluated. Retubing of the molds and minor repairs to the aids may prevent development of more serious problems.

Parents must learn about efficient use of amplification, including the physical manipulation of hearing aids, and they must become aware of environmental strategies for effective listening. They must learn about the care and maintenance of hearing aids, how to assess functioning of aids, and how to detect problems and correct them, when possible. The child who uses the aids must assume all of these responsibilities as soon as possible. There must also be in place an effective program for monitoring the hearing aids' function and regular audiologic and otologic attention to the aids and the child's hearing.

Assistive listening devices should be utilized. These include units using remote microphone technology that reduce the harmful effects of reverberation and improve signal-to-noise ratio. Others include telephone and television aids and alerting and warning devices. All possible systems should be considered in a program of complete audiologic habilitation.

References

American Academy of Audiology. (2003). Pediatric amplification protocol. Retrieved May, 2006, from www.audiology.org/NR/rdonlyres/53D26792-E321-41AF850F-CC253310FB/0/pedamp.pdf

American Speech-Language-Hearing Association. (2002). Guidelines for fitting and monitoring FM systems. Retrieved November 3, 2008, from www.asha.org/docs/html/GL2002-00010.html

American Speech-Language-Hearing Association. (2006). Preferred practice patterns for the profession of audiology. Retrieved November 5, 2008, from www.asha.org/docs/html/PP2006-00274.html

Beauchaine, K., Barlow, N., & Stelmachowicz, P. (1990). Special considerations in amplification for young children. *ASHA, 32,* 44-51.

Berger, K., Hagberg, E., & Rane, R. (1977). *Prescription of hearing aids: Rationale, procedures, and results* (4th ed.). Kent, OH: Herald.

Blair, J., Wright, K., & Pollard, G. (1981). Parental knowledge and understanding of hearing loss and hearing aids. *The Volta Review, 83,* 375-382.

Byrne, D. (1981). Clinical issues and options in binaural hearing aid fitting. *Ear and Hearing, 2,* 187-193.

Byrne, D., & Tonisson, W. (1976). Selecting the gain of hearing aids for persons with sensorineural hearing impairments. *Scandinavian Audiology, 5,* 51-59.

Carney, A., & Moeller, M. (1998). Treatment efficacy: Hearing loss in children. *Journal of Speech, Language, and Hearing Research, 41,* 61-84.

Cornelisse, L., Seewald, R., & Jamieson, D. (1995). The input/output (I/O) formula: A theoretical approach to the fitting of personal amplification devices. *Journal of the Acoustical Society of America, 97,* 1854-1864.

Cox, R. (1985). Hearing aids and aural rehabilitation: A structured approach to hearing aid selection. *Ear and Hearing, 6,* 226-239.

Dillon, H. (1999). NAL-NL1: A new procedure for fitting non-linear hearing aids. *Hearing Journal, 52*(4), 10-16.

Dillon, H., James, J., & Ginis, J. (1997). Client Oriented Scale of Improvement (COSI) and its relationship to several other measures of benefit and satisfaction provided by hearing aids. *Journal of the American Academy of Audiology, 8,* 27-43.

Downs, M. (2007). Unilateral hearing loss in infants: A call to arms. *International Journal of Audiology, 46,* 61.

Dunn, L., & Dunn, L. (1981). *Peabody Picture Vocabulary Test—Revised.* Circle Pines, MN: American Guidance Service.

Evans, W., Webster, D., & Cullen, J. (1983). Auditory brainstem responses in neonatally sound deprived CBA/J mice. *Hearing Research, 10,* 269-277.

Food and Drug Administration. (1977). Hearing aid devices—Professional and patient labeling and conditions for sale. *Federal Register, 42,* 9286-9296.

Gaeth, J., & Lounsbury, E. (1966). Hearing aids and children in elementary schools. *Journal of Speech and Hearing Disorders, 31,* 283-289.

Gelfand, S., & Silman, S. (1993). Apparent auditory deprivation in children. *Journal of the American Academy of Audiology, 4,* 313-318.

Guidelines for identification audiometry. (1985). *Asha, 28,* 49-52.

Guidelines for screening for hearing impairment and middle ear disorders. (1989). *Asha, 31,* 71-77.

Harris, F., & Muller, T. (March, 2003). *Hearing aid feedback management: Effects on gain and speech acoustics.* Paper presented to the American Auditory Society, Phoenix, AZ.

Harrison, W., & Norton, S. (1999). Characteristics of transient evoked otoacoustic emissions in normal-hearing and hearing-impaired children. *Ear and Hearing, 20,* 75-86.

Hawkins, D., Morrison, T., Halligan, P., & Cooper, W. (1989). Use of probe tube microphone measurements in hearing aid selection for children: Some initial clinical experiences. *Ear and Hearing, 10,* 281-287.

Hurley, R. (1999). Onset of auditory deprivation. *Journal of the American Academy of Audiology, 10*, 529-534.

Ireton, H., & Thwing, E. (1974). *Minnesota Child Development Inventory.* Minneapolis: Behavior Science Systems.

Jacobson, J. (Ed.). (1985). *The auditory brainstem response.* San Diego, CA: College Hill Press.

Jirsa, R., & Norris, T. (1978). Relationship of acoustic gain to aided threshold improvement in children. *Journal of Speech and Hearing Disorders, 43*, 348-352.

Kamm, C., Dirks, D., & Mickey, M. (1978). Effect of sensorineural hearing loss on loudness discomfort level. *Journal of Speech and Hearing Research, 21*, 668-681.

Kawell, M., Kopun, J., & Stelmachowicz, P. (1988). Loudness discomfort levels in children *Ear and Hearing, 9*, 133-136.

Kral, A., Hartmann, R., Tillein, S., & Klinke, R. (2000). Auditory deprivation reduces synaptic activity within the auditory cortex in a layer-specific manner. *Cerebral Cortex, 10*, 714-726.

Liden, G., & Kankkunen, A. (1969). Visual reinforcement audiometry in the management of young deaf children. *International Audiology, 8*, 99-106.

Lybarger, S. (1963). *Simplified system for fitting hearing aids.* Canonsberg, PA: Radioear.

Matkin, N. (1984). Wearable amplification: A litany of persisting problems. In J. Jerger (Ed.), *Pediatric audiology* (pp. 125-145). San Diego, CA: College Hill Press.

Matkin, N. (1986). Hearing aids for children. In W. Hodgson (Ed.), *Hearing aid assessment and use in audiologic habilitation* (3rd ed., pp. 170-190). Baltimore: Williams and Wilkins.

McCandless, G., & Lyregaard, P. (1983). Prescription of gain/output (POGO) for hearing aids. *Hearing Instruments, 34*(1), 16-21.

McKay, S. (2002). To aid or not to aid. Children with unilateral hearing loss. *Audiology Online.* Retrieved July, 2008, from http://www.audiologyonline.com/articles/article_detail.asp?article_id=357

Mindel, E., & Vernon, M. (Eds.). (1987). *They grow in silence: Understanding deaf children and adults* (2nd ed.). Boston: College Hill Press.

National Acoustic Laboratories. (April, 2001). COSI-C–Client Oriented Scale of Improvement–Children. Retrieved May, 2008, from http://www.nal.gov.au/downloads/COSI-C%20main%20document.htm

Northern, J., & Downs, M. (1991). *Hearing in children* (4th ed.). Baltimore: Williams and Wilkins.

Porter, T. (1973). Hearing aids in a residential school. *American Annals of the Deaf, 118*, 31-33.

Rintelmann, W., & Bess, F. (1977). High-level amplification and potential hearing loss in children. In F. Bess (Ed.), *Childhood deaf-ness: Causation, assessment and management* (pp. 267-293). New York: Grune and Stratton.

Seewald, R., & Ross, M. (1988). Amplification for young hearing impaired children. In M. Pollack (Ed.), *Amplification for the hearing-impaired* (3rd ed., pp. 213-271). Orlando, FL: Grune and Stratton.

Seewald, R., & Scollie, S. (1999). Infants are not average adults: Implications for audiometric testing. *Hearing Journal, 52*(10), 64-72.

Silverman, C., & Silman, S. (1990). Apparent auditory deprivation from monaural amplification and recovery with binaural amplification: Two case studies. *Journal of the American Academy of Audiology, 1*, 175-180.

Skinner, M. (1988). *Hearing aid evaluation.* Engelwood Cliffs, NJ: Prentice Hall.

Suzuki, T., & Ogiba, Y. (1961). Conditioned reflex audiometry. *Archives of Otolaryngology, 74*, 192-198.

Updike, C. (1994). Comparison of FM auditory trainers, CROS aids, and personal amplification in unilaterally hearing impaired children. *Journal of the American Academy of Audiology, 5*, 204-209.

Upfold, L. (1988). Children with hearing aids in the 1980s: Etiologies and severity of impairment. *Ear and Hearing, 9*, 75-80.

Vernon, M. (1968). Fifty years of research on the intelligence of the deaf and hard-of-hearing.

A survey of literature and discussion of the implications. *Journal of Rehabilitation of the Deaf, 1*, 1-11.

Wilson, W., & Thompson, G. (1984). Behavioral audiometry. In J. Jerger (Ed.), *Pediatric audiology* (pp. 1-44). San Diego, CA: College Hill Press.

Wolff, A., & Harkins, J. (1986). Multi handicapped students. In A. Schildroth & M. Karchmer (Eds.), *Deaf children in America* (pp. 55-82). San Diego, CA: College Hill Press.

End of Chapter Examination Questions

Chapter 6

1. **What three principles ensure effective hearing aid use for a child?**
   a.
   b.
   c.

2. **According to the chapter author, what is the foundation upon which the structure of aural habilitation is built?**

3. **(True/False) There is no causal relationship between deafness and intelligence.**

4. **What are the five advantages of two hearing aids with a bilateral hearing loss?**
   a.
   b.
   c.
   d.
   e.

5. **(True/False) Parents should turn the majority of their child's aural habilitation program over to the audiologist.**

6. **Children with profound congenital hearing loss can acquire speech through:**
   a. visual cues
   b. using their residual hearing
   c. manual communication
   d. both a and b

7. **_____ percent of hearing losses are from unknown causes.**

8. **(True/False) Cosmetics should not play a role in fitting children with hearing aids.**

End of Chapter Answer Sheet

Name _____ Date _____

Chapter 6

1. a. _____

    b. _____

    c. _____

2. _____

3. Circle one: True   False

4. a. _____

    b. _____

    c. _____

    d. _____

    e. _____

5. Circle one: True   False

6. Which one(s)?   a   b   c   d

7. _____%

8. Circle one: True   False

7

Development of Listening and Language Skills in Children Who Are Deaf or Hard of Hearing

ARLENE STREDLER-BROWN

Introduction

Language is fundamental to human communication, socialization, and learning. Language is a conventional and rule-governed symbolic system for communicating and representing thoughts and feelings. There are many ways to understand and express language. Receptively, one can understand a message by listening to it, watching someone sign it, or reading print. Expressively, one can speak, sign, or write the message. Acquiring language is the foremost challenge for a child with a hearing loss—any degree of hearing loss.

Language acquisition has critical periods, periods of time when exposure to language, or lack thereof, will have an effect on the child's language outcomes. Babies and toddlers with normal hearing learn language primarily through direct interactions with their parents and caregivers in the course of their everyday routines and activities. As they get older, children start to learn language through interactions with their peers and through incidental learning when they "overhear" conversations around them. The same principles apply to children who are learning a visual language when they are immersed in environments that have fluent users of sign language. These children learn sign language from natural interactions with their parents, caregivers, and their peers. They too acquire language through incidental learning by "overseeing" conversations.

Development of Language

Language is the orderly arrangement of linguistic symbols to convey meaning. The three basic components of language are semantic content, syntactic form, and pragmatic use.

- *Semantic Content:* Semantic content is the element of language that concerns meaning. Semantics involves much more than the acquisition of words. It also involves the meaning of words as they relate to other words in sentences. The meaning of words represents the relationship between people, actions, and objects (Bloom & Lahey, 1978).

- *Syntactic Form:* Syntax represents the grammatical rules one applies to alter words and to arrange them into meaningful sentences in an orderly fashion (Hoff, 2005). Every language has unique syntactic rules governing the order of adjectives, nouns, and verbs. All languages, spoken and signed, also have morphologic rules. Morphological inflections in spoken English (e.g., past /ed/, present progressive /ing/, plural /s/) carry a unique set of rules. In American Sign Language (ASL), morphological features are represented by specific ways to represent verb agreement, the use of classifiers (e.g., the way the hand manipulates or represents an object), and the use of specific facial expressions (e.g., to represent negation, questions, topic changes, and conditionals) (Schick, 2003).

- *Pragmatic Use:* Pragmatics represents the socially-related component of language including contextual appropriateness, functionality, and intent. Pragmatic use reflects communicative competence, which is defined by Hymes (1972) as the ability to use sentences appropriately in social interactions.

The developmental norms for language acquisition during the first 5 years of life are integral to our work with very young children with hearing loss. These norms serve as a guide for the parents, interventionist, and teacher who should be setting high expectations for language learning. The "one-for-one rule" (Deconde Johnson, 2006) sets this high expectation: for each child with hearing loss to maintain language quotients that are commensurate with their hearing peers (by chronological age or cognitive age) during the early years. At a minimum, every child who is deaf or hard of hearing, given no additional learning or language issues, should be making, on average, 1 year's growth in a 1-year period of time or, for the baby, 6 months' growth in 6 months' time. If the child is not making this rate of progress, the services should be reviewed, evaluated, and when necessary, adjusted. This goal significantly raises the expectations of interventionists, teachers, and parents from only one decade ago when one would often have a different standard for children with hearing loss and accept language delay as reasonable and customary.

There are well-established norms for language acquisition. These norms serve as established benchmarks for the development of the language of children with hearing loss. Whenever possible, norms for spoken English and ASL are presented.

Birth to 6 Months

An infant's communication starts as a cry, with the addition of other vegetative vocalizations and random body movements. Babies with hearing loss, even those with profound degrees of hearing loss, produce vocalizations (Yoshinaga-Itano, 2006). Likewise, all babies, those with hearing loss and those with normal hearing, produce random body movements.

Baby's cooing consists of recognizable syllables. Cooing is the production of pro-

longed vowels and starts when baby approaches 2 months of age.

Starting at approximately 4 months of age, a baby demonstrates vocal play (Stark, 1986) and manual play behaviors. The vocalizations include marginal babbling (a long series of sounds). Manual babbling resembles vocal babbling in some respects as it too is rhythmic and syllabically organized and shares phonological properties of ASL (Bellugi, van Hoek, Lillo-Martin, & O'Grady, 1993; Newport & Meier, 1985; Petitto, 2000).

Receptively, at approximately 5 months of age, baby will selectively respond to certain words, usually his own name (Mandel, Jusczyk, & Pisoni, 1995).

Expressively, all infants, irrespective of the exposure they receive from spoken or signed language, communicate in nonverbal ways by reaching, positioning their bodies, and directing their visual gaze. Gradually, baby adds intent to these vocalizations and body movements.

Six to 12 Months

At this stage, babies are readily babbling either vocally or manually. Vocal babbling is referred to as canonical babble (Oller, 1986; Oller & Lynch, 1992) with reduplicated, or repetitive, consonant + vowel (CV) syllables. Nonreduplicated, or variegated, babbling emerges during this stage. Nonreduplicated babble consists of more varied CV combinations and some consonant + vowel + consonant (CVC) syllables. Jargon also emerges during this stage and is characterized by nonreduplicated babble with added intonation contours. It has inflectional similarities to adult conversations, but with a noted lack of intelligible words.

Manual babble occurs from 6 to 14 months of age (Meier & Willerman, 1995; Petitto & Marentette, 1991). Manual babble resembles vocal babble in that it too is rhythmic. It shares the phonological properties of American Sign Language (ASL). The phonological characteristics of ASL include the specific handshapes that are used, the location of the hands in relation to the body, and the qualitative movement of the hands (Bellugi et al., 1993; Newport & Meier, 1985; Petitto, 2000).

Receptively, the 6-month-old child demonstrates a general contextual understanding of what is said, and this meaning is conveyed through the suprasegmental features of language (e.g., intensity, duration, pitch). By 8 months, the baby demonstrates understanding of a few phrases (e.g., "Give me a hug," "Stop it," "Come here"; Fenson et al., 1994). During this time, a baby will also start to understand the meanings of individual words. Great variability exists at 6 months of age, with children demonstrating a receptive vocabulary ranging from 11 to 154 words (Fenson et al., 1994).

Expressively, the magical milestone of first words is achieved. When using spoken language, first words emerge at 10 to 15 months of age (Benedict, 1979; Fenson et al., 1994; Huttonlocher & Smiley, 1987). These words are bound to particular and often-repeated contexts (Barrett, 1995).

For the child exposed to fluent signers, first words emerge even earlier at approximately 8 to 12 months of age (Bonvillian, 1999; Bonvillian, Orlansky, & Novack, 1983; Folven & Bonvillian, 1991; Prinz & Prinz, 1979; Schlesinger & Meadow, 1972). Bonvillian (1999) suggests the earlier appearance of signs reflects the earlier development of the motor abilities necessary to produce gestures.

During this stage, thought is extremely concrete and self-referenced. This explains why the first words that are understood, and later expressed, by the child are concrete, identify the here and now, and include labels for people and objects that are most common to baby's experiences (e.g., "mama," "dada," "baba" for bottle).

The pragmatic use of language starts to develop during this time, even before first words appear. Babies demonstrate systematic use of particular sounds and gestures to express eight different communication functions such as requests for help, directing the listener's attention, and expressing pleasure (Carter, 1978). Dore (1975) reports growth in the number of pragmatic functions that are used as first words emerge. In spoken English, these intentions are expressed with spoken intonational contours.

Twelve to 18 Months

Receptively, the average 16-month-old comprehends 92 to 321 words (Fenson et al., 1994). The toddler is practicing the suprasegmental characteristics of speech or the motoric representations of signs by readily imitating the words used by others.

Expressively, vocabulary development continues, with the 18-month-old accumulating an average inventory of 50 expressive words (Nelson, 1973).

The toddler begins to coordinate nonverbal behaviors of pointing, reaching, and looking from an object to a parent and back to the object again to communicate social intent. The toddler is starting to be a conversationalist and engages with a communicative partner by repeating, answering, and requesting.

Eighteen to 24 Months

Receptively, the toddler appears to understand more and more words each week. The toddler can identify pictures when they are named and match objects to pictures and give appropriate responses to a series of two or three simple, but related, commands. The child appears to listen to the meaning and reason of language utterances, not just to words or sounds.

The semantic focus of parents' and toddlers' verbal interactions to date has had an impact. Up until now, children make one word out of two- or three-word utterances (e.g., Idontknow, Iwant; Peters, 1986). At approximately 18 months of age, the toddler is using spontaneous two-word "telegraphic utterances" to label or describe the objects, actions, and events in the environment. Parents typically expand these telegraphic utterances, which adds syntactic and morphologic structure. The toddler is always at the ready and willing to imitate their parents' examples.

The toddler exhibits productive word combinations (Brown, 1973). Using simple two-word utterances, the toddler uses many syntactic forms such as: (a) agent + action ("daddy sit"); (b) action + object ("drive car"); (c) agent + object ("mommy sock"); (d) agent +location ("sit chair"); (e) entity + location ("toy floor"); (f) possessor + possession ("my teddy"); (g) entity + attribute ("crayon big"); (h) demonstrative + entity ("this telephone").

Once the child has acquired approximately 50 expressive words, the "word spurt" or "word explosion" is seen. Children add approximately 22 to 37 words each month to their expressive vocabulary (Benedict, 1979; Goldfield & Reznick, 1990). Babies exposed to fluent signers also start to use multisign combinations (Bellugi et al., 1993; Newport & Meier, 1985; Petitto, 2000).

The toddler demonstrates social interactions by imitating others. Imitation of common routines and gestural representations of these routines (e.g., holding a telephone to the ear, hugging a baby doll, putting a shoe to the foot) explode in the last few months of the 2nd year. This is the start of the world of make-believe or pretend play. There is an increased interest in books and pictures. Toddlers start to refer to absent objects and events that are not in the immediate environment.

Twenty-four to 48 Months

Receptively, the child demonstrates word associations and categorizes words. Conceptually and linguistically, the child understands size, shape, color, and location. The child's learning remains experience based and the range of opportunities afforded the child serve as a catalyst to learning.

During the 3rd year of life, the child uses more and varying sentence forms and increases the mean length of utterance. Most basic syntactic forms are used, although errors are frequent and telegraphic phrases may still be present.

Similar milestones are reached by children learning spoken English and those learning ASL when they are exposed to a language-rich environment (Bellugi et al., 1993; Newport & Meier, 1985; Petitto, 2000).

In developing spoken language, morphological elements (Brown, 1973) are added such as the plural /s/, the present progressive /ing/, the possessive /'s/, and articles. The child embarks on development of *wh* question forms (Brown, 1973). The child's expressive language gives clear evidence of the use of pronouns, prepositions, and articles (Brown, 1973). Prepositions come to life as the motorically coordinated and socially independent toddler goes in, under, around, and behind things.

Four to 5 Years

During the 4th and 5th years of life, the three interwoven components of language (semantic content, syntactic form, pragmatic use) are expanded and refined. Children have gleaned the generalities of form rules and applies them universally. However, they may overgeneralize these rules by saying, "I *throwed* it in the sink." The well-intentioned parent who attempts to correct form errors may say, "No, you *threw* it. *Threw*," only to have the child simply apply the same rule again by saying, "I *threwed* it in the sink!" How complex this task of language learning!

Pragmatically, a child this age is developing discourse skills and engages in more extensive dialogue with others.

Impact of Hearing Loss on Language Development

Considering the aforementioned norms, the professionals and parents set out to create a treatment program. Current trends give reasons to be optimistic about the language development of children with hearing loss. Newborn hearing screening is now common practice (Green, Gaffney, Devine, & Grosse, 2007), advanced hearing technology and cochlear implants provide better access to auditory information, and age-old arguments about the "best" communication approach are starting to be replaced with informed choices that are supported with empirical evidence (Hafer & Stredler-Brown, 2003; Stredler-Brown, in press; Stredler-Brown & Yoshinaga-Itano, 1994).

Research shows that children who are identified with hearing loss and start intervention by 6 months of age have expressive and receptive language within normal limits (± one standard deviation), whereas later-identified children demonstrate significant delays in receptive and expressive language (Mayne, Yoshinaga-Itano, Sedey, & Carey, 2000; Moeller, 2000; Yoshinaga-Itano, 2003;

Yoshinaga-Itano & Apuzzo, 1998a; Yoshinaga-Itano & Apuzzo, 1998b; Yoshinaga-Itano, Sedey, Coulter, & Mehl, 1998). An early start to intervention can mitigate the impact, so common years ago, on linguistic, social, emotional, cognitive, and academic development (Calderon, 2000; Moeller, 2000; Figure 7-1).

In addition to the opportunities afforded by earlier identification, new hearing aid technology such as digital processing strategies and early cochlear implantation provide access to sound for children with hearing loss (Geers, Nicholas, & Sedey, 2003). Better access to sound, specifically speech, can also limit the potential effects of hearing loss on language development.

Even minimal and mild degrees of hearing loss, including unilateral hearing loss, may cause delays in communication, speech, and language. Children with mild degrees of hearing loss often demonstrate academic, social, and behavioral difficulties (Bess, Dodd-Murphy, & Parker, 1998; Cho Lieu, 2004; Kiese-Himmel & Ohlwein, 2003). They may demonstrate the inability to hear speech and language adequately in typical listening situations, which interferes with speech perception (Bess, 2000; Crandell & Smaldino, 2000). Children with mild or minimal degrees of hearing loss also experience increased difficulties listening under adverse conditions, and may have less energy (Bess et al., 1998; Wake & Poulakis, 2004). An intervention program for a child with minimal or unilateral hearing loss has several purposes: (a) to provide parents with information about the potential impact of minimal and mild degrees of hearing loss on their child's development, (b) to maintain ongoing developmental assessment to determine if and when there are negative sequelae from the hearing loss, and (c) to make environmental accommodations to augment a young child's learning (Stredler-Brown, in press).

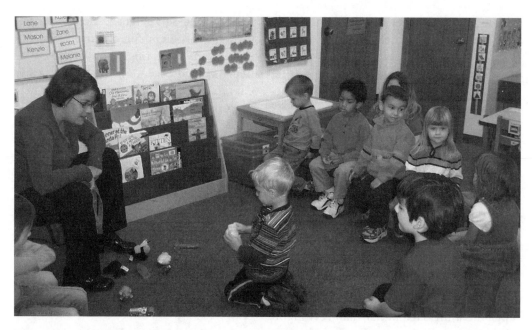

Figure 7–1. Interactions between parent and child provide enhanced speech and language development. Parents can be effective co-clinicians.

Some clinicians recommend personal amplification for children with minimal hearing loss in both ears. Amplification for children with unilateral hearing loss is being investigated with anecdotal evidence that it may prove helpful for children with moderate degrees of hearing loss in the affected ear (Kiese-Himmel, 2002; McKay, 2002).

For children with moderate, severe, and profound degrees of bilateral hearing loss, the impact of the hearing loss is always significant and likely affects all aspects of language including semantic content, syntactic form, pragmatic use, and phonologic development.

Impact of Hearing Loss on Semantic Content

Children with hearing loss typically demonstrate delays in vocabulary development (Moeller, Osberger, & Eccarius, 1986; Osberger, Moeller, Eccarius, Robbins, & Johnson, 1986). These delays may be pervasive and persistent through adulthood. They demonstrate limited understanding of metaphors, idioms, figurative language, and jokes (Culbertson, 2007). And these children generally are challenged by multiple meanings of words (e.g., "*run* the stats," "go for a *run*," "*running* water"; Culbertson, 2007).

Impact of Hearing Loss on Syntactic Form

To varying degrees, children with hearing loss exhibit a shorter mean length of utterance (MLU), they tend to use simpler sentence structures, they tend to overuse the subject-verb-object sentence pattern, and they may demonstrate infrequent use of specific word forms (e.g., adverbs, auxiliaries, conjunctions; Culbertson, 2007). Some children use inappropriate syntactic patterns (e.g., "I want you go get eat things" to convey the message, "I want you to go to the store to buy food for dinner"). They may use non-English word order (Culbertson, 2007).

Impact of Hearing Loss on Pragmatic Use

Culbertson (2007) also reports frequent errors in pragmatic use, including restricted use of communicative intents, inability to use conversational conventions (e.g., introductions, ending a conversation, interruptions), and limited use of repair strategies (e.g., repeating a message rather than revising it when it is not understood the first time.)

Impact of Hearing Loss on Phonologic Development

Speech production is affected by sounds that are not heard or not heard well when misarticulated or omitted from the child's speech. This affects speech intelligibility.

Language Stimulation: Mitigating the Impact of Hearing Loss

A primary goal of early intervention is to teach the young child's parents, caregivers, and other adults in the child's life to use stimulating, interactive behaviors with the young child with hearing loss. This goal applies to young children learning language auditorily, those learning language visually, and those learning language through both modalities.

But access to language alone does not solve the problem for children who are deaf or hard of hearing. There is a need for specialized intervention during the early years to avoid the effects hearing loss may have on the child's development of spoken and/or signed language. Early intervention teaches parents to provide their children with access to both direct and incidental language learning. Whatever language and communication system is chosen by a child's parents, access to a rich language environment (DesGeorges, Johnson, & Stredler-Brown, 2007) is the goal. The characteristics of a language-rich environment are described in Table 7–1.

Communication Approaches

The long-debated argument about which communication approach is suitable for children who are deaf or hard of hearing will not be discussed here. Rather, an alternative approach that relies on informed decisions and objective information will be presented. As a family selects the "best" approach for their child, each professional is encouraged to present all choices objectively, to honor the informed preferences of the parents, to collect objective information describing the child's developmental and communication profile, to offer their own clinical judgment based on their expertise, and to acknowledge that all approaches provide opportunities for learning (Stredler-Brown, in press). A key ingredient guiding this process is having objective information —the evidence—that is collected through assessments.

There is consensus on the specific characteristics that can make each and every

TABLE 7–1. Factors Supporting a Language-Rich Environment

1. *Capitalize on early development:* Language learning for children with hearing loss is most critical during the first months and years of a child's life (Yoshinaga-Itano et al., 1998). Knowing this, infants and toddlers need to be immersed in an environment that supports language development during this critical period.

2. *Provide immersion in a language-rich environment:* A language-rich environment is accessible, uses the child's and parent's preferred communication approach, and provides opportunities for active and consistent communication with peers and adults using the selected approach.

3. *Assure access to language stimulation:* Infants and toddlers with hearing loss may be insulated, to varying degrees, from the sounds and signs of everyday life. In order to compensate for this auditory and/or visual isolation, alternative, supplementary, and/or enhanced methods must be used to help the child access language.

4. *Provide opportunities to learn from peers:* Children learn from one another. It is essential for a child with hearing loss to be in an environment where their peers all use the same communication system or language.

5. *Make appropriate adaptations to the environment:* The learning environment must facilitate access to auditory and/or visual information. An appropriate acoustic environment promotes language and communication development by minimizing auditory distractions (background noise) and by reducing noise with carpet and other absorptive materials. Equally important are the environmental adaptations supporting visual enhancement of language. This can include appropriate lighting and reduction of visual distractions (e.g., clutter).

6. *Provide parent support:* Early intervention teaches parents about language development, the importance of ongoing, communicative interactions with their child, and specific techniques to promote and enhance their child's language development.

7. *Ensure parents have access to a multidisciplinary team:* The multidisciplinary team of qualified professionals completes evaluations at periodic intervals to assure developmental progress is being made at a satisfactory rate.

approach successful (Stredler-Brown, 1998). An approach will be successful when it is started early and when full access is provided as a child needs multiple role models to learn language, both within the family and in the community. Parental commitment goes a long way towards the child's success (Li, Bain, & Steinberg, 2003). Dedicated time needs to be given to teach parents strategies to implement the approach successfully. And it is critical for the professionals working with the family and the child to have experience and expertise using the selected approach.

A description of the communication approaches and philosophies that are most readily used in the United States is given in Table 7–2.

TABLE 7–2. Communication Approaches and Philosophies

Communication Approaches and Philosophies	Definition
Bilingual Model	A person who achieves fluency in American Sign Language and English is bilingual. ASL is often the first language with English being taught, as a second language, to develop literacy skills. English can be taught using a sign system or through print. Spoken English is not included in the bilingual model that is currently promoted by the Deaf community.
Simultaneous Communication	This is the use of signs and speech at the same time. In order to provide language in both modes simultaneously, a sign system, rather than a signed language, is used. Pidgin Signed English (PSE), Conceptually Accurate Signed English (CASE), and Manually Coded English (MCE) are examples of sign systems.
Sign-Supported Speech and Language	The use of signs to support spoken language development serves as a "bridge" to completely oral communication. Signs may be used as a back-up in certain situations such as noisy environments or when a hearing device is not in use (Lane, Bell, & Parson-Tylka, 2006).
Auditory-Oral Approach	This approach combines oral spoken language to express oneself and speechreading, accompanied by active listening, to receive information. The use of natural gestures is acceptable.
Auditory-Verbal Approach	This is an educational approach in which technology is paired with specific techniques and strategies that teach children to listen and understand spoken language. A primary emphasis is placed on access to learning through the auditory modality. This refinement of the auditory-oral approach makes a concerted effort to remove visual cues during therapy sessions so the child can develop the auditory system through directed listening practice. Speechreading is not a primary teaching strategy, and this visual information is reduced or eliminated during therapy by covering most of the face while presenting speech stimuli (Estabrooks, 1994).
Total Communication	Introduced in the 1960s by Roy Holcomb, this "philosophy" aims to make use of a number of strategies or modes of communication including sign, oral, auditory, written, and other visual aids. The choice of modalities depends on the particular needs and abilities of the child. The philosophy professes to provide whatever is needed to foster communicative success.
Cued Speech	A supplement to spoken English, Cued Speech (Cornett & Daisey, 1992) is intended to make important features of spoken language fully visible because approximately 60% of the phonemes are not visible through speechreading. This system enhances speechreading by employing phonemically-based gestures to distinguish among similar visual speech patterns.

Note. From "Intervention, Education, and Therapy for Children Who Are Deaf or Hard of Hearing," (2009), by A. Stredler-Brown, in J. Katz, L. Medwetsky, R. Burkaard, & L. Hood, (Eds.), *Handbook of clinical audiology* (pp. 934–954). Baltimore: Lippincott, Williams & Wilkins.

Focusing on Language Learning

Because children thrive in environments that are language-rich, parents are taught to use specific strategies to create a supportive and engaging environment. Stredler-Brown et al. (2006) define the elements of a language-rich environment. These concepts are described in Table 7–3.

When the child is learning to listen, it is important for the child to use properly fitted and appropriately maintained amplification during all waking hours. The parents then learn methods to enhance their child's access to auditory information and to promote the development of active listening skills. For children learning sign language, it is important for parents to commit the time and effort necessary so that each family member becomes a consistent, and ultimately

TABLE 7–3. Elements of a Language-Rich Environment

Meaningful: The child's interests and natural curiosity are used as the basis for language input. Communication is authentic; it is not contrived.

- *Constant:* The child is bathed in language during all routines, during new and exciting events, to express emotions, to comment, to share, and to discuss.

- *Responsive:* Adults follow the child's lead. The child's utterances, whether vocal or gestural, spoken or signed, are repeated by the adult and modified, as needed, to be precise and accurate linguistic utterances. This is done naturally.

- *Nurturing:* The family accepts and supports the language used by the child. At the same time, the child is challenged to use new vocabulary, complex language, and abstract ideas. Language is naturally tied to the here-and-now but also includes discussions about things that are not in the room and that happened in the past and that will happen in the future.

- *Strategic:* A variety of strategies are used to encourage communication and expand utterances. These techniques may include use of expectant pauses, rephrasing what was said or signed, adding cues to clarify the utterance, and using manipulatives to support understanding or maintain attention.

- *Social:* Children have numerous opportunities to interact with many communication partners at home and in their communities.

- *Complete:* The child is provided with fluent language models.

- *Emotional:* Family members use language to communicate their emotional availability. This provides the child with words to label and discuss feelings.

- *Thought-Provoking:* One of the most wonderful aspects of language is the ability to stimulate thought. The world is an amazing place that is full of surprises. Children need the opportunity to talk about the "whys" and "hows" of their environment.

- *Guiding:* Children are taught to use language to solve problems and to think through options with their friends and family members.

Note. From "Language Partners: Building a Strong Foundation" [DVD], by A. Stredler-Brown, M. P. Moeller, R. Gallegos, J. Corwin, & P. Pittman, 2006, Omaha, NE: Boys Town Press.

fluent, user of sign language. This provides the requisite access to both direct and incidental learning. Whatever language and method is chosen, parents can promote language development by being responsive to their baby's earliest communicative attempts and by engaging their growing child in playful and rich communicative interactions and conversations.

can develop advanced auditory skills and acquire fluent spoken language. As a result of improvements in hearing technology, and because approximately 95% of children who are deaf or hard of hearing are born to hearing parents (Mitchell & Karchmer, 2004), an increasing number of families are choosing spoken language as the mode of communication for their child.

Developing the Spoken Language of Children with Hearing Loss

The visual language approaches, specifically ASL, have been well documented by Schick (2003), Marschark et al. (2002), and Erting (2003). Likewise, the development of auditory skills, an essential component when teaching a child spoken language, has been documented (Cole & Flexer, 2008; Erber, 1982; Estabrooks, 1998; Flexer, 1999; Stout & Windle, 1992; Tye-Murray, 1992; Watkins, 1993). When parents choose to teach their child to talk, the first thing that needs to happen is to underscore the importance of teaching their child to listen. Think about it. Why do we speak the language we speak? It was learned at home. How was it learned? By listening to the native language (Werker, 2006; Winegert & Brant, 2005). One listens throughout the day and to multiple speakers. The message may be directed to the child or it may occur incidentally as adults speak to one another, when siblings talk to each other, or when the television is on.

It is important to recognize that early detection, together with recent advances in cochlear implant and hearing aid technology, has greatly increased the likelihood that even the most profoundly deaf infants

First Things First: Appropriate Hearing Technology

Although more residual hearing is beneficial to the development of auditory skills, the hearing thresholds, in and of themselves, do not afford the necessary skills to teach a child to listen. It is a child's use of, not the amount of, residual hearing that is critical to the development of functional listening.

The child's audiologist evaluates a child for amplification and other sensory devices and assistive technology (Joint Committee on Infant Hearing [JCIH[, 2007). It is now common to see a baby fit with amplification as early as the first month of life. Immediate amplification is needed to capitalize on this very critical period for auditory stimulation. Hearing aids are to be fit to both ears unless contraindicated (American Academy of Audiology [AAA], 2003).

A cochlear implant is a device that converts acoustic signals into codes that preserve the features critical to speech understanding. Cochlear implants are now approved by the Food and Drug Administration (FDA) for children 12 months of age and older. Pediatric criteria have changed over time and, no doubt, will continue to change making cochlear implants accessible to children younger than 12 months of age and, potentially, to children with less severe degrees of hearing loss. Currently, however, for children

12 to 24 months of age, cochlear implant criteria include:

- A bilateral hearing loss,
- A severe to profound degree of hearing loss,
- A demonstrated lack of progress in the development of auditory skills with the use of hearing aids,
- No medical contraindications,
- A highly motivated family,
- And access to extensive habilitation services.

Neither hearing aids nor cochlear implants "correct" or "fix" a hearing loss. Hearing aids and cochlear implants, when used consistently, can increase access to spoken language but they do not, in and of themselves, ensure typical language development. Although amplification improves hearing thresholds, a child with hearing loss needs to have amplification *and* an auditory training program to learn to listen.

Theoretical Underpinnings of Auditory Training

Hearing loss has been described as an "invisible acoustic filter" that distorts or eliminates incoming sounds (Cole & Flexer, 2008). Even with optimal amplification, the child with hearing loss experiences the world with auditorily diminished access to language. Except for children with mild degrees of hearing loss, the auditory signal is still being filtered by a less-than-perfect auditory system. This brings us to the world of auditory training—teaching a child with hearing loss to listen.

What do we know about auditory skill development? We know that auditory skills correlate directly with speech development

for children who are deaf or hard of hearing. We know that the development of auditory skills is systematic (Laughton & Hasenstab, 2000; Pollock, Goldberg, & Caleffe-Schenck, 1985) and follows an inherent hierarchy of skills. And we know that the development of auditory skills does not happen in isolation. In order to achieve optimal outcomes, specific strategies must be incorporated into all of the child's routines.

Children's optimal use of residual hearing is facilitated when the hearing loss is detected early, appropriate technology is used consistently, parents are committed to and actively engaged in the development of their child's auditory skills, and a therapeutic or educational treatment program is implemented by skilled and experienced professionals who are equally committed to the development of the child's functional auditory skills.

Establishing a Hearing Age

Having optimal amplification, paired with consistent use, defines a child's "hearing age." The hearing age may be different from the chronological age, as the hearing age starts when a child's use of technology provides access to sound and is worn during all waking hours.

Providing a Stimulating Environment

The first learning environment is the home. Auditory learning is most effective when it takes place during a child's ongoing daily activities (Erber, 1982; Simmons-Martin, 1981) (Figure 7–2). A child's integration of audition into everyday life is the ultimate goal. Strategies learned and practiced with parents at home can then generalize to other activities outside of the home. Learning to

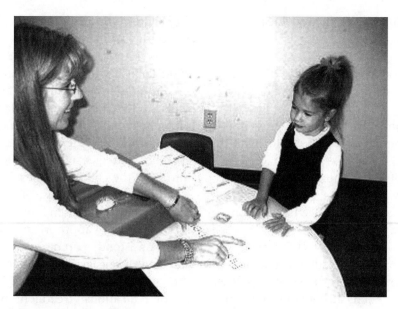

Figure 7–2. Auditory learning is most effective when it is a part of a child's everyday activities.

listen is a full-time job, a constant, never-ending process.

Parents of a child with hearing loss must start by directing their child's attention to the auditory experiences around them. Parents can enhance their infant's ability to make auditory responses by controlling the auditory distractions in their homes (e.g., the hum of a nearby dishwasher, the television, or the stereo). The parents learn to focus their child's attention on numerous common, everyday environmental sounds (e.g., the microwave, running water, the garage door, the doorbell, a cell phone, etc). Although a child with normal hearing takes these sounds for granted, a prescriptive auditory training program asks the child to acknowledge that the sound was heard. For the very young child, it is critical to associate these sounds with their source and to attribute meaning to them.

In addition to learning to listen to non-linguistic stimuli, children must learn to listen to linguistic stimuli—spoken language—as well. An optimal listening environment provides a running verbal commentary on the people, objects, and activities in the child's life. Verbal utterances should be meaningful, interesting, and repeated often. Auditory training can be incorporated into all of these routines (Rowan, 2004): child-initiated play, child-initiated routines (e.g., getting dressed, bedtime, mealtime), adult-initiated play, and adult-initiated routines (e.g., household chores, running errands, visiting people).

Receiving Guidance from Professionals

Perhaps the single most critical criterion to a child's auditory success, once consistent appropriate amplification is in place, is the ongoing interaction with parents who believe in the child's ability to listen. Professionals provide an important model for parents; they provide an attitude that expects a child with hearing loss to hear, listen, and speak. The professionals must have a broad base of knowledge about auditory skill development and speech acoustics. Furthermore, professionals must be familiar with the underpinnings of family-centered intervention so they know how to teach specific listening and speech techniques to family members so they can employ these techniques throughout the day.

Using a Progress Monitoring Tool

It is critical for the child's skills to be measured continually in order to document progress. The success of auditory skill development must be monitored rigorously and systematically according to an established hierarchy of listening skills.

Developmental Norms for Auditory Learning

The acquisition of auditory skills proceeds through the same stages for hearing children and those with hearing loss, albeit at a slower pace for the latter. Recent research by Ching (2007) provides benchmarks for the development of auditory skills in hearing children. Ching tested the auditory skills of 90 children with normal hearing using the Parent's Evaluation of Aural/Oral Performance of Children (PEACH). The results give long-awaited benchmarks for the development of functional auditory skills. Ching showed that children start to acquire auditory skills at approximately 6 months of age and these skills are near-perfect by approximately 40 months of age.

Erber's normative data (1982) associate specific listening skills with precise ages of acquisition for hearing children:

- *Birth to 3 months:* Baby startles to loud sounds, is quieted by mother's voice,

listens to soft sounds that are presented in close proximity, searches for sound, and enjoys listening to music. Even the very young baby starts to listen to his own vocalizations, which is a critical skill in order to develop an auditory feedback mechanism and can be most challenging for children with hearing loss.
- *Three to 6 months:* Baby starts to search for sound and turn in the direction of the sound. Baby may start to vocalize or stop vocalizing in response to music. Baby enjoys his own voice. Noises can be frightening and cause baby to cry.
- *Six to 9 months:* The maturing baby localizes to sounds. Baby exhibits gross vocal discrimination by responding to his own name. Baby is attentive to the conversation of others.
- *Nine to 12 months:* Baby is starting to discriminate the words of the language spoken in the home, which supports the production of first words. This phenomenon continues for the next 2 years until, at 2 to 3 years, the child has a large intelligible vocabulary.

Although acquisition of these skills is straightforward and effortless for a child with normal hearing, the acquisition of these skills for a child with hearing loss relies on prescriptive auditory training.

Models for Auditory Training

There are two different, but complementary, models for developing auditory skills (Razack, 1994): the didactic model and the generalization model. Ideally, both the didactic and generalization models are employed in the therapy plan.

As the critical period for learning is in the first 3 years of life, the provision of an optimal listening environment must not be left to chance. The didactic model teaches isolated, structured listening behaviors. It focuses on the auditory hierarchy of skills and is directed by the interventionist, therapist, teacher, or parents. Specific techniques are employed to investigate and identify effective listening routines. Although this fact-finding process is integral to the auditory training program, it is also important to generalize the skills to naturally-occurring events as the goal is to develop the child's ability to learn auditory skills independently.

Razack, then, emphasizes the importance of *auditory learning*: the need to generalize specific skills into familiar naturally-occurring routines, into language experiences, and in play. This promotes the generalization of specific auditory skills to new and novel environments.

Hierarchical Stages of Auditory Skill Development

There are many checklists and curriculums explaining the stages of auditory skill development (Ching, 2007; Erber, 1982; Estabrooks, 1998; DeConde Johnson, Benson, & Seaton, 1997; Razack, 1994; Stout & Windle, 1992; Stredler-Brown & DeConde Johnson, 2004; Tye-Murray, 1992). Although these checklists may ascribe different names to the stages of auditory training, they are essentially the same when it comes to the discrete skills that are taught.

Auditory skills typically included in various checklists will be described according to one protocol, the Functional Auditory Performance Indicators (FAPI; Stredler-Brown & DeConde Johnson, 2004). This progress monitoring tool has seven categories arranged in hierarchical order. Embedded in the categories are a total of 31 discrete skills with one to eight skills in each of the seven categories. The skills within a category are also listed in hierarchical order.

1. *Awareness and Meaning of Sounds:* The child is aware that an auditory stimulus is present. The child may demonstrate awareness of loud environmental sounds, noisemakers, music, and/or speech. The child further demonstrates that sound is meaningful by associating a variety of auditory stimuli with their sound source.

2. *Auditory Feedback and Integration:* The child changes, notices, and monitors his own vocal productions. A child may demonstrate this skill by responding to sound when amplification is turned on, by vocalizing to monitor when amplification is working, and/or by noticing his own vocalizations. Furthermore, the child uses auditory information to produce a spoken utterance that approximates or matches a spoken stimulus.

3. *Localizing Sound Source:* The child searches for and/or finds the auditory stimulus. Searching is a prerequisite skill for localizing. Children with hearing in only one ear may search for, but not be able to localize to, the sound source.

4. *Auditory Discrimination:* The child distinguishes the characteristics of different sounds as being the same or different. This includes environmental sounds, suprasegmental characteristics of speech (e.g., intensity, duration, pitch), non-true words, and true words.

5. *Auditory Comprehension:* The child demonstrates understanding of linguistic information by identifying what is said, identifying critical elements in the message, and following directions.

6. *Short-Term Auditory Memory:* The child can hear, remember, repeat, and recall a sequence of units (e.g., digits, unrelated words, sentences). This skill is developmentally appropriate when a child is 2 years of age and older.

7. *Linguistic Auditory Processing*: The child utilizes auditory information to process language. This category measures the ways in which audition is used to learn and use morphemes, to learn and use syntactic information, and to understand complex spoken messages.

A child's skill in each of the seven aforementioned domains must be considered in light of the complex listening situations that exist in the world around us. With this in mind, each skill should be practiced and measured in these dynamic listening conditions:

- Auditory stimuli that are paired with *visual cues* contrasted with responses to an *auditory stimulus alone*
- Stimuli that are presented in *close proximity* to the child contrasted with stimuli that are presented *far away*
- Auditory stimuli in a *noisy situation* contrasted with stimuli presented in a *quiet environment*
- Auditory stimuli that are observed when the child is *prompted* to listen contrasted with *spontaneous* responses to auditory stimuli
- Auditory stimuli that are presented as a *closed set* of a limited number of choices contrasted with items that are presented in an unlimited *open set*
- Words that are *familiar* to the child contrasted with *unfamiliar* words
- The use of *words* as the stimulus contrasted with *sentences* (Sentences are more difficult to listen to because of the length of the utterance)
- Stimuli that are presented when the child is in an *active listening state* contrasted with the presentation of stimuli while the child is engaged in *other activities*

It is important for a child's treatment program to have an embedded measure of accountability (Stredler-Brown, 2004). A progress monitoring tool that includes a scoring paradigm allows the early interventionist, teacher, and/or parents to quantify the improvements that are made over time and, subsequently, to measure the effectiveness of the treatment plan. The FAPI is one such tool as it has a scoring rubric. This feature provides quantitative documentation of a child's skills. Each of the 31 skills on the tool earns a value of 0 to 3 points, depending on the level to which a child has accomplished a skill. An *acquired skill* occurs 80 to 100% of the time and receives a weighted value of 3 points. A skill that is *in process* occurs 36 to 70% of the time and is assigned a value of 2 points. An *emerging skill* occurs less frequently, only 11 to 35% of the time, and receives a weighted value of 1 point. When a skill is *not present*, occurring less than 10% of the time, it receives 0 points. The profile is generated by calculating the scores for each skill, adding the weighted scores, and comparing this score to the total number of possible points. A percentage score is calculated for each skill and for each of the seven categories. The profile identifies a child's unique strengths and needs and is used to create goals for the child's individualized program.

Auditory Therapy

When working on selected listening skills, there are many accommodations that can be made to promote effective listening. These strategies fall into three categories: (a) altering the content of the message, (b) altering the phonologic characteristics of what is said, and (c) adapting the syntactic complexity of the stimulus:

- *The content of the message:* Children are most interested in the topics they choose. An informed parent or professional can integrate auditory skills into almost any activity chosen by the child.

■ *The phonologic characteristics of the message:* An utterance may be more interesting to the child when it has varied intonation contours with more rhythmic phrasing. Brief pauses between phrases and sentences make the message more discrete and, therefore, more easily understood. Repetition of the message gives the listener a second or third opportunity to understand what was said.

■ *The syntactic complexity of the message:* Shorter utterances are easier to listen to. This includes spoken utterances with fewer clauses and fewer structure or function words (e.g., auxiliary verbs, noun markers or articles, and bound morphemes). Note that although it is often advantageous to adjust the syntactic complexity of a message in order for the listener to understand it, it is also critical for a child to hear typical running speech.

Summary

All degrees and all types of hearing loss can have an impact on the development of a child's speech, communication, and language. The effects may be in the characteristics of semantic content, syntactic form, and/or pragmatic use. With the advent of newborn hearing screening, and the potential for early intervention, it is possible to mitigate the effects of hearing loss. Despite the common effect of hearing loss on language learning, children with hearing loss are not a homogeneous group when it comes to language acquisition. To accommodate the individuality of children and the unique qualities of their families, there are many communication approaches available. Selection of a communication approach should be based on informed choice, associated counseling, and empirical evidence.

For families who select an oral approach to language learning, there must be a prescriptive auditory training program in place. This approach has become increasingly popular and increasingly successful. The success of the auditory approaches reflects the opportunities made possible by early identification, early intervention, and excellent hearing technology. There are prescribed procedures to develop the listening skills of a child with hearing loss that are based on emerging developmental norms, provision of services by trained professionals, use of prescriptive curriculums, and utilization of a progress monitoring tool.

One day, hopefully in the not-too-distant future, children with hearing loss will demonstrate developmental progress similar to their hearing peers. It is possible.

References

American Academy of Audiology. (2003). *Pediatric amplification protocol.* Reston, VA: American Academy of Audiology. Available at http://www.audiology.org/professional/positions/pedamp.pdf

Barrett, M. (1995). Early lexical development. In P. Fletcher & B. MacWhinney (Eds.), *The handbook of child language* (pp. 83–109). Oxford, UK: Blackwell.

Bellugi, U., van Hoek, K., Lillo-Martin, D., & O'Grady, L. (1993). The acquisition of syntax and space in young deaf signers. In D. Bishop & K. Mogford (Eds.), *Language development in exceptional children* (pp. 132–150). Hove, UK: Erlbaum.

Benedict, H. (1979). Early lexical development: Comprehension and production. *Journal of Child Language, 6,* 183–200.

Bess, F. H. (2000). Classroom acoustics: An overview. *The Volta Review, 101,* 1-14.

Bess, F. H., Dodd-Murphy, J., & Parker, R. A. (1998). Children with minimal sensorineural hearing loss: Prevalence, educational performance, and functional status. *Ear and Hearing, 19*(5), 339-354.

Bloom, L., & Lahey, M. (1978). *Language development and language disorders.* New York: John Wiley & Sons.

Bonvillian, J. D. (1999). Sign language development. In M. Barrett (Ed.), *The development of language* (pp. 54-82). East Sussex, UK: Psychology Press.

Bonvillian, J. D., Orlansky, M. D., & Novack, L. L. (1983). Developmental milestones: Sign language acquisition and motor development. *Child Development, 54,* 1435-1445.

Brown, R. (1973). *A first language: The early stages.* Cambridge, MA: Harvard University Press.

Calderon, R. (2000). Parent involvement in deaf children's education programs as a predictor of child's language, reading, and social-emotional development. *Journal of Deaf Studies and Deaf Education, 5*(2), 140-155.

Carter, A. (1978). The development of systematic vocalizations prior to words: A case study. In N. Waterson & C. E. Snow (Eds.), *The development of communication* (pp. 134-168). Chichester, UK: Wiley.

Ching, T. Y. C. (2007). The Parents' Evaluation of Aural/Oral Performance of Children (PEACH) Scale: Normative data. *Journal of the American Academy of Audiology, 18,* 220-235.

Cho Lieu, J. E. (2004). Speech-language and educational consequences of unilateral hearing loss in children. *Archives of Otolaryngology and Head & Neck Surgery, 130,* 524-530.

Cole, E. B., & Flexer, C. (2008). *Children with hearing loss: Developing listening and talking birth to six.* San Diego, CA: Plural.

Cornett, R. O., & Daisey, M. E. (1992). *The cued speech resource book.* Raleigh, NC: National Cued Speech Association.

Crandell, C. C., & Smaldino, J. J. (2000). Classroom acoustics for children with normal hearing and with hearing impairment. *Language, Speech, and Hearing Services in Schools, 31,* 362-370.

Culbertson, D. S. (2007). Language and speech of the deaf and hard of hearing. In R. L. Schow & M. A. Nerbonne (Eds.), *Introduction to audiologic rehabilitation* (pp. 197-217). Boston: Pearson Education.

DesGeorges, J., Johnson, C. D., & Stredler-Brown, A. (2007). Natural environments: A call for policy guidance for infants and toddlers (0-3) who are deaf/hard of hearing. *Hands & Voices Communicator, 10*(4), 1-6.

Dore, J. (1975). Holophrases, speech acts, and language universals. *Journal of Child Language, 2,* 20-40.

Erber, N. P. (1982). *Auditory training.* Washington, DC: Alexander Graham Bell Association for the Deaf.

Erting, C. J. (2003). Signs of literacy: An ethnographic study of American Sign Language and English literacy acquisition. In B. Bodner-Johnson & M. Sass-Lehrer (Eds.), *The young deaf or hard of hearing child: A family-centered approach to early education* (pp. 142-161). Baltimore: Paul H. Brookes.

Estabrooks, W. (1994). *Auditory-verbal therapy.* Washington, DC: Alexander Graham Bell Association for the Deaf.

Estabrooks, W. (1998). Auditory-verbal ages and stages of development. In W. Estabrooks (Ed.), *Cochlear implants for kids* (pp. 74-92). Washington, DC: Alexander Graham Bell Association for the Deaf.

Fenson, L., Dale, P. S., Reznick, J. S., Bates, E., Thal, D. J., & Pethick, S. J. (1994). Variability in early communicative development. *Monographs of the Society for Research in Child Development, 59* (Serial No. 242).

Flexer, C. (1999). *Facilitating hearing and listening in young children.* San Diego, CA: Singular.

Folven, R. J., & Bonvillian, J. D. (1991). The transition from nonreferential to referential language in children acquiring American Sign Language. *Developmental Psychology, 27,* 806-816.

Geers, A., Nicholas, J., & Sedey, A. (2003). Language skills of children with early cochlear implantation. *Ear and Hearing, 24,* 46-58.

Goldfield, B. A., & Reznick, J. S. (1990). Early lexical acquisition: Rate, content, and the vocabulary spurt. *Journal of Child Language, 17,* 171-184.

Green, D. R., Gaffney, M., Devine, O., & Grosse, S. D. (2007). Determining the effect of newborn hearing screening: An analysis of state hearing screening rates. *Public Health Reports, 122*(2), 198–205.

Hafer, J. C., & Stredler-Brown, A. (2003). Family-centered developmental assessment. In B. Bodner-Johnson & M. Sass-Lehrer (Eds.), *The young deaf or hard of hearing child: A family-centered approach to early education* (pp. 126–151). Baltimore: Paul H. Brookes.

Hoff, E. (2005). *Language development.* Belmont, CA: Wadsworth Thomson Learning.

Huttonlocher, J., & Smiley, P. (1987). Early word meanings: The case of object names. *Cognitive Psychology, 19*, 63–89.

Hymes, D. H. (1972). Models of the interaction of language and social life. In J. Gumperz & D. Hymes (Eds.), *Directions in sociolinguistics: The ethnography of communication* (pp. 97–128). New York: Holt, Rinehart & Winston.

DeConde Johnson, C. (2006). One year's growth in one year, expect no less. *Hands & Voices Communicator, 9*, 3.

DeConde Johnson, C., Benson, P. V., & Seaton, J. B. (1997). *Educational audiology handbook.* San Diego, CA: Singular.

Joint Committee on Infant Hearing. (2007). Year 2007 position statement: Principles and guidelines for early hearing detection and intervention programs. *Pediatrics, 102*(4), 893–921.

Kiese-Himmel, C. (2002). Unilateral sensorineural hearing impairment in childhood: Analysis of 31 consecutive cases. *International Journal of Audiology, 41*, 57–63.

Kiese-Himmel, C., & Ohlwein, S. (2003). Characteristics of children with permanent mild hearing impairment. *Folia Phoniatrica et Logopaedia, 55*(2), 70–79.

Lane, S., Bell, L., & Parson-Tylka, T. (2006). *My turn to learn: A communication guide for parents of deaf or hard of hearing children.* British Columbia, Canada: Bauhinea Press.

Laughton, J., & Hasenstab, S. M. (2000). Auditory learning, assessment, and intervention with school-age students who are deaf or hard-of-hearing. In J. Alpiner & P. McCarthy (Eds.), *Rehabilitative audiology: Children and adults* (pp. 178–225). Baltimore: Lippincott, Williams and Wilkins.

Li, Y., Bain, L., & Steinberg, A. G. (2003). Parental decision making and the choice of communication modality for the child who is deaf. *Archives of Pediatric Adolescent Medicine, 157*(2), 162–168.

Mandel, D. R., Jusczyk, P. W., & Pisoni, D. B. (1995). Infants' recognition of the sound patterns of their own names. *Psychological Science, 6*, 314–317.

Marschark, M., Lang, H. G., & Albertini, J. A. (2002). *Educating deaf students: From research to practice.* New York: Oxford University Press.

Mayne, A. M., Yoshinaga-Itano, C., Sedey, A. L., & Carey, A. (2000). Expressive vocabulary development of infants and toddlers who are deaf or hard of hearing. *The Volta Review, 100*, 1–28.

McKay, S. (2002). To aid or not to aid: Children with unilateral hearing loss. Retrieved August 20, 2007, from http://www.audiologyonline.com

Meier, R. P., & Willerman, R. (1995). Prelinguistic gesture in deaf and hearing infants. In K. Emmorey & J. Reilly (Eds.), *Language, gesture, and space* (pp. 137–153). Hillsdale, NJ: Lawrence Erlbaum Associates.

Mitchell, R. E., & Karchmer, M. A. (2004). Chasing the mythical ten percent: Parental hearing status of deaf and hard of hearing students in the United States. *Sign Language Studies, 4*(2), 138–163.

Moeller, M. P. (2000). Early intervention and language development in children who are deaf and hard of hearing. *Pediatrics, 106*(3), 1–9.

Moeller, M. P., Osberger, M. J., & Eccarius, M. (1986). Receptive language skills: Language and learning skills of hearing-impaired students. *ASHA Monographs, 231*, 41–54.

Nelson, K. (1973). Structure and strategy in learning to talk. *Monographs of the Society for Research in Child Development, 38* (1 and 2, Serial No. 149).

Newport, E. L., & Meier, R. P. (1985). The acquisition of American Sign Language. In D. I. Slobin (Ed.), *The cross-linguistic study of language acquisition: Vol. 1. The data* (pp. 881–938). Hillsdale, NJ: Erlbaum.

Oller, D. K. (1986). Metaphonology and infant vocalizations. In B. Lindbloom & R. Zetterstrom (Eds.), *Precursors of early speech* (pp. 21–35). New York: Stockton Press.

Oller, D. K., & Lynch, M. P. (1992). Infant vocalizations and innovations in infraphonology: Toward a broader theory of development and disorders. In C. A. Ferguson, L. Menn, & C. Stoel-Gammon (Eds.), *Phonological development: Models, research, implications* (pp. 509–536). Timonium, MD: York Press.

Osberger, M. J., Moeller, M. P., Eccarius, M., Robbins, A. M., & Johnson, D. (1986). Expressive language skills. In M. J. Osberger (Ed.), Language and learning skills of hearing-impaired students. *ASHA Monographs* (Vol. 23, pp. 54–65). Washington, DC: American Speech, Language, Hearing Association.

Peters, A. M. (1986). Early syntax. In P. Fletcher & M. Garman (Eds.), *Language acquisition* (pp. 307–325). Cambridge, UK: Cambridge University Press.

Petitto, L. A. (2000). The acquisition of natural signed languages: Lessons in the nature of human language and its biological foundations. In C. Chamberlain & J. P. Morford (Eds.), *Language acquisition by eye* (pp. 41–50). Mahwah, NJ: Erlbaum.

Petitto, L. A., & Marentette, P. F. (1991). Babbling in the manual mode: Evidence of the ontogeny of language. *Science, 251,* 1493–1496.

Pollock, D., Goldberg, D. M., & Caleffe-Schenck, N. (1985). *Educational audiology for the limited hearing infant and preschooler: An auditory-verbal program.* Springfield, IL: Charles C. Thomas.

Prinz, P. M., & Prinz, E. A. (1979). Simultaneous acquisition of ASL and spoken English (in a hearing child of a deaf mother and hearing father). Phase I: Early lexical development. *Sign Language Studies, 25,* 283–296.

Razack, Z. (1994). *The development of listening function.* Ontario, Canada: The Waterloo County Board of Education.

Rowan, L. (2004). Natural environments and routines. In S. Watkins, D. Johnson Taylor, & P. Pittman (Eds.), *SKI-HI curriculum: Family-centered programming for infants and young children with hearing loss* (pp. 835–870). North Logan, UT: Hope, Inc.

Schick, B. (2003). The development of American Sign Language and manually coded English systems. In M. Marschark & P. E. Spencer (Eds.), *Oxford handbook of deaf studies, language,* *and education* (pp. 219–231). New York: Oxford University Press.

Schlesinger, H. S., & Meadow, K. P. (1972). *Sound and sign: Childhood deafness and mental health.* Berkeley: University of California Press.

Simmons-Martin, A. (1981). Acquisition of language by under-fives including the parental role. In A. M. Mulholland (Ed.), *Oral education today and tomorrow* (pp. 253–273). Washington, DC: Alexander Graham Bell Association for the Deaf.

Stark, R. E. (1986). Prespeech segmental feature development. In P. Fletcher & M. Garman (Eds.), *Language acquisition* (pp. 15–32). Cambridge, UK: Cambridge University Press.

Stout, G. G., & Windle, J. V. E. (1992). *The developmental approach to successful listening.* Englewood, CO: Resource Point.

Stredler-Brown, A. (1998). Early intervention for infants and toddlers who are deaf and hard of hearing: New perspectives. *Journal of Educational Audiology, 6,* 46–49.

Stredler-Brown, A. (2004). Documenting functional benefit from FM technology. In D. Fabry & C. DeConde Johnson (Eds.), *ACCESS: Achieving clear communication employing sound solutions 2003* (pp. 203–206). UK: Immediate Proceedings Limited.

Stredler-Brown, A. (2009). Intervention, education, and therapy for children who are deaf or hard of hearing. In J. Katz, L. Medwetsky, R. Burkard, & L. Hood (Eds.), *Handbook of clinical audiology* (pp. 934–954). Baltimore: Lippincott, Williams & Wilkins.

Stredler-Brown, A., & DeConde Johnson, C. (2004). *Functional auditory performance indicators: An integrated approach to auditory development.* Boulder: Department of Speech, Language and Hearing Science, University of Colorado at Boulder.

Stredler-Brown, A., Hulstrom, W. J., & Ringwalt, S. S. (2008). Early intervention. *Seminars in Hearing, 29*(2), 178–195.

Stredler-Brown, A., Moeller, M. P., Gallegos, R., Corwin, J., & Pittman, P. (2006). *Language partners: Building a strong foundation* [DVD]. Omaha, NE: Boys Town Press.

Stredler-Brown, A., & Yoshinaga-Itano, C. (1994). The FAMILY assessment: A multidisciplinary evaluation procedure. In J. Roush & N. Matkin

(Eds), *Infants and toddlers with hearing loss* (pp. 133-161). Baltimore: York Press.

Tye-Murray, N. (1992). *Cochlear implants and children: A handbook for parents, teachers and speech and hearing professionals.* Washington, DC: Alexander Graham Bell Association for the Deaf.

Wake, M., & Poulakis, Z. (2004). Slight and mild hearing loss in primary school children. *Journal of Pediatric & Child Health, 40*(1-2), 11-13.

Watkins, S. (1993). *The SKI*HI resource manual.* North Logan, UT: Hope, Inc.

Werker, J. (2006, May). *Infant speech perception and early language acquisition.* Paper presented at the Fourth Widex Congress of Pediatric Audiology, Ottawa, Canada.

Winegert, P., & Brant, M. (2005, August). Reading your baby's mind. *Newsweek, 15*, 33-39.

Yoshinaga-Itano, C. (2000). Development of audition and speech: Implications for early intervention with deaf and hard-of-hearing infants. *The Volta Review, 10*(92), 213-236.

Yoshinaga-Itano, C. (2003). Early intervention after universal neonatal hearing screening: Impact on outcomes. *Mental Retardation and Developmental Disabilities Research Reviews, 9*, 252-266.

Yoshinaga-Itano, C. (2006). Early identification, communication modality, and the development of speech and spoken language skills: Patterns and considerations. In M. Marschark & P. E. Spencer (Eds.), *Advances in the spoken language of deaf and hard-of-hearing children* (pp. 298-327). New York: Oxford University Press.

Yoshinaga-Itano, C., & Apuzzo, M. (1998). Identification of hearing loss after age 18 months is not early enough. *American Annals of the Deaf, 143*, 380-387.

Yoshinaga-Itano, C., & Apuzzo, M. (1998). The development of deaf and hard of hearing children identified early through the high risk register. *American Annals of the Deaf, 143*, 416-424.

Yoshinaga-Itano, C., Sedey, A. L., Coulter, D. K., & Mehl, A. L. (1998). The language of early- and later-identified children with hearing loss. *Pediatrics, 102*(5), 1161-1171.

End of Chapter Examination Questions

Chapter 7

1. **There are many different communication approaches that can be used with a child with hearing loss. Identify the characteristics of a communication approach that make it successful:**
   a. The approach should complement the degree of hearing loss.
   b. The approach should start early and full access should be provided.
   c. The approach should be available in the child's local school district.
   d. All of the above

2. **The "one-for-one rule" (DeConde Johnson, 2006) is a standard for language learning. Characteristics that describe the one-for-one rule include all of the following *except*:**
   a. The one-for-one rule raises the expectations of interventionists and parents.
   b. The one-for-one rule is not appropriate for a young child with hearing loss as developmental progress should not be based on the same standard as children with normal hearing.
   c. The one-for-one rule expects each child to maintain language quotients that are commensurate with their hearing peers.
   d. The one-for-one rule expects an infant or toddler who is deaf or hard of hearing, given no additional learning or language issues, to make 6 months' growth in 6 months' time.

3. **More families are now choosing an auditory communication approach for their child with hearing loss because:**
   a. there have been many improvements in hearing technology, which provides improved access to sound.
   b. auditory approaches are more accessible than visual approaches.
   c. hearing parents, who comprise more than 90% of the parents of children with hearing loss, tend to want their children to use spoken language.
   d. a and c
   e. all of the above

4. **Ching (2007) published norms for the acquisition of auditory skills by hearing children. The hearing children in her sample acquired near-perfect auditory skills by:**
   a. 30 months of age.
   b. 36 months of age.
   c. 40 months of age.
   d. 60 months of age.

5. **The didactic model of auditory training includes all of these techniques** *except*:
    a. teaches isolated listening behaviors
    b. practices generalization of listening behaviors to other situations
    c. creates a structure for developing skills using specific auditory techniques
    d. is directed by the therapist

6. **Auditory learning is distinguished from auditory training because it:**
    a. generalizes specific skills to familiar routines and language experiences.
    b. measures the skills that are learned.
    c. promotes good speech.
    d. documents the acquisition of skills on the auditory hierarchy.

7. **In order to measure the progress a child is making in the acquisition of auditory skills, the therapist can:**
    a. use a protocol that provides quantitative scores.
    b. conduct a team meeting to discuss progress.
    c. corroborate the acquisition of auditory skills by comparing auditory performance to the audiogram.
    d. all of the above

8. **To facilitate auditory access to the message, one can:**
    a. alter the content of the message.
    b. alter the phonologic characteristics of what is said.
    c. adjust the syntactic complexity of the stimulus.
    d. all of the above

End of Chapter Examination Answer Sheet

Name _____ Date _____

Chapter 7

1. Which one(s)?   a   b   c   d

2. Which one(s)?   a   b   c   d

3. Which one(s)?   a   b   c   d   e

4. Which one(s)?   a   b   c   d

5. Which one(s)?   a   b   c   d

6. Which one(s)?   a   b   c   d

7. Which one(s)?   a   b   c   d

8. Which one(s)?   a   b   c   d

8

Speech Development for Children Who Are Hearing Impaired

DANIEL LING

Chapter Outline

Introduction

For several centuries, children with various degrees of hearing impairment, including many who were totally deaf, have been taught to communicate through the use of spoken language. Nowadays, speech development is included on the curricula of most special schools and classes for hearing-impaired children. The extent to which such teaching succeeds depends not only on the characteristics of the children enrolled, but also on the importance assigned to speech in any given educational program and on the relative competence of the professionals undertaking the work (Markides, 1983).

Until the years immediately preceding World War II, speech development among children with hearing impairment was promoted mainly by teachers of the deaf in the course of their classroom work. Among the most famous of such teachers was Alexander Graham Bell (1916), who contributed many specific speech teaching techniques to the field. In more recent years, speech-language pathologists and, to a lesser extent, audiologists have become increasingly involved in developing spoken language skills, often working in clinical settings with very young children and their parents.

Speech as a Sensory-Motor Process

Speech acquisition is a perceptual as well as an oral process. Perception pervades speech communication. For people to understand the speech addressed to them, they must, through the ears, the eyes, and/or the skin, be able to detect, discriminate, and identify sufficient information in the spoken message to permit them to comprehend it. For acquiring accuracy of expression, a talker also requires some form of sensory feedback involving conscious or unconscious awareness of the sensations generated in the act of talking. The sensory modalities that are most appropriate for the development of speech vary from one child to another, mainly according to the degree of hearing impairment and the type of educational or habilitation program that has been or is being followed (Boothroyd, 1982; Ling, 1988; Reed, 1984).

The work of teachers of speech for those with hearing impairment up to about 50 years ago was based almost exclusively on speechreading, the use of tactile cues, and awareness of internal feedback cued by kinesthesia (Silverman, 1983). Now, as a result of research and the technology developed during the past few decades, much more is known about spoken language and its acquisition. Hearing impairment can be identified at birth or even before birth and speech communication skills can be enhanced by working with parents and their hearing-impaired children during the earliest stages of infancy. Modern speech development procedures are supported by ever-more sophisticated devices and strategies to measure hearing and to provide amplification. One can now, through the use of cochlear implants, stimulate the neural receptors in the inner ear of children who would formerly have had to function as totally deaf individuals, thus permitting many of them to perceive a great deal of spoken language and other acoustic stimuli in their environments. During recent years it has also become possible to transmit speech to the skin through wearable vibrotactile and electrotactile devices (Blamey & Clark, 1985; McGarr, 1989; Proctor, 1984;). As a result, we are now in a much better position than at any other time in history to promote the development of speech communication skills among hearing-impaired children (Lauter, 1985).

The Rationale for Promoting Spoken Language

Speech skills are strongly associated with superior educational achievements (Jensema & Trybus, 1978); and educational achievements, in turn, are strongly influenced by how effectively children can read and use English (Hanson, Liberman, & Schankweiler, 1984). In reviewing the evidence relating to speech and memory, Quigley and Paul (1984) concluded that "speech recoding is important to reading development" and that "faithful representation of English structure seems to be particularly sensitive to speech recoding" (p. 50) At a more general level, it is clear that individuals with hearing impairment who can communicate through the use of spoken language, whether or not they also use signs, have many advantages. They can interact more freely with other members of society, most of whom talk. They can, therefore, function more independently in most of the everyday situations that they are likely to meet in employment, leisure, and family life (Subtelny, 1980).

Legislation and social awareness have improved the lot of most hearing-impaired people in Western societies, but, even so, the advantages lie with those who can talk. With spoken language, opportunities for higher education are less restricted, a more extensive range of careers is open, and there is greater security of employment. Those who can talk also face fewer limitations in the personal and social aspects of their lives (Silverman, 1983). To talk poorly rather than well can, however, be disadvantageous to individuals with hearing impairment in their employment. Doggett (1989), for example, found that there was a high correlation between employers' ratings of the comprehensibility of speech and their ratings of a person's independence, likeability, and competence. Her hearing-impaired subjects received poorer ratings than those who were native or foreign speakers, and the poorest ratings were given to the poorest speakers.

The Speech Achievements of Children with Hearing Impairment

The speech of children with moderate (50–70 dB HL) or severe (70–90 db HL) hearing impairment usually reflects the quality of their auditory management. Such children, when appropriately aided and stimulated, are able to acquire much of their spoken language spontaneously through the use of their residual hearing (Ling, 1988). The speech of profoundly (> 90 dB HL) hearing-impaired children tends to reflect not only the type of information provided by the device(s) a child is using (hearing aid, cochlear implant, and/or tactile aid), but also the amount and quality of systematic teaching received (Figure 8-1). The more profoundly hearing impaired the child, the more difficult it is to acquire speech spontaneously. In general, the more profound the degree of hearing impairment, the greater the amount of formal speech teaching a child will require to acquire spoken language (Markides, 1983).

Various levels of speech and spoken language achievement by children with impaired hearing have been reported in the literature. On the one hand, the many advantages of early perceptual-oral treatment have led some profoundly hearing-impaired children to acquire normal or near-normal speech (Ling & Ling, 1978; Ling & Milne, 1981). On the other hand, several large-scale demographic studies have shown that, overall, there has been scant improvement in the average standards of speech production

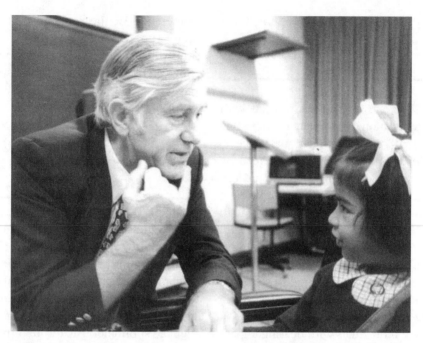

Figure 8–1. The quality of speech of a child with impaired hearing reflects not only the device worn, but also the systematic level of teaching.

by hearing-impaired school children during recent years despite technical and educational advances in speech science and allied fields (Wolk & Schildroth, 1986). There is clearly a great deal of unrealized potential for better speech and language among children who are hearing impaired.

Speech in the Context of Spoken Language

The traditional method of teaching speech to children with hearing impairment has been to develop the production of sound patterns largely in isolation and then to combine them to form syllables, words, and sentences. But, during the last few decades, authors such as Calvert and Silverman (1975, 1983); Ewing and Ewing (1964), and Vorce (1974), among others, have recognized that some speech skills can, under conditions that favor speech reception and language learning, usually be acquired spontaneously by many such children. Accordingly, authors such as Clark (1989), Cole (1990), and the writer (Ling, 1988) have advocated a greater focus on promoting the acquisition of speech in the context of spoken language as it is used in natural communication. Their views are strongly supported by numerous other writers in the Volta Bureau's 1992 monograph on speech production in hearing-impaired children and youth edited by Stoker and Ling (1992).

Individual differences among children with hearing impairment are often greater than those among children who hear normally because degree and age at onset of hearing impairment are additional and important variables affecting development. Consequently, no one type of speech development program can possibly suit the needs of all such children. Some, with appropriate parental participation and professional support, can learn to hear (and even overhear) people talking to them and around them and, by this means, acquire most of their speech and spoken language skills much as normally hearing children do Others require highly organized training to develop effective speech communication (see Ling, 1976, 1988; Stone, 1988). Most require at least some remedial help to gain mastery over the production of certain sound patterns, for abnormalities commonly develop in the speech of children whose hearing impairment is severe (about 70–90 dB HL) or profound (>90 dB). Remedial help is usually focused on particular speech patterns and on strategies for their carryover into everyday communication practices.

Carryover from lessons to life is least difficult to orchestrate when speech lessons and speech-language therapy closely relate to real-life conditions. It is most difficult to manage effectively when lessons or therapy are organized around the use of devices and procedures that are not part and parcel of everyday communication (Ling, 1988, pp. 250–255). If inappropriate devices are used extensively and exclusively in formal teaching or therapy, generalization problems facing children who are hearing impaired can, therefore, become even more serious than those facing normally hearing children who have language deficits. A far-reaching analysis of issues affecting generalization from lessons to life has been undertaken by various writers in a clinical forum section of *Language, Speech and Hearing Services in Schools* (Fey, 1988).

Factors Affecting Speech Development

Both intrinsic and extrinsic factors influence the acquisition of speech skills among children who have hearing impairment. Factors that are intrinsic to each child cannot, in general, be changed or greatly improved through direct intervention. These include unaided sensorineural hearing levels, age at onset of hearing impairment, visual acuity, integrity of or damage to the central nervous system, integrity of or damage to the peripheral speech mechanisms, and so on.

Extrinsic factors may be defined as devices, procedures, people, and life experiences that, either by design or chance, affect the development of children's communication skills. They include hearing aids, cochlear implants, tactile aids, glasses, socioeducational practices and experiences, environmental communication modes, parents' management skills, teacher/clinician competence, availability of support personnel, and the extent and type of children's contacts with peers (Ling, 1988). Orchestration of such extrinsic factors so that they operate most effectively to enhance the development of spoken language skills should be regarded as an extremely important part of any speech development program. To be optimally effective, developmental and remedial speech training programs for children who have hearing impairment cannot be confined within the walls of a clinic or classroom or to professionals' involvement within their normal working hours.

Crucial Bases for Optimal Speech Development

Early Detection of Hearing Impairment

During the past few decades, the use of computers has become widespread in the fields of speech, language, and hearing (Curtis, 1987). They have allowed development of the various forms of electrophysiological hearing tests that are now in widespread clinical use, not only as diagnostic tools, but also for screening the hearing of children at birth (Jerger, 1984). Further relatively recent and highly significant contributions to tests of hearing in early infancy have been the development of the immittance battery (Popelka, 1981) and visual response audiometry (Wilson & Thompson, 1984). Such tests, together with the use of probe-tube microphone systems in hearing aid selection, permit the effective use of hearing aids or other sensory aids with more and more children from a few months of age (Jerger, 1984; Stelmachowicz & Seewald, 1990).

When spoken language development begins in the first year of life rather than later, children cannot only be provided with more natural exposure to their mothers' spoken commentaries on objects and events that interest them, but can monitor and preserve the quality of much of the reflexive vocalization and repetitive babble they produce during that first year (Oller, Eilers, Bull, & Carney (1985). Such auditory or alternative sensory access to their own early utterances promotes the children's production of an extended range of vocalization (Mischook & Cole, 1986). It also provides them with the essential foundations for feedback on the quality of their voices and the accuracy of the spoken language that they will later acquire (Ling & Ling, 1978). The ultimate development of children's spoken language has long been known to be most effectively triggered by appropriate stimulation during the first few years of life (Friedlander, 1970; Fry, 1966; Lenneberg, 1967; Studdert-Kennedy, 1984). Music and song, well within the perceptual capacity of most children who have hearing impairment, are a recommended part of such stimulation (Estabrooks & Birkenshaw-Fleming, 1994).

The acoustic environment of most homes approaches the ideal for speech acquisition by children under a year of age. With carpets on the floors, relatively little noise is created by movement. With drapes at the windows and soft furnishings around the house, reflection and reverberation of sounds are at minimal levels in most rooms. Most important, however, is that mothers are usually quite close to their infants when they are talking to them. Conditions that predominate in most homes thus make for clear speech signals at babies' ears—signals that are not degraded by background noise. Speaking while a child is within earshot is clearly an essential for auditory learning (Ling, 1981).

After their first year, children's acoustic environments are less stable. As they become able to move over considerable distances without help from or contact with their mothers, they tend to have less speech addressed to them at close quarters. Nevertheless, young children are more frequently at home in good acoustic conditions than out and in noise. The emphasis in early speech habilitation over the past few decades has, therefore, shifted to the guidance of parents rather than direct intervention with infants. Descriptions of exemplary programs having such emphasis have been provided by the several contributors to a book edited by the writer (Ling, 1984a). Many ways in which parents can be involved in the aural habilitative process are discussed by Atkins in this volume (see Chapter 5).

Provision of Appropriate Sensory Aids: Devices and Speech

The three senses through which we can gather information about speech are audition, vision, and touch. When aided hearing does not provide adequate sensory information about speech, vision and touch can be used as supplementary or alternative sensory channels. Cochlear implants and tactile aids, both of which became generally available as recently as the 1980s, are now quite frequently prescribed as alternatives to hearing aids for children who have little or no residual hearing over all or part of the frequency range of speech. Either type of instrument can be of single- or multichannel design, and both vibro- and electrotactile devices are available. No currently available cochlear implant or tactile device can compensate fully for severe, profound, or total deafness so, like hearing aids, they are most effective when used to supplement speechreading (DeFilippo, 1984; Pickett & McFarland, 1985).

Some children use both a hearing aid and a cochlear implant, and many children who hear nothing beyond 1000 Hz find that a multichannel tactile device or frequency transposition will supplement aided audition in speech perception. These devices and what they can contribute to children's speech and spoken language acquisition have been presented in detail in a book by the writer (Ling, 1988), and are also discussed by others in this volume. The selection of appropriate sensory aids (hearing aids, cochlear implants, and tactile devices) will depend on the needs of individual children. To use any one of them to the utmost effect in developing speech skills, the teacher/clinician must be thoroughly familiar with the acoustic properties of speech, know exactly what speech patterns a given sensory aid can be expected to provide for each particular child, ensure that the sensory aids for each child have been appropriately selected and adjusted, and see that the devices are consistently used under good acoustic conditions.

Vision and Speech

Speechreading is the art of understanding the visual cues that occur as talkers move their tongues, lips, and jaws and produce related facial expressions and body postures in the act of speaking (Ijsseldijk, 1988). Unfortunately, only comparatively degraded information on speech production is available through speechreading. This is because there are no visible correlates of some speech patterns. For example, vocalization (the use of voice), prosody, and nasality cannot be perceived through speechreading alone, because adjustments and positions of the larynx, tongue, and velum are partially or completely obscured by the lips and the teeth. Thus, there are severe limitations to learning speech through visual imitation. Also, several other sounds share visual patterns and, on this account, are frequently confused (see DeFilippo & Sims, 1988; Dodd & Campbell, 1987).

Although speechreading by itself provides a very impoverished signal, it is nevertheless a natural and often effective supplement to hearing in the development of spoken language. This is because the cues that speechreading provides, such as those relating to place of consonant production, can usefully augment a message that is heard only in part (see Erber, 1972). Many of the sensory aids such as tactile devices and cochlear implants produced in recent years serve or have been designed to supplement speechreading. If vision is to be used in helping children who have hearing impairment to talk, the teacher or clinician must know exactly what components, if any, of a given speech pattern can be clearly seen and how such components complement the information provided by the sensory aid or aids used by each individual.

Numerous visual aids, some involving sophisticated technology, have been produced to enhance children's speech production in the course of clinical training. However, there are at least three major problems inherent in their use. First, visual displays that represent the complete speech signal are hard to perceive, whereas simpler displays poorly represent the dynamic nature of communicative speech. Second, because they provide information that is quite unlike that required for communication in everyday life, it becomes essential for the teacher or clinician to design and supervise an extensive range of generalization procedures to ensure that speech skills acquired through the use of such devices are carried over into children's meaningful use of spoken language. Third, teaching through reference to a visual representation of only part of the normally complex speech signal has to be done under the close supervision of a professional, if one skill is not to be learned to the detriment of another. Although one can easily show that children can learn particular skills through the use of visual speech training aids (and it is on this account that they are recommended), there have been no convincing studies demonstrating that the use of such devices leads to improved speech communication abilities in the everyday lives of children. It is difficult to promote the carryover of speech skills into everyday life when they are learned through strategies that are not primarily based on interpersonal communication (Perigoe & Ling, 1986).

Early Intervention

To be optimally effective in developing perceptual-oral communication, professionals and parents must adopt developmental strategies for speech perception and speech production that differ according to each child's unique sensory capacities and needs. Special attention to such needs should, ideally, be initiated from the first few months of life. Such early intervention, in which parents become the primary agents in the process of fostering their children's development, is discussed in Chapter 5, Chapter 7, and Chapter 10 in this volume.

Topics such as audition, speechreading, hearing aids, speech development, language development, technology, education, parent guidance, and early intervention inevitably tend to be discussed in separate chapters. Unfortunately, this gives many readers the false impression that activities related to such topics may also be treated as distinct when helping children develop speaking skills. Nothing could be further from the truth. Programs that do not integrate all aspects of habilitation can impede rather than encourage progress in the acquisition of perceptual-oral communication.

Children can acquire optimal speech communication skills only when they use personal hearing aids and/or other selected sensory aids during all waking hours. A further requirement is that the speech addressed to children relates closely to their cognitive levels, motor development, self-help skills, and personal and social experiences. Such experiences normally abound in the meaningful situations that pervade the activities of everyday living (Grant, 1987; Ling & Ling, 1978). Early speech development should not be based initially on the formal teaching of particular speech patterns, but on children's desire to communicate through speech and on their approximations to adult sentence patterns in the various areas of discourse—conversation, narration, questions, explanation, and description (Ling, 1988).

The first step in the process of learning speech informally will usually result in vocalizations in which desirable intonation contours rather than consonants or vowels are imitated. Appropriate perception and production of segmental features are likely to follow naturally under such circumstances if, according to their individual needs, children are using acoustic hearing aids, more than one sort of sensory information, or another sort of sensory aid. Even with children who start their program somewhat later—for example at age 3 or 4—developing speech through the meaningful use of spoken language in interactive situations is likely to result in later speech skills that are superior to those developed through more formal teaching (Ling, 1988).

Systematic Programming

Many different levels of skill have to be acquired before intelligible words can appear (Murry & Murry, 1980). Just as a variety of vocalizations and canonical (repetitive) babbling patterns precedes speech in normally hearing babies, so do such prespeech patterns help to lay the foundations for the speech of children who have hearing impairment. Just as control of a wide range of vowels and diphthongs precedes mastery of most consonants and blends in the speech of normally hearing children, so do they create a similar groundwork for consonant production in those with hearing impairment. The order of speech pattern development presented in the model described and discussed by Ling (1988) appears to be optimal for both informal and (the later) formal development and remediation of speech among children with hearing impairment. The model suggests that speech development should be promoted in seven somewhat overlapping sequential stages, progressing from control of vocalization, to production of prosodic patterns, vowels and diphthongs, consonants differing in manner, consonants differing in place, consonants differing in voicing, to consonant blends (clusters). Such organization can save substantial amounts of time and increase efficiency, because systematic programming ensures that behaviors that are prerequisites for the production of any given pattern are already present and that new skills can be developed that relate to skills that have been previously acquired. For example, children who, on account of their hearing impairment, have failed to develop a /g/ spontaneously can, as explained by Ling (1988), more easily learn to produce the sound through reference to the production of /b/ and /d/ than through description, direct imitation, or any other strategy (see following discussion).

Evaluation

Children's potential for learning to talk should, particularly during the early stages of habilitation, be assessed mainly through ongoing evaluation in the course of treatment in a program that features wholehearted commitment to the development of spoken language. Many factors contribute to young children's speech acquisition and, apart from a relatively few essentials such as hearing levels and basic oral-peripheral function, the aspects cannot be assessed simply through formal clinical evaluation. For example, it is only following parental counseling, education, and support services that one can determine the extent to which they are able to help their children. Also, it is only when children have sufficient experience of speech reception through an appropriate sensory aid that their capacities for speech recognition can be assessed. In short, diagnostic training under optimal conditions is a prerequisite for a valid prognosis and the planning of therapy or teaching (Cole & Gregory, 1986).

Evaluation of both speech reception and speech production is an essential aspect of any program directed toward children's speech development. Tests of either aspect can be norm-referenced (designed and standardized to permit comparisons) or criterion-referenced (designed to determine what skills a particular child has acquired). The latter tests provide the most appropriate guides for therapy or teaching. To evaluate speech reception abilities, one must have tests that determine if children can detect, discriminate, and identify the elements of speech (prosodic features, vowels and consonants) as well as tests that determine how well running speech is perceived. Audiological tests of these types have been discussed by Beasley (1984) and by Bess (1988). Such tests, as currently performed, however, can provide but part of the necessary information, as speech reception measures must also encompass appraisal of children's performance not only with hearing aids, but with cochlear implants, tactile aids, speechreading, or a combination of these (see Geers & Moog, 1989).

Various tests of speech production are available, and procedures that measure speech intelligibility through listener judgments and rating scales are commonly used in research studies (Subtelny, 1980; Wolk & Schildroth (1986). For therapy and teaching purposes, however, one needs to use tests that permit the assessment of each child's ability to produce both the elements of speech (vocalization, suprasegmental features, vowels, and consonants) and to use speech meaningfully in everyday discourse. Only if one can identify the precise deficits in place, can one select the most appropriate remedial measures to overcome them. The Ling (1976) Phonetic Level and Phonologic Level Evaluations are criterion-referenced tests designed to provide the necessary diagnostic information for effective speech development, and the program of which they are part is also in widespread use (Cole & Mischook, 1985). An adaptation of this test, the Phonetic-Phonologic Speech Evaluation Record, was designed by Ling (1991) to permit comparison of pre- and post-training results with different types of sensory aids and teaching strategies.

Teaching and Learning: Some Strategies

Informal and Formal Procedures

Informal speech development procedures can be defined as those that involve activities with children (particularly young ones) that are largely unplanned by adults, that are primarily determined by the children's interests and needs, and that lead to the spontaneous acquisition of spoken language. Informal procedures usually involve parents, caregivers, and/or peers to a greater extent than professionals. Formal procedures are those in which learning and teaching activities are deliberately planned and carried out in accordance with a predetermined program of speech development, usually by teachers or clinicians (Ling, 1988).

The basic techniques, tactics, and tools involved in the teaching and learning of speech communication by children who have hearing impairment are summarized in Table 8–1. The content of this table is illustrative rather than exhaustive. It simply lists the major elements of effective speech development programs that are discussed in this chapter and details the somewhat sequential nature of the techniques and strategies that can be applied. Note that the tools of greatest importance are sensory aids —primarily hearing aids, but also cochlear implants or tactile devices for some children.

Whether speech acquisition programs are formal or informal, perception must either precede or accompany production. Speech addressed to, used in the presence of, or produced by children with hearing impairment must be processed through devices that permit the child (as Hirsh, 1940, put it) to detect, discriminate, identify, and comprehend as much as possible of an utterance. Among the most important cues for

TABLE 8–1. Techniques, Tactics, and Tools Involved in Teaching and Learning Spoken Language

Techniques	Tactics	Tools
Informal learning (enhancement of early childhood experiences and events)	**Focus on:** Early intervention Early detection Parental involvement Speech reception Speech production Communication Personal-social growth	Appropriate diagnostic technology, sensory aids, everyday objects.
Informal teaching (enhancement of care giving practices)	**Focus on:** Context based spoken language Perception of message Refinement of dialogue Perception of meaning Clarity of expression Spontaneous discourse Integration of personal-social skills	Tools as above
Formal Teaching (initiated only following optimal exposure to informal techniques)	**Focus on:** Evaluation of sensory aids Systematic programming Development of specific skills Remediation of specific faults Use of anticipatory set Training to automaticity Programming generalization Promoting carryover Developing discourse skills Extending communicative competence	Appropriate and selected materials
Formal learning (school-age through adult life)	**Focus on:** Conscious and deliberate acquisition of knowledge and skills by an individual	Tools as above

the acquisition and maintenance of speech by children who have hearing impairment are the tactile and kinesthetic sensations that are produced as they, themselves, talk. Just as every speech pattern in the language sounds different to a normal listener, so does every such pattern feel different to a normal talker. It is the tactile and kinesthetic codes that are established in the course of speech acquisition that permit older children who lose all of their hearing to maintain most, if not all, of their speech skills. Being sure that children who are (or become) hearing impaired encode accurate tactile and kinesthetic patterns to guide their speech production must be treated as an essential part of informal or formal learning and teaching (Ling, 1976).

Informal Learning

Informal learning takes place as children receive stimuli from their environments and try to derive meaning from them. Speech is normally addressed to (or used within earshot of) children in the context of activities that permit them to derive meaning from what has been said. The effective use of appropriate sensory aids, supplemented or not by speechreading, provides optimal opportunities for children who have hearing impairment to learn a great deal about speech reception and speech production in much the same way as their normally hearing peers (Wood, Wood, Griffiths, & Howarth, 1986).

Informal Teaching

Informal teaching is usually provided by parents in the course of everyday activities around the home, where repetitive situations such as daily dressing, food preparation, feeding, and housework, as well as caregiving, supervision, and play activities, contribute abundant opportunities for both children and parents to initiate spoken language and for the children to acquire speech perception and speech production skills. With appropriately selected sensory aids, children who have hearing impairment can be

encouraged to interact effectively and verbally with parents, caregivers, siblings, and peers. Informal teaching of children by others in the home can be enhanced through parent guidance work and, even with children whose hearing impairment is profound, can at least result in approximations to adult forms of speech that provide the ideal base for more formal teaching.

Informal teaching is not only a part of parent guidance programs. It can also be provided in the course of therapy or education in which the principal purpose of the play or other activity is to promote the acquisition of spoken language through interaction and the encouragement of increasingly complex vocalizations and spontaneous approximations to mature forms of speech. Informal teaching procedures strongly feature the positive reinforcement of involuntary sound patterns, such as those in crying ("boo-hoo"), laughing ("ha-ha"), giggling ("hee-hee"), and babbling. This is done with a view to enhancing awareness and feedback of such sounds through the sensory aid(s) that have been selected. Groundwork can thus be provided for the voluntary production of such sound patterns and their inclusion in speech.

Formal Teaching

Formal teaching involves an adult's planned instruction to a child. The purpose of such instruction is to develop knowledge or skills that the child has not previously acquired (Figure 8–2). Most schoolwork and a great deal of therapy is of this type. Formal teaching of speech may be considered as a remedial procedure that has two major objectives: first, helping children to produce particular sounds or sequences of sounds that, even after extensive and appropriate stimulation, have not been acquired through informal procedures, and second, the correction of

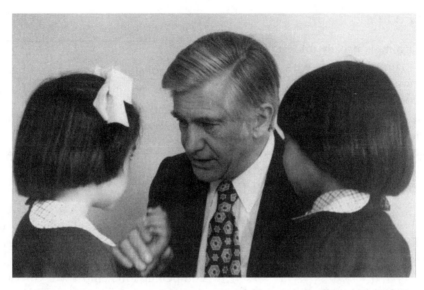

Figure 8–2. Formal teaching is used to develop knowledge or skills the child has not previously acquired.

errors. Formal teaching is not appropriate as the first step in promoting children's acquisition of speech skills. Further, if formal teaching of speech is begun before a child is using sentence approximations consisting of at least two or three words to communicate, the development of natural sounding speech may be inhibited. Every opportunity should, therefore, be afforded for children to acquire a wide range of speech patterns spontaneously through the use of suitable sensory aids before formal work is attempted.

The extent to which children acquire speech skills spontaneously depends largely on the degree to which the sensory aids selected for them compensate (with or without speechreading) for their hearing impairment. It follows that when particular patterns have not emerged (or have emerged in a distorted form) following extensive informal teaching, devices and procedures other than those previously used will be required to elicit the patterns.

Because there are only three sensory modalities through which speech can be perceived—hearing, vision, and touch—and because the use of hearing and vision (and possibly tactile devices) will already have been promoted in the course of informal teaching, the direct use of touch will clearly have to be the basis of much formal speech teaching. Indeed, many tactile strategies are available for guiding speech production. They include having the children feel vibration of the chest when vocalizing, the movement of the larynx as intonation changes, and the duration, intensity, and temperature of the breath stream as different vowels, fricatives, and plosives are produced. A finger tap on the hand or a finger drawn slowly or quickly along the arm can be used to signal durational cues that a given child can neither hear nor see, such as the difference between /m/ and /b/. Care should, of course, be exercised to ensure that the children receive such cues without feeling that the clinician or teacher is invading their personal space.

Formal Learning

Formal learning is usually undertaken only by quite mature children with a peer or adult to monitor production, because feedback on correctness is an important aspect of formal learning in speech acquisition. If sufficiently accurate feedback is not directly available to a child, then it must be provided through an external source. Analytical feedback provided by a skilled listener is preferable to that derived through instrumental analysis, because whether or not speech patterns are perceived as acceptable or "correct" depends largely on how they interact with other sounds (i.e., coarticulation) in the context in which they are produced.

The Process of Learning and Teaching Speech

The most natural and effective process in learning and teaching speech is to ensure that children acquire new patterns as an extension of those that are already mastered. Indeed, all children proceed from one stage of development to the next using previously established skills that, in many instances, are actually prerequisites for new behaviors. For example, control over vocalization has to precede controlled production of prosodic patterns and vowels. The production of vowels, in turn, has to precede the mastery of consonants, because consonants in the dynamic stream of speech are, by and large, merely different ways of initiating, interrupting, or releasing vowels. Encouraging the development of speech through formal teaching based on the recognition of natural ordering has long been advocated (see McDonald, 1964).

The Anticipatory Set

The use of anticipatory set is a strategy based on both natural ordering and the propensity of human beings to anticipate required future responses on the basis of immediately preceding stimuli. To provide an example of such anticipation, ask literate people to pronounce the two letters *i* and *g* as a syllable and they will say "ig." Then ask them what they call an artificial head of hair and they will say "wig." Finally, ask them to name a large piece of wood broken from a tree and, because anticipatory set is such a compelling force, most will say "twig," even though a response such as "branch" would be more accurate.

Anticipatory set can be applied at all stages of speech development. To apply it to the development of consonants, for instance, first establish manner of consonant production with an early-occurring speech sound, and then through the use of anticipatory set elicit the other consonants, sharing that manner of production one by one. Thus, first have a child produce /b/ in repeated syllables such as /ba/, /bi/, and /bu/. This establishes an anticipatory set for manner of production. Then, by reference to /b/, establish /d/. Once this can be easily produced, sufficient anticipatory set is usually established, so that when asked to make a sound like /d/ with a finger placed behind the teeth, children will produce a /g/. Similarly, for unvoiced fricatives, establish the /´/ first, then have the children draw their tongues back slowly over either their top or bottom teeth and the likelihood is that /s/ will be produced. When the /s/ can be produced with ease, repeating the procedure but taking the tongue back further will usually elicit the /ʃ/. Eliciting sound patterns in this way is, of course, a formal teaching procedure and one that has to be followed up by a generalization program to ensure the necessary transfer of training from lessons to life. Detailed procedures for using anticipatory set in the development of these and numerous other speech patterns are provided by Ling (1988).

One can usually capitalize on the use of residual audition in using and generalizing from early-occurring speech patterns, because most children with impaired hearing have better hearing levels for the lower frequencies—those that carry the most salient cues relating to vocalization, prosodic elements, vowels and diphthongs, and manner of consonant production. In contrast, cues on place of consonant production are carried in the frequency range above 1500 Hz, for which most such children have less, if any, hearing. Because many children with severe and profound hearing impairment are quite unable to hear unvoiced fricatives or cues on place of production, formal teaching that employs both direct touch and the use of anticipatory set is recommended for those who have difficulty with these aspects of speech (Calvert & Silverman, 1983; Ling, 1976, 1988).

Essentially, a seven-step program is needed to ensure the effectiveness of formal teaching. These steps are:

1. Ensure the presence of prerequisite behaviors;
2. Decide on the set to be used;
3. Select a child's most appropriate sense modality;
4. Choose the strategies to be used;
5. Achieve production of the targeted speech sound;
6. Provide reinforcement of the behavior; and
7. Generalize production to other contexts, including spoken language.

Automaticity

The ability to concentrate on what one is saying rather than on how one is saying it is an essential aspect of spoken language. Speech should, therefore, be developed to be produced automatically—that is, without conscious effort. Speech patterns are acquired by children over at least five distinct stages, with (a) production at first being novel (and difficult), then (b) variable (but easier), (c) controlled, (d) practiced, and finally (e) habitual. Effective formal teaching ensures the development of speech skills through all of these five stages.

To ensure the automaticity of acceptable, coarticulated speech patterns in the variety of contexts in which they occur in spoken language, they must, if taught formally, be developed so that their production meets four basic criteria: (a) accuracy, (b) speed, (c) economy of effort, and (d) flexibility. Accuracy is the first requirement, as rehearsal of an inaccurate pattern can lead to a habitual speech problem. The rate at which a speech pattern can be repeated or alternated with others is important to a child's ability to integrate it appropriately into the stream of speech. Speech patterns produced with economy of effort do not unduly involve extraneous musculature and are not exaggerated. Thus, they provide a better base for developing further speech patterns and lead to more normal-sounding speech. Flexibility in the production of speech has been acquired only when children can produce spoken language patterns appropriately in any context (see Ling, 1976).

Generalization and Carryover

When children have learned a skill in one situation and then applied it in another, they are said to have generalized that skill. Generalization and carryover are not serious problems when speech is acquired as a result of informal learning, because most such learning occurs in the context of spoken language communication in everyday situations. The less formal the intervention, the more closely lessons and real life are related. This is not the case when speech is acquired through formal teaching.

Consider the production of a /g/ as described. When it is elicited through formal teaching in one vowel context, such as /a/, children will usually have to be helped to generalize its production to other vowel contexts, particularly those in which the /g/ has to be produced with the high-back and high-front vowels /u/ and /i/. This is because the point of contact between tongue and palate shifts according to vocal tract configuration for the vowels.

To ensure that such generalization occurs, children should repeat several syllables, first with /a/, as in /gagaga/, and then repeat the sound with each of the intervening vowels, one by one, moving gradually further and further away from the /a/, until /gugugu/ and /gigigi/ can be produced with ease. Production of such syllables may be a necessary speech skill, but unless it is deliberately carried over into real-life usage through integration into words, sentences, and discourse, it will remain far from an effective tool in communication (Calvert & Silverman, 1983; Fey, 1988; Perigoe & Ling, 1986).

Prevention and Remediation of Faults

The most all-embracing statement on deviant speech due to hearing impairment must be that of Black (1971, p. 156) who wrote, "The speech of deaf children differs from normal speech in all regards." The literature since that date indicates that Black's statement still holds true for the majority of children with hearing impairment, in spite of the technological advances that have been made during the past 20 years (Hochberg, Levitt, & Osberger, 1983). Nevertheless, in the writer's experience, the application of current knowledge about speech and language acquisition, present day technology, and up-to-date educational practices would prevent many of the speech faults that are widely reported among children with hearing impairment (Ling, 1984a; Ling & Milne, 1981). In this section, various faults that led Black to make his statement are examined and this writer's suggested treatments and expectations for higher level expectations are discussed.

Vocalization and Voice Patterns

One of the primary requirements for controlled vocalization is adequate breathing. Among speakers with hearing impairment, voice production tends to be begun at, rather than sufficiently above, lung resting level (Forner & Hixon, 1977). Audition is not required for feedback on speech breathing. Sufficient tactile and kinesthetic cues are available for control of breathing patterns in the act of speech production. This fault is not, therefore, an inevitable outcome of hearing impairment. Instead, it appears to be a product of inappropriate speech development procedures. Such faults occur when a great deal of formal teaching of isolated speech patterns or single words is undertaken. The faults are less likely to occur when sufficient approximations to mature forms of speech based on multiword utterances have been developed through informal strategies.

Voices characterized by pharyngeal tension, abnormal pitch and prosody, and hypernasality are commonly associated with hearing impairment (Hochberg et al., 1983; Monsen, 1979). Such problems are, indeed, likely when there is lack of auditory perception and auditory feedback, along with insufficient appropriate teaching or therapy. However, because the harmonics associated with voicing and the nasal murmur are in the low frequency range (250 Hz plus or minus a half-octave), they should be rendered audible in spite of even profound hearing impairment by the use of appropriately fitted hearing aids. These components of speech are also relatively simple to transmit through other forms of sensory aids. It follows that such abnormalities would be reduced or avoided for many children, if more attention were given to the selection and application of suitable devices to improve the reception of these components. Indeed, such abnormalities are less frequently found in the voices of children who have used appropriate sensory aids in the development of spoken language from an early age (Ling, 1988).

Vowel Production

The most common faults with vowel production by children who have hearing impairment are neutralization, prolongation, diphthongization, and exaggeration (Calvert & Silverman, 1983). Residual audition that extends up to at least 2500 Hz is required for the auditory detection of the first two formants of all vowels. On the other hand, the first formants of all vowels can be detected if there is residual audition to about 1000 Hz and most can be identified if speechreading is used. Many fewer vowel errors are likely, if adequate use is made of residual hearing, multichannel cochlear implants, or multichannel tactile aids (Carney & Beachler, 1986) if necessary, in conjunction with speechreading (Ling, 1989). An over-strong focus on speechreading can, however, lead to these faults rather than prevent them, because the problems are mainly from tongue movements that cannot be clearly seen. Neutralization (the predominant use of a central vowel), diphthongization (moving toward a central vowel from other vowels), and prolongation can be from inadequate feedback, inappropriate teaching, or both. Exaggeration is almost always due to inappropriate teaching of static rather than dynamic strategies.

All four problems can be overcome by focusing remedial speech work on nonvisual feedback, increased tongue and reduced jaw movements, and the rapid alternation of different vowels, as well as syllables and words containing different vowels (Ling, 1976).

Consonant Production

In addition to normal developmental errors, the major faults in consonant production among children with hearing impairment are reported to be omission, substitution, and distortion, voiced-voiceless confusions, and implosion of stops. Such problems were reported more than half a century ago by Hudgins and Numbers (1942) and have been reported to persist, but to a much smaller extent, in the phonology of orally taught children today. In the group studied by Abraham (1989), the best levels of correct consonant production were found among the children who had the best hearing levels at 2000 Hz. This finding is, of course, not surprising in view of the fact that place cues are available in, but not below, the octave band centered on 2000 Hz.

The acquisition of acceptably produced consonants can be enhanced through the effective use of hearing aids by those who have useful residual hearing for frequencies over 1500 Hz. It can also be augmented by other sensory aids that provide relevant information, such as cochlear implants (Owens & Kesler, 1988) and tactile devices (Weisenberger, 1989). When sensory aids do not provide sufficient information for the development of certain consonants, systematic formal teaching of the type described by Ling (1976, 1988) can usually lead to their acquisition.

Future Trends

Prosthetic Devices and Programs

With advances in technology, new and improved sensory aids that can lead to better perception and production of speech will become available. It follows that one may expect a greater amount of research to be devoted to assessing the potential and the limitations of various sensory aids in the development of speech. One can, on the basis of recent advances in technology, reasonably predict a trend towards greater use of various devices in promoting the acquisition of speech among children with impaired hearing. The extent of that trend will depend not only on how well future sensory aids can be designed to transmit information, but on the number of educational programs committed to the development of spoken language.

There is every reason for the variety of programming that currently exists to be preserved. Paradoxically, however, during recent years, when technology has offered greatly improved opportunities for successful acquisition of spoken language, there has been a trend toward the increased use of sign language and this is likely to continue. Indeed, it has been suggested that American Sign Language programs should now begin to replace both oral and total communication programs (Johnson, Liddell, & Erting, 1989). Such a development would certainly receive widespread support from members of the Deaf community (see Sacks, 1989). However, less than 3% of children who have hearing impairment are born to parents who are deaf (Jung, 1989), and the majority of parents will probably continue to press for programs that develop spoken language as the primary mode of communication, so that their children can learn to speak.

The trend towards the use of multi-channel as compared with single-channel sensory aids may be expected to continue because, by and large, they appear to yield superior results (Pickett & McFarland, 1985). The thrust in hearing aid design with digital processing and better hearing aid selection procedures involving children will continue. Accordingly, it is likely that productive strategies for the otologic and audiological management of young children will become more widespread and thus permit more children to acquire much of their speech more naturally, particularly through the use of cochlear implantation. Because the means are now at hand, detection and diagnosis of hearing impairment can be carried out at an earlier age. More extensive application of current practices should lead to the expansion, if not proliferation, of parent-infant treatment programs in which children's speech will be more frequently developed within the first few years of life (Cole & Gregory, 1986).

Personnel

In recent years, the focus on training teachers of the deaf in simultaneous communication has reduced the pool of educational personnel who are skilled in developing all aspects of spoken language (Ling, 1984b). At the same time, more audiologists and speech-language pathologists have become involved with spoken language development among children with hearing impairments, either as support personnel or as case managers.

There is a definite need for more personnel who are able to provide auditory-verbal programs, and this need is more likely to be met through the recruitment of audiologists and speech-language pathologists to this area of work than through the training of more educators to work with parents and their children. Teacher training programs are more strongly geared to work with school-age children. Regardless of their children's age and the types of professionals engaged in promoting their speech communication skills, parents will continue to create the strongest demand and to be the greatest resource for speech development in children with impaired hearing.

Acknowledgement. Thanks are due to Richard Seewald and Kevin Munhall, University of Western Ontario, who read and suggested revisions to the first draft of this chapter.

References

Abraham, S. (1989). Using a phonological framework to describe speech errors of orally trained, hearing-impaired school-agers. *Journal of Speech and Hearing Disorders, 54,* 600–609.

Beasley, D. S. (Ed.). (1984). *Audition in childhood.* San Diego, CA: College Hill Press.

Bell, A. G. (1916). *The mechanism of speech.* New York: Funk and Wagnalls.

Bess, F. H. (Ed.). (1988). *Hearing impairment in children.* Parkton, MD: York Press.

Black, J. W. (1971). Speech pathology for the deaf. In L. E. Connor (Ed.), *Speech for the deaf child: Knowledge and use* (pp. 154–169). Washington DC: Alexander Graham Bell Association for the Deaf.

Blamey. P. J., & Clark, G. M. (1985). A wearable multiple-electrode electrotactile speech processor for the profoundly deaf. *Journal of the Acoustical Society of America, 77,* 1619–1621.

Boothroyd, A. (1982). *Hearing impairments in young children.* Englewood Cliffs, NJ: Prentice-Hall.

Calvert, D. R., & Silverman, S. R. (1975). *Speech and deafness.* Washington, DC: Alexander Graham Bell Association for the Deaf.

Calvert, D. R., & Silverman, S. R. (1983). *Speech and deafness* (2nd ed.). Washington, DC: Alexander Graham Bell Association for the Deaf.

Carney, A. E., & Beachler, C. R. (1986). Vibrotactile perception of suprasegmental features of speech: A comparison of single-channel and multichannel instruments. *Journal of the Acoustical Society of America, 79,* 131–140.

Clark, M. (1989). *Language through living.* Toronto, Canada: Hodder and Stoughton.

Cole, E. B. (1990). *Listening and talking: A guide to promoting spoken language in young, hearing-impaired children.* Washington, DC: Alexander Graham Bell Association for the Deaf.

Cole, E. B., & Gregory, H. (Eds.). (1986). *Auditory learning.* Washington, DC: Alexander Graham Bell Association for the Deaf.

Cole, E. B., & Mischook, M. (1985). Survey and annotated bibliography of curricula used by oral preschool programs. *The Volta Review, 87,* 139–154.

Curtis, J. F. (1987). *An introduction to microcomputers in speech, language, and hearing.* Boston: Little Brown.

DeFilippo, C. L. (1984). Laboratory projects in tactile aids to lipreading. *Ear and Hearing, 5,* 211–227.

DeFilippo, C. L., & Sims, D. G. (Eds.). (1988). *New reflections on speechreading.* Washington, DC: Alexander Graham Bell Association for the Deaf.

Dodd, B., & Campbell, R. (Eds.). (1987). *Hearing by eye: The psychology of lip-reading.* Hillsdale, NJ: Erlbaum.

Doggett, G. (1989). Employers' attitudes toward hearing-impaired people: a comparative study. *The Volta Review, 91*, 269–281.

Erber, N. P. (1972). Auditory, visual and auditory-visual recognition of consonants by children with normal and impaired hearing. *Journal of Speech and Hearing Research, 15*, 413–422.

Estabrooks, W., & Birkenshaw-Fleming, R. (1994). *Hear and listen! Talk and sing!* Toronto, Canada: Arisa.

Ewing, A. W. C., & Ewing, E. C. (1964). *Teaching deaf children to talk*. Manchester, UK: Manchester University Press.

Fey, M. (1988). Generalization issues facing language interventionists: An introduction. *Language, Speech and Hearing Services in Schools, 19*, 272–281.

Forner, L. L., & Hixon, T. J. (1977). Respiratory kinematics in profoundly hearing-impaired speakers. *Journal of Speech and Hearing Research, 20*, 373–408.

Friedlander, B. Z. (1970). Receptive language development in infancy: Issues and problems. *Merrill-Palmer Quarterly of Behavior and Development, 16*, 109–122.

Fry, D. B. (1966). The development of the phonological system in the normal and the deaf child. In F. Smith & G. A. Miller (Eds.), *The genesis of language* (pp. 128–159). Cambridge, MA: MIT Press.

Geers, A. E., & Moog, J. S. (1989). Evaluating speech perception skills: Tools for measuring the benefits of cochlear implants, tactile aids and hearing aids. In E. Owens & D. K. Kessler (Eds.), *Cochlear implants in young deaf children* (pp. 227–256). Boston: College Hill Press.

Grant, J. (1987). *The hearing-impaired: Birth to six*. Boston: Little Brown.

Hanson, V. L., Liberman, I. Y., & Schankweiler, D. (1984). Linguistic coding by deaf children in relation to beginning reading success. *Journal of Experimental Child Psychology, 37*, 378–393.

Hirsh, I. J. (1940). Acoustical bases of speech perception. *Journal of Sound and Vibration, 27*, 111–122.

Hochberg, I., Levitt, H., & Osberger, M. (Eds.). (1983). *Speech of the hearing-impaired: Research, training and personnel preparation*. Baltimore: University Park Press.

Hudgins, C. V., & Numbers, F. C. (1942). An investigation of the intelligibility of the speech of the deaf. *Genetic Psychology Monographs, 25*, 289–392.

Ijsseldijk, F. J. (1988). Speechreading tests for the deaf. *Journal of the British Association of Teachers of the Deaf, 12*, 3–15.

Jensema, C. J., & Trybus, R. H. (1978). *Communication patterns and educational achievement of hearing-impaired students*. Washington, DC: Office of Demographic Studies.

Jerger, J. (Ed.). (1984). *Pediatric audiology*. San Diego, CA: College Hill Press.

Johnson, R. E., Liddell. S. K., & Erting, C. J. (1989). *Unlocking the curriculum: Principles for achieving access in deaf education* (Gallaudet Research Institute Working Paper 89-3). Washington, DC: Gallaudet University.

Jung, J. H. (1989). *Genetic syndromes in communication disorders*. Boston: College Hill Press.

Lauter, J. L. (Ed.). (1985). Proceedings of the Conference on the Planning and Production of Speech in Normal and Hearing-Impaired Individuals: A seminar in honor of S. Richard Silverman. *ASHA Reports, 15*.

Lenneberg, E. H. (1967). *Biological foundations of language*. New York: John Wiley and Sons.

Ling, D. (1976). *Speech and the hearing-impaired child: Theory and practice*. Washington, DC: Alexander Graham Bell Association for the Deaf.

Ling, D. (1981). Keep your child within earshot. *Newsounds, 6*, 506.

Ling, D. (Ed.). (1984). *Early intervention for hearing-impaired children: Oral options*. San Diego, CA: College Hill Press.

Ling, D. (Ed.). (1984). *Early intervention for hearing-impaired children: Total communication options*. San Diego, CA: College Hill Press.

Ling, D. (1988). *Foundations of spoken language for hearing-impaired children*. Washington, DC: Alexander Graham Bell Association for the Deaf.

Ling, D. (1991). *The phonetic-phonologic speech evaluation record*. Washington, DC: Alexander Graham Bell Association for the Deaf.

Ling, D., & Ling, A. H. (1978). *Aural habilitation: The foundations of verbal learning in hearing-impaired children.* Washington, DC: Alexander Graham Bell Association for the Deaf.

Ling, D., & Milne, M. (1981). The development of speech in hearing-impaired children. In F. Bess, B. A. Freeman, & J. S. Sinclair (Eds.), *Amplification in education* (pp. 99–108). Washington, DC: Alexander Graham Bell Association for the Deaf.

Markides, A. (1983). *The speech of hearing-impaired children.* Manchester, UK: Manchester University Press.

McDonald, E. T. (1964). *Articulatory testing and treatment: A sensory-motor approach.* Pittsburgh, PA: Stanwix House.

McGarr, N. S. (Ed.). (1989). Research on the use of sensory aids for hearing-impaired people (Monograph of *The Volta Review*, *91*, No. 5). Washington, DC: Alexander Graham Bell Association for the Deaf.

Mischook, M., & Cole, E. (1986). Auditory learning and teaching of hearing-impaired infants. *The Volta Review*, *88*(5), 67–82.

Monsen, R. B. (1979). Acoustic qualities of phonation in young hearing-impaired children. *Journal of Speech and Hearing Research*, *22*, 270–288.

Murry, T., & Murry, J. (Eds.). (1980). *Infant communication.* Houston, TX: College Hill Press.

Oller, D. K., Eilers, R. E., Bull, D. H., & Carney, A. E. (1985). Prespeech vocalizations of a deaf infant: A comparison with normal metaphonological development. *Journal of Speech and Hearing Research*, *28*, 47–63.

Owens, E., & Kessler, D. K. (1988). *Cochlear implants in young deaf children.* Boston: Little, Brown.

Perigoe, C. B., & Ling, D. (1986). Generalization of speech skills in hearing-impaired children. *The Volta Review*, *88*, 351–366.

Pickett, J. M., & McFarland, W. (1985). Auditory implants and tactile aids for the profoundly deaf. *Journal of Speech and Hearing Research*, *28*, 134–150.

Popelka, G. R. (1981). *Hearing assessment with the acoustic reflex.* New York: Grune and Stratton.

Proctor, A. (1984). Tactile aids for the deaf: A comprehensive bibliography. *American Annals of the Deaf*, *129*, 409–416.

Quigley, S. P., & Paul, P. V. (1984). *Language and deafness.* San Diego, CA: College Hill Press.

Reed, M. (1984). *Educating hearing-impaired children.* Milton Keynes, UK: Open University Press.

Sacks, O. (1989). *Seeing voices.* Berkeley, CA: University of California Press.

Silverman, S. R. (1983). Speech training then and now: A critical review. In I. Hochberg, H. Levitt, & M. J. Osberger (Eds.), *Speech of the hearing-impaired* (pp. 1–20). Baltimore: University Park Press.

Stelmachowicz, P. G., & Seewald, R. C. (1990). *Probe-tube microphone measures in children. Seminars in hearing.* New York: Thieme-Stratton.

Stoker, R. G., & Ling, D. (1992). *Speech production in hearing-impaired children and youth: Theory and practice.* Washington, DC: Alexander Graham Bell Association for the Deaf.

Stone, P. (1988). *Blueprint for developing conversational competence.* Washington, DC: Alexander Graham Bell Association for the Deaf.

Studdert-Kennedy, M. (1984). Early development of phonological form. In C. von Euler, H. Forssberg, & H. Lagercrantz (Eds.), *Neurobiology of early infant behavior* (pp. 82–96). New York: Stockton Press.

Subtelny, J. D. (Ed.). (1980). *Speech assessment and speech improvement for the hearing impaired.* Washington, DC: Alexander Graham Bell Association for the Deaf.

Vorce, E. (1974). *Teaching speech to deaf children.* Washington, DC: Alexander Graham Bell Association for the Deaf.

Weisenberger, J. (1989). Tactile aids for speech perception and production by hearing-impaired people. *The Volta Review*, *91*, 79–100.

Wilson, W. R., & Thompson, G. (1984). Behavioral audiometry. In J. Jerger (Ed.), *Pediatric audiology* (pp. 1–44). San Diego, CA: College Hill Press.

Wolk, S., & Schildroth, A. N. (1986). Deaf children and speech intelligibility. In A. N. Schildroth & M. A. Karchmer (Eds.), *Deaf children in*

America (pp. 139–156). San Diego, CA: College Hill Press.

Wood, D., Wood H., Griffiths, A., & Howarth, I. (1986). *Teaching and talking with deaf children.* New York: John Wiley and Sons.

End of Chapter Examination Questions

Chapter 8

1. **Fifty years ago speech for those with hearing impairment was generally based on:**
   a. Speechreading and tactile clues
   b. Sign language
   c. No particular focus
   d. Speechreading

2. **Which of the following would be considered the most significant hearing loss as it relates to language, learning, and social/emotional behaviors?**
   a. Profound
   b. Mild
   c. Severe
   d. Moderate

3. **The most efficient use of visual clues in speech understanding also requires:**
   a. Excellent vision
   b. Even minimal levels of hearing
   c. Good receptive vocabulary
   d. The use of both vision and hearing

4. **According to the author of this chapter, what is necessary for a child to produce spoken language patterns appropriately in context?**
   a. Vocalization
   b. Accuracy
   c. Flexibility
   d. Production

5. **What are the advantages for individuals who have hearing impairment who use both sign and spoken language?**

6. **Contrast and compare the intrinsic and extrinsic factors that influence acquisition of speech.**

7. **List or describe the context and the people involved in the formal and informal procedures of teaching and learning.**

8. **Discuss the advantages and disadvantages of signing. Briefly state your opinion.**

End of Chapter Answer Sheet

Name _____ Date _____

Chapter 8

1. Which one(s)?   a   b   c   d

2. Which one(s)?   a   b   c   d

3. Which one(s)?   a   b   c   d

4. Which one(s)?   a   b   c   d

5. _____

_____

_____

6. _____

_____

_____

7. _____

_____

_____

8. _____

_____

_____

9

Cochlear Implantation in Children

THOMAS C. KRYZER

Introduction

A severe or profound sensorineural hearing loss usually causes a significant disruption of education, employment, and interpersonal relationships. In postlingually deafened adults, the loss of the ability to orally communicate often leads to drastic changes in the person's employment and social relationships and can lead to social isolation. A European study showed that deaf and hard-of-hearing workers are twice as likely to become unemployed when compared to their normally hearing coworkers, and finding work was harder because of their hearing loss (Royal Institute of Deaf People in the UK, 2000). Parents of children with newly diagnosed hearing impairment experience the loss of their child's expected future. Their educational and professional expectations for that child have effectively been lost. These parents now must face the process of coping with this loss in their child's new, altered life expectations. This can realization can evolve into a grieving process as they come to terms with being the parents of a disabled child. As 90% of deaf children have two normal hearing parents, isolation within the family becomes a very real possibility if some form of communication is not developed between them and their hearing-impaired child.

The societal cost of deafness is staggering. There is an estimated cost of $122 billion in lost earnings due to hearing loss and an additional estimated $18 billion lost from decreased work force paid taxes (Kochkin, 2005). Another $2 billion on equal access for the disabled deaf is spent annually (NIH Consensus Statement, 1992). Overall, there may be a lifetime cost of over $1,000,000 per patient with untreated or unrecognized hearing in educational and lost work force costs (Mohr et al., 2000).

In a study using patients' self-ratings and comparing all disabilities, deafness had the lowest marks for educational level, the lowest marks for percentage working, and the lowest self-assessment of well-being of all assessed disabilities (Harris, Anderson, & Novak, 1995).

Efforts to identify hearing loss early in childhood have been ongoing for years. Although the number of children with severe-to-profound hearing loss has remained between 1 and 3 out of every 100,000 births, earlier identification has allowed aural rehabilitation to be initiated sooner than it would have just a few years ago. Hearing loss in children has been associated with delayed receptive and expressive language skills and lower educational achievement (Joint Committee on Infant Hearing Screening, 2000). Earlier identification of infants does lead to earlier intervention. Earlier intervention improves both receptive and expressive language skills when compared to children identified later in childhood (Kennedy et al., 2006).

The advent of cochlear implantation for postlingually deafened adults (1984) and prelingually deafened children (1992) has forever changed the landscape of treatment and rehabilitation for these patients. For adult patients where hearing aids are no longer appropriate and profoundly deafened children receiving no benefit from hearing aids, cochlear implants offer a return to the hearing world. Permanent isolation, educational delay, and reduced employment opportunities are no longer absolutes. Hearing loss is the most common sensory deficit. By successfully treating patients with the most severe form of hearing loss, their future quality of life can be markedly improved.

History of Electrical Stimulation of the Ear

The history of electrical stimulation of the ear began in the late 1790s when Alessandro Volta, developer of the electrolytic cell or battery, experimented in delivering electricity to areas of the head. After stimulating the muscles of the face and optic nerve he turned his attention to the ear. Delivering a 50 V stimulus to his own ear he described " . . . a kind of crackling with shocks, as if some paste or tenacious matter had been boiling." The disagreeable sensation and his apprehension of causing a "shock in the brain" prevented him from repeating the experiments (Shah, Chung, & Jackler, 1997).

The first reported direct stimulation of the cochlear nerve for production of sound was in 1957 by Djourno and Eyries (Djourno, Eyries, & Vallencien, 1957). Andre Djourno, a physiologist, and Charles Eyries, an otolaryngologist, teamed to implant an induction coil in a deafened patient. They placed electrodes near the frayed ends of the cochlear nerve in a patient deafened from bilateral cholesteatomas. The patient received extensive postoperative rehabilitation and was able to perceive environmental and some speech sounds. Speech understanding was not possible and the implant failed after a few months due to an electrode fracture. This patient represents the first implant for the production of sound.

In 1961, William House, an otologist, learned of Djourno and Eyries's work when a deaf patient presented him with the translated paper. He implanted two patients later that year, one with an electrode near the round window and one with an electrode in the scala tympani. These single-channel implants yielded some speech perception and limited speech understanding. Later in

the 1960s, both single-channel and multiple-channel implants were being developed and placed in patients at Stanford University and the University of San Francisco. These early implant efforts were followed closely by the beginning of a neural prosthesis program in 1970 funded by the National Institutes of Health (Hannaway, 1996). This program, initially designed to help studies in treating blindness, gave legitimacy to the research and allowed for greater funding of cochlear implant development.

Graham Clark, at the University of Melbourne, realized early the importance of multichannel stimulation of the cochlea. His research focused on integrating all the parts necessary for the multichannel, non-simultaneous stimulation of the cochlear nerve. With funding from Australian private and public sources he was able to develop a safe and minimally traumatic surgical procedure with a well-tolerated, long-lived implant electrode. He implanted his first patient in 1978 and by 1981 had patients that were able to show open set speech recognition without visual aids (Clark, Tong, & Marting, 1981).

This Australian device would become the Nucleus multichannel cochlear implant. The FDA granted approval for the House/3M single-channel device in 1984, by which time several thousand devices had been implanted during trials. In 1985 the Nucleus multichannel device gained FDA approval for postlingually deafened adults. Children above the age of 2 were added in 1990. Due to the rapid success and continuing improvement in patient results, especially with children, approval expanded in 1998 to adults with severe-to-profound hearing loss and children to 1 year of age with profound hearing loss. Cochlear implants are now compact, implantable devices with multiple channels to stimulate the cochlear nerve along much of the cochlear turns (Figure 9–1 and Figure 9–2). There are now three cochlear implants with FDA approval: Nucleus, Cochlear Corporation, Australia; HiRes 90K, Advanced Bionics, Sylmar, California; and Tempo+, Med-El, Austria.

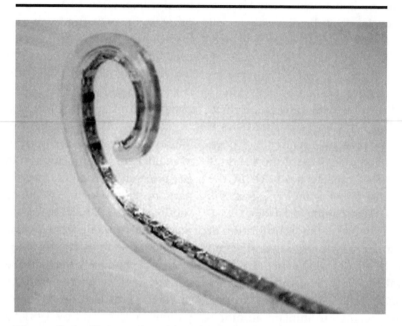

Figure 9–1. Picture of cochlear implant electrode set.

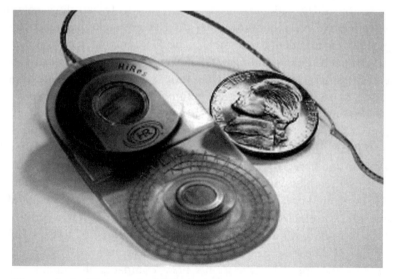

Figure 9–2. Picture of cochlear implant receiver.

Cochlear Implantation

Preoperative Evaluation

Preoperative medical and radiological evaluation of the cochlear implant patient is often standardized but may be altered and customized as dictated by the patient's medical and social history. The evaluation process tries to identify patients who are not only candidates for surgery but also identify any factors that might influence outcome.

Medical Evaluation

The medical evaluation is usually concerned with the patient's ability to tolerate a 1.5- to 3-hour surgical procedure. Very young patients (less than a year) should weigh more than 8 kilograms (16 pounds) and be cleared for surgery by the managing pediatricians. Many of these children are graduates of intensive care units and have multiple medical problems that need to be managed. All children with a profound hearing loss should have an electrocardiogram to exclude the diagnosis of Jervell-Lange-Nielson syndrome, which is characterized by certain electrocardiographic abnormalities and sudden cardiac death (Siem et al., 2008). Although cochlear implantation has been a safe procedure in patients 1 year of age and older (Hoffman, 1997), the safety in operating on patients as young as 6 to 8 months of age remains to be seen.

Older adults often have many medical problems that need to be managed in the preoperative period. Seldom are these medical problems of the magnitude that would contraindicate surgery. Severely reduced cardiac performance and very poor pulmonary function are the most common reasons for medical denial. Age alone is not a disqualifying factor. Patients in their 80s can often be expected to live well into their 90s. A family history of longevity can be helpful to determine cochlear implant candidacy of octogenarians.

Psychological aspects of hearing loss and cochlear implantation can be enormous for patients and families. Psychological evaluation for patients and families of pediatric patients can expose patient and family dynamics that may prove to be hurdles to rehabilitation after surgery. It is always better to ensure that appropriate expectations for surgery and rehabilitation are present before surgery rather than after.

Radiologic Evaluation

Usually, patients are evaluated with a high-resolution CT scan of the temporal bones in both the axial and coronal planes. This study gives vital information on the anatomy of the mastoid, facial nerve, and cochlea and its patency. Some developmental abnormalities of the cochlea require different insertion techniques or different implant electrodes. In cases of postmeningitic deafness, the cochlea may be filled with reactive bone called labyrinthitis ossificans. In these cases, an MRI can help to determine if the cochlea is patent or obliterated with the reactive bone (Nair, Abou-Elhamd, & Hawthorne, 2000). This process can happen quite quickly after meningitis and, if it has occurred, presents the surgeon with difficult challenges to implant insertion. Post-implant radiologic evaluation is generally used only in situations where there are questions regarding implant function or patient performance.

CT scans expose the patents to radiation. In young patients, often with intensive care unit stays, this radiation exposure is not insignificant. Every effort should be taken to reduce the number of scans and radiation exposure for these patients.

Audiologic Evaluation

The initial audiologic evaluation serves to determine the severity of the hearing loss and "shape" of the audiogram. Typically, this involves unaided air and bone conduction thresholds and speech discrimination and speech reception thresholds. In young children and infants, auditory brainstem response (ABR) testing is used to confirm hearing thresholds because they are prelingually deafened. The FDA guidelines for cochlear implant candidacy have changed over the years. With consistent evidence of increasing benefit from cochlear implants, the most recent guidelines are more lenient than earlier FDA criteria. In very young children where speech reception testing may not be possible, the benefit from amplification is assessed with questionnaires. The Meaningful Auditory Integration Scale (MAIS) or the infant-toddler version (IT-MAIS) is helpful in determining any benefit received from hearing aids (Robbins, Renshaw, & Berry, 1991). In older children a score of less than 40% on the Multi-Lexical Neighborhood Test (MLNT) is an indication that little or no benefit is received from hearing aids (Kirk, Pisoni, & Osberger, 1995). Candidacy criteria are likely to change in the future as results from cochlear implants improve and with better testing of early language development.

Adult Candidacy Criteria

- Bilateral severe-to-profound sensorineural hearing loss (70 dB or greater threshold)

- Speech discrimination of less than 60% on common sentences in the HINT (Hearing in Noise Test) under best-aided conditions
- Limited benefit from appropriately fitted hearing aids

Pediatric Candidacy Criteria

- At least 12 months of age with a profound sensorineural hearing loss
- 24 months of age with a severe-to-profound sensorineural hearing loss
- Lack of progress on developmental auditory skills despite adequate hearing aid use in children younger than 4 years, defined as:
  - Lack of spontaneous response to name in quiet or environmental sounds, as measured by the MAIS or the IT-MAIS, or
  - Less than 40% correct on the MLNT in soundfield under best-aided conditions
- Three- to 6-month trial of appropriately fitted hearing aids
- High motivation of family and family support structures
- Placement of the child in an educational program that emphasizes auditory skills

Surgical Procedures

The surgical procedure for children and adults is generally the same. The important structures of the cochlea, middle ear, and facial recess are essentially of adult size shortly after birth (Hoffman, 1997). The length of the electrode array accommodates any growth in the mastoid and skull. It is a 2- to 3-hour procedure performed under general anesthesia and often on an outpatient basis. Very old and very young patients are usually observed overnight in the hospital as a precaution.

The incision is a curvilinear postauricular incision of varying length, depending on the surgeon's preference and patient's needs (Figure 9–3). A mastoidectomy is performed by removing the cortical mastoid bone directly behind the external auditory canal. Once the mastoid cavity is opened, the area of the facial recess is identified and opened. This area is bounded by the facial nerve, chorda tympani, and the lateral process of the incus. The facial recess allows access to the posterior middle ear space and a direct route to the round window niche.

At this point a circular well, or seat, is drilled in the posterior temporal bone about an inch behind the mastoid cavity (Figure 9–4). This allows the internal cochlear stimulator to lie below the bone and not project too much into the skin. Small suture passing holes are drilled above and below the seat to allow the stimulator to be sutured in place and keep it from migrating. A shallow groove is then drilled to connect this well to the mastoid cavity (see Figure 9–4) for the electrode array to travel from the implant to the middle ear.

After the well for the stimulator is drilled, attention returns to the round window niche. The opening into the cochlea, or cochleostomy, is made by removing bone from the anterior and inferior edge of the round window niche. The scala vestibuli is then opened and the opening enlarged in the inferior direction. The entire basal turn of the cochlea is then seen and identifies the cochlea. Each implant has a slightly different insertion technique, but ideally the electrode array is inserted in an atraumatic way that allows the electrodes to lie closely to the modiolus. If the cochlea is filled with scar tissue or bone (labyrinthitis ossificans) from meningitis, the basal turn is drilled to a depth of about 8 mm and the electrodes inserted as deeply as possible. The scala vestibuli may also be implanted in difficult cases either directly across from the round

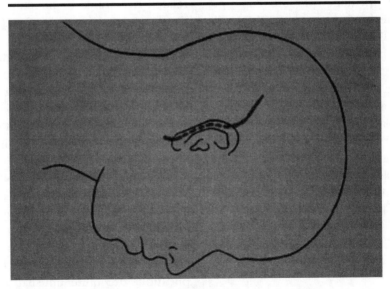

Figure 9–3. Position and curvilinear nature of incision.

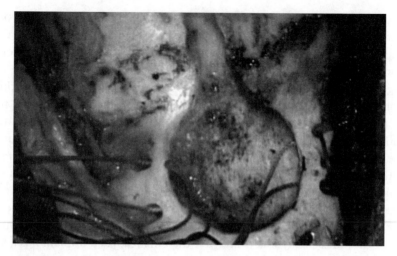

Figure 9–4. The well (or seat) for the implant in the posterior temporal bone.

window or by using a split electrode array. The electrode array is then gently coiled in the mastoid cavity to take up the extra length of the electrodes (Figure 9-5).

Once the electrodes are inserted and the stimulator is sutured in place, small pieces of tissue are placed in the cochlear opening to seal the opening with soft tissue, preventing a leak of inner ear fluid into the middle ear. This tissue also presumably keeps middle ear purulent material from entering the cochlea during episodes of acute otitis media. The postauricular wound is then closed and a dressing applied. The dressing is kept in place for 24 hours and the patient examined 1 week after surgery to remove the Steri-Strips (children) and staples (adults). The ear is allowed to heal for 1 month before the patient is allowed to wear the external device and be initially programmed.

Surgical Complications

Surgical complications are the same as those for all ear surgery: infection, hematoma, facial nerve paralysis, cerebrospinal fluid leak, meningitis, and need for further surgery. Fortunately, these risks are unusual and patients are generally expected to have an uneventful postoperative recovery (Roland, 2000).

The most common problem, which occurs in 6 to 10% of cases, is a wound-related hematoma or infection. Failure of the wound to heal with subsequent exposure of the implant is very unusual and is avoided by proper surgical technique and planning of the incision. Cerebrospinal fluid leak after implantation can occur secondary to leak though the round window area and is more likely in patients with a congenitally malformed cochlea. This is most easily dealt with during surgery by placing small pieces of tissue in the cochleostomy to seal this area. Dural injury during creation of the seat for the stimulator may also cause a leak of spinal fluid. This can usually be repaired using a small piece of fascia at the time of the initial surgery. These complications are quite unusual and can be avoided during the initial procedure with proper care and planning.

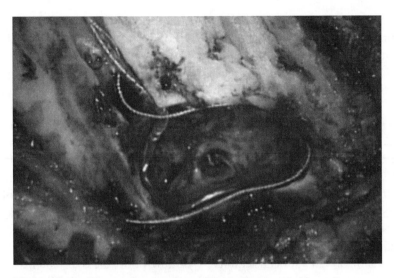

Figure 9–5. Electrode array is coiled in the mastoid cavity.

Meningitis in cochlear implant patients has been a concern from the very beginning. In June of 2002 there seemed to be a sudden increase in the cases of meningitis. A survey of implant centers (O'Donoghue et al., 2002) and an inquiry from the Federal Drug Administration (FDA) and Centers for Disease Control (CDC) led to a public health warning being issued regarding meningitis in children with cochlear implants (Reefhuis et al., 2003). Although small, there was an increased number of meningitis cases among implant recipients. It was quickly realized that most of the meningitis patients had a type of implant that had a positioner placed to help keep the electrodes in a perimodiolar position. That insertion technique was immediately abandoned and strict adherence to closing the cochleostomy with soft tissue emphasized. The FDA also recommended that all implant patients receive vaccinations for pneumococcal bacteria. Now that positioners are no longer used, patients' progress has been followed and the incidence of meningitis is still slightly above the rate for non-implanted peers.

Clinicians need to be vigilant regarding the diagnosis and treatment of ear infections after cochlear implantation and must ensure that all implant patients are up to date in the pneumococcal vaccine prior to surgery.

Surgery to replace nonfunctioning implants amounts to about 2% in pediatric populations (Cullen, Fayad, Luxford, & Buckman, 2008). Implants fail for several reasons. Reasons for failure include internal electronic failure, traumatic fracture, and unknown or "soft failure." Protecting the implant from trauma such as a blow to the head is important and patients should be counseled regarding such trauma. Electrostatic charge can also damage an implant, and therefore the external device should not be worn when playing on plastic playground equipment. Reimplantation surgery is safe and reliable, with expected results similar to the patient's previous functional level.

MRI examinations can be done with some precautions to avoid damage to the internal magnet of the implant. Movement of the electrodes in the MRI field is not significant in low-strength magnetic fields.

Medical and surgical procedures may be safely performed, but no monopolar electro-cautery should be used above the shoulders in any patient with an implant; otherwise, damage to the internal components of the internal device is likely.

Outcomes

Outcomes in adults and adolescent patients who are postlingually deafened concentrate more on speech perception and receptive language skills because expressive language skills have presumably already been acquired. Most of these patients achieve proficiency in the use of their implant within 6 to 12 months of implantation. Early results indicate the average adult after implantation will understand about 80% of sentences without the aid of visual cues (Staller et al., 1997). Many have much better results than this, and the number able to regularly use the telephone is growing. These results are generally age-independent, in that an 80-year-old patient may perform as well as a 50-year-old implant user. As language results have continued to improve, studies on music perception in cochlear implant recipients are now looking to better understand the nature of cochlear stimulation (Cooper, Tobey, & Loizou, 2008; Looi, McDermott, McKay, & Hickson, 2008).

Prelingually deafened children, on the other hand, can exhibit devastating delays in all aspects of their language development. Receptive and expressive language skills and academic achievement are significantly delayed in prelingually profoundly deaf children despite advances in hearing aid technology and tactile aids. Because literacy is strongly based on language skills, children with severe language delay also have a severe delay in their reading and writing skills

(Boothroyd, Geers, & Moog, 1991; Geers & Moog, 1994; Holt, Traxler, & Allen, 1997). Therefore, outcomes for cochlear implants in prelingually deafened children must take into account all aspects of language development, receptive and expressive.

Early studies in speech performance in post-implant children showed that the ability to imitate speech sounds improved in 66% of patients and speech intelligibility improved in 62% of patients (Tobey, Angelette, Murchison, Nicosia, Spraque, et al., 1991). This study was based on both older and younger children with varying length of time of deafness. In 2003, a study of 181 prelingually deafened children implanted by age 5 showed that more than half of these patients were similar to age-matched peers on a language battery (Geers, Nicholas, & Sedey, 2003). Another study of 47 children implanted by age 18 months found significantly better language development than those implanted after 18 months (Hammes et al., 2002). Furthermore, those implanted before 18 months made a full transition to oral communication, despite being predominately users of total communication prior to implantation. Several studies have shown that the usual child after implantation acquires 1 year's language in 1 year's time (Bollard, Chute, Popp, & Parisier, 1999; Robbins, Svirsky, & Kirk, 1997). This is true for children implanted at a younger age, especially under 2 years of age. Therefore, any delay in language present before cochlear implantation will persist unless these children can learn language faster than their normal hearing peers; many do just that.

The advantage of early implantation is translated to prelinguistic skills. Children implanted between 7 and 15 months of age with 2 to 6 months of implant experience performed similarly to normal-hearing peers on the preferential looking paradigm assessing preword learning skills (Houston, Ying, Pisoni, & Kirk, 2003). In addition, children implanted between 5 and 20 months were assessed through the entire babbling period. Inventories of consonants and vowels and consonant-vowel combinations were acquired with video tape. The qualitative characteristics were similar between the early implanted children and the normal-hearing infants (Schauwers, Gillis, & Govaerts, 2008). The phonetic complexity of prelinguistic vocalizations correlates significantly with global language abilities at 4 years of age (Walker & Bass-Ringdahl, 2008).

Prelingually deafened children implanted before the age of 2 are twice as likely of being mainstreamed into a traditional educational setting. This is in direct contrast with their nonhearing and nonspeaking counterparts who experience a much more limited educational experience.

One area where speech perception studies dominate is that of bilateral cochlear implantation. Multiple studies have shown an improvement in sound localization in children and adults after bilateral implantation (Grantham et al, 2007; Murphy & O'Donoghue, 2007). Detection of sound direction also seems to enhance speech intelligibility in noise for bilateral cochlear implanted patients. Improved hearing and speech understanding in noise are exactly what these children need to navigate the rigors of a mainstream education. It appears that not only early implantation but bilateral implantation readies these children to enter a mainstream educational setting and maximize their educational opportunities.

Much has been studied regarding various factors that may influence the outcome of implantation. The age of onset and duration of deafness have long been known to be factors in implant outcome. Early identification of infants with hearing loss and

intervention may not be enough. Even when children are identified, enrolled in language intervention, and appropriately aided, those who are implanted at an earlier age perform better than their later implanted peers (Hammes et al., 2002). Therefore, early intervention and aiding may not be enough in trying to produce age-appropriate language in deaf infants. In addition, the type of learning environment, oral (OC) versus total (TC), seems to have an effect on the language development, with the oral communication group performing much better on expressive language tests (Miyamoto, Osberger, Robbins, Myres, & Kessler, 1993).

In adults, the length of time spent with a profound hearing loss also affects overall performance. Usually, the ear that has been deaf the shortest amount of time is implanted or the last ear to hear is implanted. As results have improved, the best ear is often implanted to gain the best results.

Cost-utility analysis is a method of determining the cost effectiveness of a particular medical treatment. The results are usually reported in cost per quality-adjusted-life-year (QALY). Multiple studies have shown that cochlear implants in profoundly deafened children and adults significantly improve the quality of life of these patients. And when the medical costs of surgery and rehabilitation are factored in, cochlear implants compare favorably with medical procedures such as heart transplantations, hip replacement, and kidney dialysis (Cheng & Niparko, 1999; Wyatt, Niparko, Rothman, & deLissovoy, 1996).

The cause of deafness does not seem to be an important factor, with a few exceptions. Meningitis can cause an inflammatory response to the cochlea, resulting in ossification of the scala vestibuli. If the cochlea is ossified, then complete insertion of the electrode array may not be possible. The prospect of cochlear ossification and limited insertion often leads to a quick decision to implant the postmeningitis patient and forego a 6- month hearing aid trial. There is also little chance of spontaneous resolution of hearing loss after meningitis.

Patients with auditory neuropathy/dyssynchrony generally seem to have guarded expectations from implants. These patients have associated cochlear nerve abnormalities and generally perform more poorly after implantation than their age-matched peers (Rance & Barker, 2008; Walton, Gibson, Sanli, & Prelog, 2009). Although these patients may derive some benefit from cochlear implantation, their expectations should perhaps be lower than other groups. Children with multiple medical neurologic deficits are also likely to perform more poorly after receiving a cochlear implant.

In contrast, children who have their deafness as a result from a mutation in the gene gap junction beta-2 (GJB2) may have an advantage. The GJB2 gene mutation alters the normal connexin 26 (Cx26) protein that leads to abnormal discrete cochlear dysfunction and leaves the cochlear nerve and spiral ganglion area normal. These patients generally have an excellent outcome for cochlear implants (Bauer, Geers, Brenner, Moog & Smith, 2003). Therefore, the test for the GJB2 gene may be useful to families as a prognostic indicator for cochlear implantation.

Summary

Cochlear implantation and rehabilitation is a highly technical and time-consuming process that has been undergoing changes and improvements for over 20 years. Both adults and young children receive significant benefits that greatly increase the quality of their lives and improve their educational and economic opportunities. Cochlear implants now offer a therapeutic option for those patients not otherwise helped with conventional hearing aid technology.

References

Bauer, P. W., Geers, A. E., Brenner, C., Moog, J. S., & Smith, R. S. (2003). The effect of GJB2 allele variants on performance after cochlear implantation. *Archives of Otolaryngology-Head Neck Surgery, 113*, 2135–2140.

Bollard, P. M., Chute, P. M., Popp, A. C., & Parisier S. (1999). Specific language growth in young children using the CLARION cochlear implant. *Annals of Otology, Rhinology and Laryngology, 117*(Suppl.), 119–123.

Boothroyd, A., Geers, A. E., & Moog, J. S. (1991). Practical implications of cochlear implants in children. *Ear and Hearing, 12*(Suppl. 4), 81S–89S.

Cheng, A. K., & Niparko, J. K. (1999). Cost-utility of the cochlear implant. *Archives of Otolaryngology-Head Neck Surgery, 125*, 1214–1218.

Clark, G. M., Tong, Y. C., & Marting, L. F. (1981). A multiple-channel cochlear implant: An evaluation using open-set CID sentences. *Laryngoscope, 91*, 628–634.

Cooper, W. B., Tobey, E., & Loizou, P. C. (2008). Music perception by cochlear implant and normal hearing listeners as measured by the Montreal Battery for Evaluation of Amusia. *Ear and Hearing, 29*, 618–626.

Cullen, R. D., Fayad, J. N., Luxford, W. M., & Buckman, C. A. (2008). Revision cochlear implant surgery. *Otology and Neurotology, 29*, 214–220.

Djourno, A., Eyries, C., & Vallencien, B. (1957). De l'excitation életrique du nerf cochleaire chez l'homme, par induction à distance, àl'aide d'un micro-bobinage inclus à demeure. *CR Soc Biology* (Paris), *151*, 423–425.

Geers, A., & Moog, J. (1994). Spoken language results: Vocabulary, syntax and communication. *The Volta Review, 96*, 131-150.

Geers, A., Nicholas, J., & Sedey, A. L. (2003). Language skills of children with early cochlear implantation. *Ear and Hearing, 24*, 46S-58S.

Grantham, D. W., Ashmead, D. H., Ricketts, T. A., Labadie, R. F., & Haynes, D. S. (2007). Horizontal-plane localization of noise and speech signals by postlingually deafened adults fitted with bilateral cochlear implants. *Ear and Hearing, 28*, 524-541.

Hammes, D. M., Novak, M. A., Rotz, L. A., Willis, M., Edmondson, D. M., & Thomas, J. F. (2002). Early identification and cochlear implantation: Critical factors for spoken language development. *Annals of Otology, Rhinology and Laryngology, 111*, 74-78.

Hannaway, C. (1996). *Contributions of the National Institutes of Health to the development of cochlear prosthesis.* Bethesda, MD: National Institutes of Health.

Harris, J. P., Anderson, J. P., & Novak, R. (1995). An outcome study of cochlear implants in deaf patients. *Archives of Otolaryngology-Head and Neck Surgery, 121*, 398-404.

Hoffman, R. (1997). Cochlear implant in the child under two years of age: Skull growth, otitis media and selection. *Otolaryngology-Head and Neck Surgery, 117*, 217-219.

Holt, J., Traxler, C., & Allen, I. (1997). *Interpreting the scores: A user's guide to 9th edition Stanford Achievement test for educators of deaf and hard-of-hearing students.* Gallaudet Research Institute Technical Report 97-1. Washington, DC: Gallaudet University.

Houston, D. M., Ying, E., Pisoni, D. B., & Kirk, K. I. (2003). Development of pre-word-learning skills in infants with cochlear implants. *The Volta Review, 103*, 303-326.

Joint Committee on Infant Hearing Screening. (2000). Year 2000 position statement: Principles and guidelines for early hearing detection and intervention programs. *Pediatrics, 106*(4), 798-817.

Kennedy, C. R., McCann, D. C., Campbell, M. J., Law, C. M., Mullee, M., Petrou, S., et al. (2006). Language ability after early detection of permanent childhood hearing impairment. *New England Journal of Medicine, 354*(20), 2131-2141.

Kirk, K. I., Pisoni, D. B., & Osberger, M. J. (1995). Lexical effects on spoken word recognition by pediatric cochlear implant users. *Ear and Hearing, 16*, 470-481.

Kochkin, S. (2005). *The impact of untreated hearing loss on household income.* Alexandria, VA: Better Hearing Institute.

Looi, V., McDermott, H., McKay, C., & Hickson, L. (2008). Music perception of cochlear implant users compared with hearing aid users. *Ear and Hearing, 29*, 421-434.

Miyamoto, R. T., Osberger, M. J. Robbins, A. M., Myres, W. A., & Kessler, K. (1993). Prelingually deafened children's performance with the Nucleus multichannel cochlear implant. *American Journal of Otology, 14*, 437-445.

Mohr, P. E., Feldmann, J. J., Dunbar, J. L., McConkey-Robbins, A., Niparko, J. K., Rittenhouse, R. K., et al (2000). The societal cost of severe to profound hearing loss in the United States. *International Journal of Technology Assessment in Health Care, 16*, 1120-1135.

Murphy, J., & O'Donoghue, G. (2007). Bilateral cochlear implantation: An evidence-based medicine evaluation. *Laryngoscope, 117*(8), 1412-1418.

Nair, S. B., Abou-Elhamd, K. A., & Hawthorne, M. (2000). A retrospective analysis of high resolution computed tomography in the assessment of cochlear implant patients. *Clinical Otolaryngology, 25*(1), 55-61.

NIH Consensus Statement. (1992). Early identification of hearing impairment in infants and young children. *NIH Consensus Statement, 11*(1), 1-12.

O'Donoghue, G., Balkany, T., Cohen, N., Lenarz, T., Lustig, L., & Niparko, J. K., (2002). Meningitis and cochlear implantation. *Otology and Neurotology, 23*, 823-824.

Rance, G., & Barker, E. J. (2008). Speech perception in children with auditory neuropathy/ dyssynchrony managed with either hearing aids or cochlear implants. *Otology and Neurotology, 29*, 179-182.

Reefhuis, J., Honein, M. A., Whitney, C. G., Chamay, S., Mann, E. A., Biernath, K., et al, (2003). Risk of bacterial meningitis in children with cochlear implants. *New England Journal of Medicine, 349*, 435–445.

Robbins, A. M., Renshaw, J. J., & Berry, S. W. (1991). Evaluating meaningful auditory integration in profoundly hearing-impaired children. *American Journal of Otology, 12*(3), 144–150.

Robbins, A. M., Svirsky, M., & Kirk, K. I. (1997). Children with implants can speak but can they communicate? *Otolaryngology-Head and Neck Surgery, 117*, 155–160.

Roland, J. T. (2000). Complications of cochlear implant surgery. In S. B. Waltzman & N. L. Cohen (Eds.), *Cochlear implants* (pp. 171–175). New York: Thieme.

Royal National Institute of Deaf People in the UK. (2000, May). 15% of people who are deaf or hard-of-hearing are unemployed. Available at http://press.hear-it.org/page.dsp?page=1787

Schauwers, K., Gillis, S., & Govaerts, P. J. (2008). The characteristics of prelexical babbling after cochlear implantation between 5 and 20 months of age. *Ear and Hearing, 29*, 627–637.

Shah, S. B., Chung, J. H., & Jackler, R. K. (1997). Lodestones, quackery and science: Electrical stimulation of the ear before cochlea implants. *American Journal of Otology, 18*, 665–670.

Siem, G., Fruh, A., Leren, P., Heimdal, K., Teig, E., & Harris, S. (2008). Jervell and Lange-Nielsen syndrome in Norwegian children: Aspects around cochlear implantation, hearing and balance. *Ear and Hearing, 29*, 261–269.

Staller, S., Menapace, C., Domico, E., Mills, D., Dowell, R. C., Geers, A., et al. (1997). Speech perception abilities of adult and pediatric Nucleus implant recipients using the spectral peak (SPEAK) coding strategy. *Otolaryngology-Head and Neck Surgery, 117*, 236–242.

Tobey, E. A., Angelette, S., Murchison, C., Nicosia, J., Sprague, S., Staller, S., et al. (1991). Speech production performance in children with multichannel cochlear implants. *American Journal of Otology, 12*(3), 165–173.

Walker, E. A., & Bass-Ringdahl, S. (2008). Babbling complexity and its relationship to speech and language outcomes in children with cochlear implants. *Otology and Neurotology, 29*, 225–229.

Walton, J., Gibson, W. P. R., Sanli, H., & Prelog, K. (2008). Predicting cochlear implant outcomes in children with auditory neuropathy. *Otology and Neurotology, 29*, 302–309.

Wyatt, R. J., Niparko, J. K., Rothman, M., & de-Lissovoy, G. (1996). Cost utility of the multichannel cochlear implant in 258 profoundly deaf individuals. *Laryngoscope, 106*, 816–821.

End of Chapter Examination Questions

Chapter 9

1. The author of this chapter specifies the societal cost of deafness. What is it estimated to be?

2. The lifetime cost of untreated or unrecognized hearing loss is estimated to be _____ per patient.

3. The first known electrical stimulation surgery was conducted in the late _____s (give estimated year).

4. The first reported direct stimulation of the cochlear nerve was in what year?

5. Candidacy of children for cochlear implantation is based on six criteria. What are *four* of those?
   a.
   b.
   c.
   d.

6. For children, the primary benefit of cochlear implantation is _____.

End of Chapter Answer Sheet

Name _____   Date _____

Chapter 9

1. $_____.

2. $_____.

3. _____ (year)

4. _____ (year)

5. a. _____

  b. _____

  c. _____

  d. _____

6. _____

10

Educational Management of Children with Impaired Hearing

MOLLY POTTORF-LYON

Chapter Outline

Introduction

The purpose of this chapter is to acquaint the reader with the numerous and complex issues surrounding the education of children with impaired hearing, which are intricately intertwined, and often philosophically opposed. There are varying perspectives in working with children with impaired hearing in an educational system. These perspectives vary across many professional fields, including but not limited to deaf education, speech-language pathology, medicine, and audiology. Professionals from each of these fields approach educational issues with different orientations and experiences. Our ultimate goal is to ensure the highest educational outcomes for children with hearing impairment, which requires the professionals from each of these fields to work collaboratively in a positive direction to address the many and varied needs of individual children.

This chapter is written by an educational audiologist. The orientation is toward maximizing the hearing capabilities of children with hearing impairment and ensuring children have the opportunity to optimally use audition across a wide array of listening environments. This is no small feat, as the challenges are great, but the ultimate reward of successfully preparing a student to be an independent and productive citizen is even greater. This chapter will address the multifaceted issues and challenges we face in the educational management of children with impaired hearing.

Definitions and Terminology

What is impaired hearing? Who are we talking about? One would think it would be simple to define *hearing impairment* as one who doesn't hear normally. But, what is "normal" hearing? An adult who at one time had normal hearing and acquired hearing loss has a solid language base and an entire life of experiences to assist in accurately deciphering partially heard speech utterances. An English-speaking adult does not need to hear every /s/ sound to correctly understand the intent of a spoken message because of preexisting knowledge of English syntax and vocabulary. An adult also knows, almost intuitively, that the environment affects the ability to hear and knows how to manipulate the listening environment in order to facilitate improved hearing. An adult will also know how to accurately judge the quality of assistive listening devices because a standard for normal speech and sounds has already been established. These are skills that have been acquired through life's experiences.

The examples given above provide clues to the problems associated with working with children who have impaired hearing. A child has no life experiences, no preexisting knowledge of speech and the world of sound. What children hear, whether complete or not, becomes the standard of normal. Young children will accept the quality of assistive listening devices (hearing aids, FM systems, cochlear implants) without question, and often only complain if the sound is overly loud or physically uncomfortable. Normal hearing therefore could be defined as the hearing levels required to successfully fulfill the communication needs at different stages of our lives. For the purpose of acquiring normal speech and language skills, young children require hearing levels no poorer than 15 dB HL across all the frequencies as recorded on an audiogram.

The current terminology used to describe hearing loss in children is worrisome because the terms are apt to minimize the problems associated with hearing impairment in children. Hearing loss is generally categorized as follows:

    0–15 dB = Normal hearing

    15–25 dB = Slight hearing loss

    25–40 dB = Mild hearing loss

    40–55 dB = Moderate hearing loss

    55–70 dB = Moderately-severe hearing loss

    70–90 dB = Severe hearing loss

    > 90 dB = Profound hearing loss

In a study by Haggard and Primus (1999), 30 parents were asked to compare their listening impressions of speech filtered to simulate slight, mild, and moderate hearing losses to that of an unfiltered or unattenuated speech signal. The parents used descriptors such as "difficult" and "handicapping" to describe even a slight hearing loss. The parents estimated the percent of hearing loss they experienced to be 46%. Ironically, this same slight hearing loss represents a 2% loss using adult standards established by the American Academy of Otolaryngology. The motivation of a parent or a physician to resolve a hearing loss may be poor simply because the term *slight* significantly minimizes the urgency of care the child requires.

Research has consistently found that hearing levels of 20 dB (slight loss), inconsequential for most adults, have a profound impact on a young child's ability to hear and develop age-appropriate language skills (Bess, Dodd-Murphy, & Parker, 1998). Some audiologists have suggested that instead of reporting a "slight" or "mild" loss, it should be stated that any degree of hearing loss places a child "at risk" for educational achievement and to avoid using terms that may be counterproductive to seeking proper follow-up

care. The challenge is to successfully convey the true meaning of a slight hearing loss to parents and other professionals to ensure timely and appropriate treatment.

Facilities and Personnel

Programs designed to provide for the educational needs of students with impaired hearing must address the fundamental questions of who, what, and where, and must provide for a continuum of services from identification to rehabilitation. School districts must determine if audiological and educational services for deaf and hard-of-hearing students will be provided by the local school district (local education authority or LEA), or whether to contract for these services with outside agencies. Smaller districts may find it more cost effective to join educational cooperatives in order to pool limited financial resources.

Hearing screening programs are costly, both for initial start-up, as well as for the provision for annual calibrations, maintenance, and replacement of obsolete audiometric equipment. Many larger school districts and educational cooperatives employ educational audiologists who are able to provide and/or supervise hearing screening programs and provide a full spectrum of audiological services. Basic hearing screening is often completed by school nurses or other trained audiometric technicians. Appropriate training and supervision must be provided to individuals who are not audiologists who provide hearing screening services.

Disastrous results may occur if personnel conducting hearing screenings are not properly trained and supervised. As an example, an inexperienced school nurse "passed" a newly enrolled kindergarten student and allowed the staff to believe that his inability to comply with classroom rules was due to behavior. Eighteen months later, a second nurse completed another hearing screening and correctly made a referral to the educational audiologist, who identified a bilateral moderate hearing loss. The student was mislabeled, lost valuable learning time, and developed inappropriate coping strategies; he did not know he could not hear like all the other students. Locating an appropriate screening location is often one of the greatest challenges because the screening environment must meet standards for allowable noise levels, sometimes nearly impossible to find in many schools. There are specific standards set forth by the American National Standards Institute, which clearly state the allowable noise levels that must be obtained in order to accurately identify students with hearing loss (American National Standards Institute [ANSI], 1991).

Identification and Rehabilitation

School screening programs are designed to identify students who do not have hearing within normal limits—at least on the one day hearing screening is administered. True prevalence of hearing loss is difficult to determine, but recent figures suggest that its prevalence in school-age children is between 11.3% and 14.9% (Adams, Hendershot, & Marano, 1999), with an average of 131 of every 1000 school-age children having some degree of hearing loss that can potentially affect communication and academic achievement. Mass screening has its limitations, as many students pass because the hearing screening was administered on a day when, for example, a student who has chronic ear infections did not happen to have an infec-

tion, or a student who typically has normal hearing had impacted earwax. The possibility for erroneous findings and inaccurate data is endless. When a teacher or parent is told that a particular student passed the hearing screening, it may be wrongly assumed that hearing will be "within normal limits" all year long, and that hearing could not possibly be a factor as to why a student does not attend well in class.

Children with hearing loss at only certain frequencies, or who have normal hearing in only one ear, are at risk for speech, language, and academic challenges. Studies have found that children with unilateral hearing losses repeat a grade at a rate three times that of students with normal hearing in each ear (Bess, 1986; Bess et al., 1998), and many students require additional academic and/or speech or language assistance. Ear-specific or frequency-specific hearing losses are not readily observable, and it is not unusual to find that no accommodations are made for children who seem to "hear just fine." Children are not aware of what they do not hear and often assume that everyone else hears what they hear. It is a rare child who can identify the presence of a hearing loss and ask for assistance. It was surprising when a second grade student with a mild high-frequency hearing loss reported that he could not hear the difference between the spelling words, *oil*, *foil*, and *soil*. It was later found that he had a 130 IQ, which helped explain his ability to listen with a discerning ear.

The educational management of children with minimal hearing loss is under adult control, and Herculean efforts are required to educate parents and teachers on the effects of minimal hearing loss and, more importantly, how to optimize the auditory learning environment at home and at school. In-service presentations and demonstrations simulating different degrees and configurations of hearing loss have generally been found to be effective ways to increase the probability for appropriate educational management. Problems arise, however, because there are no visible signs reminding adults of the presence of a slight or mild hearing loss. Best intentions fade with time, and, sadly, it is not unusual for teachers and parents to forget about the existence of a hearing loss because it is "invisible" to most observers.

Many students have a permanent hearing loss of greater degree and have additional challenges to face. These students often require some type of assistive listening technology in the form of hearing aids, FM systems, and/or cochlear implants. Adult support is needed to help manage this specialized equipment, ensure its proper functioning, and, just as they do for peers with lesser degrees of hearing loss, ensure optimal acoustic access in the learning environment. The challenges in audiological management transform from convincing individuals that a hearing loss exists, to one of convincing teachers to consistently and effectively use the technology the student must have in order to access instruction. If a student with hearing loss is in regular education and requires special accommodations, a 504 plan may be written under the guidelines set forth in the Americans with Disabilities Act (ADA, 1990). In education, a 504 plan is a nonfunded mandate in which schools are required to provide reasonable accommodations that are necessary to address hearing or other difficulties in the learning environment. These accommodations may include such things as the need for teacher in-service, preferential positioning, the consistent use of assistive technology, the use of note-takers, the need for face-to-face instruction, the need for slower paced instruction, extra time on tests, and other modifications that have little to no financial burden.

Listening Environment

This may be the most challenging factor affecting children with impaired hearing, as the listening environment is dynamic—constantly changing throughout the day. If children could be individually taught in a sound booth from birth through age 18, fewer children with hearing impairment would have language or academic difficulties (although social adjustment would surely be affected!). Educational audiologists assess different listening environments and make suggestions to improve the acoustic characteristics of an environment. Factors evaluated include size and shape of a learning space, number of students in a class, noise sources, and the acoustical treatment of the learning environment in terms of the building materials of the ceiling, walls, and floor. These factors change every time the child moves to a different room, or when the teacher simply opens a window, leaving the assumption that a child in question hears just fine.

A child's ability to respond due to a hearing loss may vary across superficially identical situations causing adults to misinterpret a child's behavior. Adults may get frustrated and accuse the child of willfully disobeying. For example, a child in kindergarten with a 30 dB hearing loss may easily turn to his name in the classroom and the teacher interprets this to mean that the child has normal hearing (a poor test of hearing, but unfortunately one that many teachers use). When the child fails to respond to his name on the playground, the teacher asserts that he needs "structure" to comply with the rules, and refers him for further evaluation to address his noncompliant behavioral concerns. The teacher failed to realize that the child, standing upwind of her on a windy spring day with his attention intently focused on successfully crossing the jungle gym, could not possibly have heard her! His inconsistent behavior could easily be explained when examining his hearing abilities across listening environments. Children with hearing loss are victims of the listening environment and adults should be mindful of all the factors that impact acoustic access.

Standards for Schools

In 1998, the U.S. Access Board joined with the Acoustical Society of America (ASA) to support the development of a classroom acoustics standard. Their efforts resulted in the development of ANSI/ASA S12.60-2002, *Acoustical Performance Criteria, Design Requirements and Guidelines for Schools* (ANSI, 2002). The standard sets specific criteria for maximum background noise and reverberation time for unoccupied classrooms, a baseline that can easily be replicated. The standard remains voluntary; however, a few states have opted to officially endorse the standards by writing them into regulation, whereas other states have taken the initiative to require compliance in the development of new construction. These standards are urgently needed as it has been repeatedly shown that poor classroom acoustics affects the learning of all students, but even more so that of students with hearing impairment.

Acoustical measurements in many classrooms built before ANSI/ASA S12.60-2002 exceed the levels set forth in the standards. The current criterion for maximum background noise is 35 dB and reverberation time or "echo" of 0.6 to 0.7 seconds for unoccupied classrooms. Whether the background noise is from internal sources, such as HVAC units or overhead projector fans, or external sources, such as hallway noise and highway traffic, the effects of noise significantly impact the ability of all children, whether they possess impaired or normal hearing, to clearly discriminate all speech sounds and maintain auditory attention. Poorly maintained or inexpensive HVAC units are the most common source of excessively high noise levels in classrooms. High reverberation times also adversely affect speech discrimination abilities due to the masking of soft, high-frequency speech sounds by the reflections of the more prominent, louder, low-frequency speech sounds. In addition, low-frequency sounds are more likely to be reflected and continue to propagate, whereas high-frequency sounds tend to be absorbed, which further compounds the already disproportionate balance of high- and low-frequency speech sounds.

Speaking Habits of Teachers

Another variable that affects children's ability to hear and process instruction are the actual speaking habits of the speaker. Most normal hearing adults can quickly and easily adjust to a wide variety of speaker characteristics. Children, on the other hand, who are still in the stages of learning the rules of speech and language, need special attention paid to the speech model. When talking to children, adults and teachers should focus on using speech that is clear, audible, and well paced, critically important for students who have any degree of hearing loss, and for students who possess normal hearing (Hull, 2008). A speaking rate that is appropriate for children, however, is almost tedious to many adults. A good example of an ideal speech rate for children was Mr. Rogers, the star of the top rated children's show, who spoke at a rate of approximately 124 words per minute. Children seemed to be mesmerized by his delivery of rambling dialogue that was simple, slow, and clear.

When children are actively engaged in listening, the development of speech and language is optimized. Common sense would tell us that a child with a hearing loss needs to have speech presented louder. Efforts have been made to train teachers to "just talk louder," but even after continual speech training, many teachers seem not to be able to maintain more than a slight increase in vocal intensity. On the surface, this appears to be a good solution, and possibly is in some listening environments. However, in a large classroom with poor acoustics and high noise levels, simply using a louder voice tends to distort the speech signal because the discrepancy between voiced and voiceless speech sounds becomes even wider. For example, the vocal tract can make a voiced vowel sound, such as *ah* much louder than a low-intensity, high-frequency speech sound as in *f*.

Educational Placement

The Special Education Law, or the 2004 Individuals with Disabilities Education Act (IDEA), specifies the requirements for the provision of educational services for children with disabilities, including those with hearing impairment. Part H of IDEA sets forth the regulations for children under the age of 3, whereas Part B addresses the needs of school-age children between the ages of 3 and 21. Under these laws, children are guaranteed a free and appropriate education (FAPE). In providing for a FAPE, it is the intent of IDEA to maintain children in the least restrictive environment, or LRE, which for most children is in a regular education setting in a neighborhood school. Anytime a child receives services "away from the ordinary," placement becomes more restrictive and the need for special services must be substantiated. If a child's hearing impairment is such that she cannot fully participate in regular education, the child receives a comprehensive evaluation to first determine the presence of a handicapping condition, and secondly determine if there is a need for special services.

This comprehensive evaluation is multidisciplinary and includes parents, administrators, teachers, speech pathologists, audiologists, psychologists, social workers, school nurses, and other professionals as needed as team members. The team determines to what extent the child qualifies and needs special education services. These services are described through the development of an individual family service plan (IFSP) for children below the age of 3, or an individual educational plan (IEP) if the child is school age. Due to the young age of the child, an IFSP is family focused and provides the family with support and information, monitors the child's development, and provides the family with appropriate community resources. An IFSP also helps to ensure a smooth transition to the school setting and the writing of the first IEP. Based on the results of a comprehensive evaluation, goals and objectives are written, and educational placement is determined. Efforts are made to maintain the student in the least restrictive environment as possible, and the need for support services is determined. Support services may include audiology, speech and language services, occupational and physical therapy, adaptive physical education, nursing, and so forth.

Educational placements vary greatly and many factors enter into the decision-making process. School personnel must consider academic levels, cognitive abilities, communication needs, social needs, and cultural issues before recommending a placement for a student. Educational placements range from attending a neighborhood school with no special services to a full-time residential placement. An evaluation recently took place for a seventh grade student who just moved to the United States with his family from Mexico. The family did not speak English, and he was enrolled in his neighborhood middle school, which had a large Hispanic student population. The student had a moderately-severe hearing loss that was identified when he was a toddler, but the parents could not afford hearing aids for him. The family tried to compensate by always speaking loudly, and spoke very close to him. Hearing aids were fitted as quickly as possible and a comprehensive evaluation was completed. Evaluation results identified some mild language delays in his native language, but normal intellectual abilities. With appropriate amplification, he was able to hear speech within normal limits. It was determined that the LRE would be his neighborhood school because with amplification he could hear classroom instruction and remain in a bilingual (Spanish/English) environment. In addition, he would receive services through a teacher of the deaf and hard of hearing in a consultative model (which meant the teacher would consult with regular education teachers to ensure his continued academic growth), continue to receive intensive instruction through the program for English for other Language Learners (ELL), and receive audiology services to ensure his hearing aids were functioning properly. After the team determined placement and services, goals and objectives were written to address the mild language delay.

A second example illustrates that the LRE is not necessarily a neighborhood school, which is the case with a culturally Deaf student. There are situations when the LRE is one that shares a common communicative mode, as for a child who communicates through sign language. The LRE for a cultur-

ally Deaf child may be one that would provide barrier-free communication with teachers and peers, which may be found in a state or private school for the deaf. The LRE requirements of IDEA must be interpreted thoughtfully and the needs of each individual student carefully and fully assessed.

Technology

Staying technologically current is one of the greatest challenges in providing for the auditory needs of children with hearing impairment in the educational setting. Children enroll in schools with personal hearing aids and listening devices fit from a myriad of fitting sources, particularly in large urban school districts. The educational audiologist must be familiar with a multitude of brands and models of hearing aids and assistive technology that are currently on the market. The educational audiologist must ensure that the hearing instrument meets the listening demands of students in the school setting and ensure that students have acoustic access to instruction throughout the day. This is not a simple task, as neither teachers nor students stay in one place. Students are required to listen from distances from 2 feet to 100 feet and, as has already been discussed, in extremely noisy listening environments.

The need for FM technology is becoming unquestionably apparent and parents and educators are rightfully demanding this technology be provided. There is no "one size fits all" approach as listening requirements vary. The audiologist must consider the age of the student, how many students are in the class, the clustering of students, the number of teachers, the size and construction of the classroom, the need for portability, the listening demands for each setting, and the learning style of the student. Armed with this information, a recommendation for specific FM or infrared (IR) technology can be made. It is then necessary to determine the specific type of receiver to be used by the child, such as a personal earmold, a set of earphones, or a telecoil neckloop, and the type of teacher microphone to be used, such as a lapel microphone, boom microphone, earpiece, or lavaliere microphone. And lastly, and possibly most importantly, what the student and teacher are willing to use must be considered.

To illustrate, a student in the seventh grade with a moderately-severe hearing loss may do well using a personal FM system in school, a system that the student can wear throughout the day in a variety of listening situations. On the other hand, a student in first grade with a slight hearing loss, too minimal of a loss to require amplification, and who remains in one class the majority of the day, may receive appropriate benefit from a free-field sound system. This second example was a fairly straightforward decision until the teacher announced she would not use a boom microphone, the style the school was accustomed to, because she had "big hair" and couldn't easily put it on or take it off. She did thankfully agree to use a lapel microphone.

Free-field sound systems are becoming increasingly common in the school setting. The systems are designed to provide equal distribution of a teacher's voice across a classroom, and provide a consistent 6 to 10 dB signal-to-noise ratio (teacher's voice louder than background noise). After using a sound distribution system, teachers report improved student achievement and attention, and a reduction in fatigue and vocal strain. Many administrators have been convinced that the one-time cost of a sound distribution system, usually around $1000 per classroom, is minimal when compared to the benefit the systems provide students. Recently, the state of Ohio mandated sound distribution systems be installed in all new school construction, and several other states are considering passing similar mandates. Even though sound distribution systems have been found to be beneficial in educational settings, they are not designed to meet the amplification needs for children with impaired hearing.

Children with Cochlear Implants

There is little doubt that cochlear implants have had the greatest impact on the education of deaf and hard-of-hearing students than any other technological advancement. In the early 1990s, it was rare to find a child with a cochlear implant. The early implants, with single electrode insertion, provided little more than what a powerful conventional hearing aid or a tactile aid could provide. However, only a few years later, with the advent of multichannel implants, the auditory potential of deaf children has skyrocketed, and now children with cochlear implants can be found in nearly every school district across the country. Teachers of the deaf, audiologists, and speech-language pathologists have had to scramble to find continuing education opportunities in order to address the needs of our first generation of "hearing deaf children," and deaf education teacher training programs are finding it necessary to modify curriculums to meet these new demands for oral deaf education. Cochlear implants, digital hearing aid technology, and the use of FM and/or IR technology in the schools are advancing so rapidly that this may represent the greatest current challenge in the education of children with hearing impairment.

Communication Mode

In addressing the educational management of children with impaired hearing, a discussion on communication mode is necessary, but it is a topic that often carries a heavy emotional load. Several professionals, including teachers of the deaf, speech-language pathologists, sign language interpreters, audiologists, and physicians, are all stakeholders in the education of children with hearing loss. Each professional receives specialized training and each comes with personal experiences that shape individual perspectives.

Historically, communication modes have included those that are founded on using all possible residual hearing to develop speech and oral language, and the belief that the education of deaf children should focus on the use of the stronger, unimpaired visual sensory system via sign language. The continuum of communication options continues to exist, but with the arrival of cochlear implants, there is renewed interest in oral deaf education options. All perspectives should be understood and respected, and it is not the intent of this chapter to promote or denounce the different philosophies. Rather, a few guiding principles are offered to help the decision-making process that IDEA requires of a multidisciplinary team.

IDEA requires the thoughtful consideration of the communication needs of a child who is deaf or hard of hearing, and many states have implemented a communication plan to further address and clarify the communication needs of students with impaired hearing. This process is directed toward ensuring an objective evaluation of the child by the team of educators and parents who are responsible for optimizing the learning opportunities for each child, and is guided by *five principles*. Those are:

■ *Principle 1: Ability to use residual hearing to access spoken language.* On the surface this seems definable and easily measurable via hearing thresholds (usually aided or implanted) on the audiogram, speech threshold, and word recognition scores. However, a student's ability to use residual hearing, as we have seen, varies across educational settings. It would be misleading to assume that a child's performance in a sound booth, which represents optimal auditory capabilities, is duplicated in a classroom setting. The question becomes, Can the student successfully access spoken language across educational settings by using assistive technology and other supportive measures? What type of technology would be the most beneficial? What support does the student require to efficiently use the technology?

■ *Principle 2: Ability to support an effective visual communication mode, i.e., sign language.* No child will be academically successful if the quality and quantity of sign language is poor. When children require the use of sign language, either as the sole mode of communication, or as a support to spoken language, they are entitled to a clear and consistent visual vocabulary and syntax. What system is in place to ensure signing competency from the teaching and sign language interpreting staff? What measures are taken to ensure family members are utilizing the same signing vocabulary and syntax? What opportunities are there for children to experience barrier-free communication with peers and adult role models who also use sign language?

■ *Principle 3: Impact of Deaf culture.* If the child has deaf parents who utilize

American Sign Language (ASL), how will this language be utilized to facilitate literacy and written language skills? What measures are in place to ensure positive peer relationships across languages and communicative modalities? How will positive adult role models who use ASL be provided?

■ *Principle 4: Communication mode supported and used by the family.* It is important to assess the communication mode used at home by the family, as well as the communication mode the family requests be used at school. It is important for families to understand the importance of providing a consistent initial language, especially for young deaf and hard-of-hearing students. A consistent communication mode should be used at home and at school, and this open dialogue should occur routinely at all IFSP or IEP meetings and recorded on the child's communication plan.

■ *Principle 5: Rate of language acquisition.* Procedural safeguards should be in place to ensure the child's rate of language acquisition is commensurate with learning potential or intelligence quotient (IQ). It is often accepted, and even expected, for deaf and hard-of-hearing students to have deficient language abilities. Many deaf and hard-of-hearing students have the same intellectual capacity as their normal hearing counterparts, and to passively accept deficient language abilities is indefensible. Standardized language assessments should be administered systematically to ensure adequate growth. If a child does not make expected gains, additional support should be provided, and it may involve an inspection of the current communication mode. Is too much of the auditory signal lost? Is the

child not accessing visual communication? Is academic instruction being presented above the child's language level? Is the learning environment acoustically well designed? Does the family have adequate support to become proficient in the chosen communication mode? It is dangerous to believe that a deaf or hard-of-hearing student can "catch up" once academic and language delays are identified, because normal hearing peers do not stop learning to allow this to happen. It is preferable that a specific schedule for periodic assessment should be in place to prevent delays from initially occurring, and to monitor the degree of deficiency if one is already present.

Special Populations

Students may have handicapping conditions in addition to hearing loss that further complicate their educational management. Thorough multidisciplinary team evaluations are required in order to determine the impact of each individual disability on the educational profile of the student. It is often necessary to administer multiple assessments to accurately determine IQ, learning style, sensory processing, and current academic levels, which are critical pieces to determining special education placement. Multidisciplinary teams are required to determine the impact of each handicapping condition and how they interact, and then an appropriate IEP must be developed.

In recalling experiences with students with multiple handicaps, one student in particular pushed the team's knowledge, experience, and creativity to the limits. A once-healthy, active 10-year-old contracted a near-fatal virus that resulted in the loss of legs, one hand, three fingers on the second hand, speech, and language—including reading and most of the hearing. With loss of speech and inability to write, how is knowledge assessed? With loss of hearing and no alternative communication established, how is instruction provided? With absent and limited use of limbs, how are mobility issues addressed? How can an appropriate peer group be provided? An IEP was written with input from a host of professionals all having to think "outside the box" in order to develop appropriate educational services for this student.

The Final Challenge

Every aspect of the educational management of children who are deaf and hard of hearing is complex and requires thoughtful deliberation every step of the way. From screening programs to IEPs, the importance of knowledgeable professionals, parent involvement, and supportive administrators is essential throughout the educational process. Hearing impairment is difficult to manage. It is easy to hide or deny its existence. It is the only handicapping condition that varies in severity from appearing to be nearly nonexistent to profoundly disabling, depending on the listening environment and the speaker, which can vary throughout the day.

The descriptors of hearing loss work against the professionals attempting to obtain proper treatment, and the rapid advancements in technology can easily leave students using "last year's model." And finally, the philosophical debate of methodology leaves many stakeholders so threatened that "do nothing, say nothing" may be their only safe harbor. None of these challenges represents appropriate ends. However, they should be considered opportunities for professionals to earnestly collaborate and learn from each other. They represent the need to challenge ourselves to find the solutions to meet the learning potential of each deaf and hard-of-hearing student who crosses our educational threshold.

References

Adams, P. F., Hendershot, G. E., & Marano, M. A. (1999). Current estimates from the National Health Interview Survey, 1996. *Vital and Health Statistics, 10*(200).

American National Standards Institute. (1991). *Maximum permissible ambient noise levels for audiometric test rooms* (ANSI S3.1-1991). New York: Acoustical Society of America.

American National Standards Institute. (2002). *Acoustical performance criteria, design requirements, and guidelines for schools* (ANSI S12.60-2002). Melville, NY: Acoustical Society of America.

American Speech-Language-Hearing Association. (1993). Guidelines for audiology services in schools. *Asha, 35*(Suppl. 10), 24–32.

American Speech-Language-Hearing Association. (2002). *Guidelines for fitting and monitoring FM systems.* Rockville, MD: Author.

American Speech-Language-Hearing Association. (2005). *Guidelines for addressing acoustics in educational settings.* Rockville, MD: Author.

Americans with Disabilities Act of 1990—P.L. 101-336, 42 USC §§ 12101 et seq. (1990).

Bess, F. H. (1986). The unilaterally hearing-impaired child: A final comment. *Ear and Hearing, 7,* 52–55.

Bess, F. H., Dodd-Murphy, J., & Parker, R. A. (1998). Children with minimal sensorineural hearing loss: Prevalence, educational performance, and functional status. *Ear and Hearing, 19*(5), 339–354.

Crandell, C. (1991). Effects of classroom acoustics on children with normal hearing: Implications for intervention strategies. *Educational Audiology Monograph, 2,* 18–38.

Crandell, C., & Smaldino, J. (1996). Sound field amplification in the classroom: Applied and theoretical issues. In F. Bess, J. Gravel, & A. Tharpe (Eds.), *Amplification for children with auditory deficits* (pp. 229-250). Nashville, TN: Vanderbilt Bill Wilkerson Center Press.

Crandell, C., Smaldino, J., & Flexer, C. (1995). *Sound field FM amplification: Theory and practical applications.* San Diego, CA: Singular.

Davis, J. (1974). Performance of young hearing-impaired children on a test of basic concepts. *Journal of Speech and Hearing Research, 17,* 342-351.

Davis, J. (1990). *Our forgotten children: Hard-of-hearing pupils in the schools.* Washington, DC: U.S. Department of Education.

Finitzo-Hieber, T. (1988). Classroom acoustics. In R. Roeser (Ed.), *Auditory disorders in school children* (2nd ed., pp. 223-257). New York: Thieme-Stratton.

Flexer, C. (1994). *Facilitating hearing and listening in young children.* San Diego, CA: Singular.

Gravel, J. S., & Wallace, I. F. (1998). Audiological management of otitis media. In F. Bess (Ed.), *Children with hearing impairment: Contemporary trends* (pp. 221-227). Nashville, TN: Vanderbilt Bill Wilkerson Center Press.

Haggard, R. S., & Primus, M. A. (1999). Parental perceptions of hearing loss classification in children. *American Journal of Audiology, 8,* 83-92.

Hull, R. H. (2008). How to talk to children. A. Banotai (Interview). *Advance for Speech-Language Pathologists and Audiologists, 18,* 6-9.

Individuals with Disabilities Education Act-Reauthorization 1997, 20 USC §§ 1400 et seq.

Nelson, P. B., & Soli, S. (2000). Acoustical barriers to learning: Children at risk in every classroom. *Language, Speech and Hearing Services in Schools, 31*(4), 356-361.

Oyler, R. F., Oyler, A. L., & Matkin, N. D. (1988). Unilateral hearing loss: Demographics and educational impact. *Language, Speech and Hearing Services in Schools, 19,* 201-209.

The Rehabilitation Act of 1973—P.L. 93-112, 29 USC § 794, Section 504. (1973).

Seep, B., Glosemeyer, R., Hulce, E., Linn, M., & Aytar, P. (2000). *Classroom acoustics.* Melville, NY: Acoustical Society of America.

End of Chapter Examination Questions

Chapter 10

1. **It is advisable to carefully use the descriptive terms of "slight" or "mild" when categorizing hearing loss in children because:**
    a. It is difficult to obtain insurance coverage for this minimal degree of hearing loss.
    b. Parents may overreact and make unnecessary demands on school districts.
    c. The terms minimize the hearing difficulties, which is counterproductive to receiving adequate treatment.
    d. It is acceptable to only use these terms if the hearing loss is permanent.
    e. Schools using these terms may be required to reimburse parents for medical treatment.

2. **The American National Standards Institute has established which of the following standards in regards to hearing screening in the schools?**
    a. Maximum allowable ambient room noise
    b. The number of students to be screened per hour
    c. The minimum competencies of an individual administering hearing screening
    d. Hearing referral criteria
    e. The frequency of hearing screenings from birth through age 21

3. **Which of the following factors has the least impact on acoustic access?**
    a. Background noise
    b. Distance
    c. Reverberation
    d. Rate of speech
    e. Female voices

4. **Which of the following is not a component of IDEA?**
    a. Free and appropriate public education
    b. Individual education plan
    c. Individual family service plan
    d. Rehabilitation 504 plan
    e. Least restrictive environment

5. **In developing a communication plan for deaf and hard-of-hearing students, which factor would be least likely to be addressed?**
    a. Degree of hearing loss and ability to "hear" spoken language
    b. Communication method chosen by the family
    c. Socioeconomic status of the family
    d. Availability of deaf role models and interpreters
    e. Family's ability to receive opportunities to develop adequate signing skills.

End of Chapter Answer Sheet

Name _____   Date _____

Chapter 10

1. Which one?   a   b   c   d   e

2. Which one?   a   b   c   d   e

3. Which one?   a   b   c   d   e

4. Which one?   a   b   c   d   e

5. Which one?   a   b   c   d   e

PART III

Introduction to Aural Rehabilitation: Adults Who Are Hearing Impaired

11

Aural Rehabilitation for Adults: Theory and Application

RAYMOND H. HULL

Introduction

One of the basic premises in serving adults who possess impaired hearing is that some form of rehabilitative service should accompany the discovery of a hearing loss. The most successful approaches to aural rehabilitation appear to be those that address and incorporate procedures that specifically address the short-term and long-term objectives of the patient, planned jointly with the audiologist. Even though this chapter addresses a number of avenues and approaches to aural rehabilitation, it must be remembered that the complexities observed in individual adults with impaired hearing require a patient-oriented approach to treatment. Using a "method" without considering the specific needs of patients will probably result in inadequate treatment.

Techniques for Improving Communication for Adults Who Are Hearing Impaired: Past and Present

Before addressing current issues involved in the process of aural rehabilitation for adults, a review of issues and early approaches is appropriate.

Early Approaches to Serving Adults with Impaired Hearing

Lipreading

Most people do not find total reliance on the visibility of the phonemes of speech to be sufficient for purposes of communication. However, it has been difficult over the years to extinguish the term *lipreading* from its connotation of a vision-only mode of communication, and, for some laypersons, from the process of aural rehabilitation.

Early definitions of lipreading, such as Bruhn (1949), stressed the eye as literally taking the place of the ear. She believed that the eye could be trained to distinguish the visible characteristics of the movements of the speech mechanism. Such descriptions of lipreading have been passed on through the years, and the term still tends to denote a strict concentration on the visualization of speech.

Other early methods of lipreading stressing the primary use of vision were those of Bunger (1961), Kinzie & Kinzie (1931), and Nitchie (1950). In the early to middle part of the last century, however, it was undoubtedly more necessary to emphasize the visual mode in communication when providing therapy for hearing-impaired adults. As stated by McCarthy and Alpiner (1983), the visual-only methods stressed in early attempts at aural rehabilitation were necessary because of lack of efficient amplification systems.

Even though they are used very infrequently today, a review of those early methods is appropriate for historical purposes, as it is from these that our more current procedures have either evolved or deviated. For a more in-depth look at various early approaches to lipreading instruction, French-St. George and Stoker (1988) have presented a concise historical discussion of that topic.

The Mueller-Walle Method

Martha Bruhn introduced the Mueller-Walle method in 1902. This method was strictly analytic in its approach. It stressed the development of lipreading skills through kinesthetic awareness of the movements involved in speech production. It involved rapid, rhythmic syllable drills, as it was believed that the syllable is the basic unit of words and in turn compose sentences, and they should be subconsciously recognized. Bruhn viewed lipreading as training the eye as well as the mind and believed that it involved visual, auditory, and motor memory. Her plans for lipreading lessons were divided into four parts:

1. Definition of the movement(s) of the new sound to be studied, contrasting the movements of the new sound with the ones previously studied;
2. Written work;
3. A story or talk that incorporated the new sounds; and
4. Group practice, or a period of questions.

Jena Method

Anna Bunger and Bessie Whitaker introduced the Jena method of lipreading. The method was originally developed by Karl Brauckmann of Germany. Bunger (1944, 1961) outlined Brauckmann's method, which emphasizes the audible, visible, movement, mimetic, and gesture forms of communication, including syllables and rhythm. The movement form was thought of as being complete for all persons, no matter what the level of hearing, as not all movements of the muscular system for speech are completely visible. The mimetic form was viewed as incomplete, but an important component of communication. Brauckmann also believed that the gesture form is not complete, but that it complements all others. Bunger (1961) states that the first aim of persons who desire to learn lipreading is to develop awareness of the movements of speech and to learn how they feel. This was called *kinesthetic awareness*, which was then to become a substitute for audition.

The Jena method included an explanation of the formation and composition of syllables. The consonants were presented and classified under the categories of production, including lips, tongue, and tongue-soft palate. The consonants were combined with words for practice. The consonants were said aloud by the clinician and then the patient said them. Patients were asked to concentrate on the manner of articulation for their production and to categorize consonants in accordance with the three areas of production.

The rhythmic component of this method included a basic pattern that was established to accompany the syllable drills, such as hand clapping, tapping, or ball bouncing. The aim of this aspect was to alert the patient to the feeling of speech movements as he talks and to imitate visible speech movements as another person is speaking. The materials used included syllable exercises, grammatical forms, and stories and conversations.

The Nitchie Approach

In 1903, Edward Nitchie introduced an approach that was intended to break away from the more analytic approaches. His method advocated a "whole thought" approach to lipreading by emphasizing a working relationship between mind and eye. This mode of thinking paved the way toward a more psychological-synthetic basis for lipreading. Stress was placed on grasping the whole of a message when not all auditory information was available. This was in contrast to the philosophies of Bruhn and Bunger, which stressed working with the analytic components of speech. Elizabeth Nitchie (1950), Edward's wife, later revised his materials and added additional ones. However, the integrity of Edward's holistic approach was retained. Ordman and Ralli (1957) utilized Nitchie's approach and, with the aid of Elizabeth Nitchie, developed "lifelike" materials for use in lipreading lessons. The result was a book of lessons entitled, *What People Say*.

The Kinzie Approach

The Kinzie sisters, Cora and Rose (1931), designed a lipreading approach and materials that evolved from a philosophy that incorporated portions of those by Mueller-Walle and Nitchie; it is considered a synthetic approach. Their method involved a graded sequence of lipreading lessons based on varying levels of lipreading ability for both children and adults. The grading of the lessons was included so that individuals could progress from one level of skill to the next at their own rate.

In the development of their materials, several rules were established:

1. Sentences that were definite should be used.
2. Sentences should be natural in structure.
3. Word selection should also be natural.
4. Sentences should be interesting, pleasing, and rhythmic.
5. All sentences must be dignified.

For their story sections, the Kinzies chose items that were short and humorous. They felt that these held the greatest value for beginners and intermediates. They also chose stories about famous people for these two levels. They felt that higher level literary selections were most appropriate for advanced patients.

As part of their lessons, explanations of articulatory movements for sound production were made, including sample words that contained those sounds, along with contrasting words. Vocabulary lists preceded sentence work. More advanced lessons included stories and accompanying ques-

tions. Mirror work in relation to sound production was advocated during lipreading practice. They also stressed the use of voice during lessons to aid patients in the use of their residual hearing. Their materials for adults included 36 lessons on movements of sounds, 36 lessons with stories, and 18 lessons utilizing homophonous words.

Discussion of Early Approaches

The methods reviewed above were generally administered to patients in strict, unalterable ways. When patients had progressed through the lessons to the point of completing them or had advanced in their lipreading skills to their apparent maximum, they were dismissed. The actual success rate is still unknown, although many patients apparently felt that they benefitted. And some probably did. In one way or another, they were perhaps better able to understand the speech of others, or at least attend to the visual aspects of speech with greater efficiency in spite of the fact that they did not have the advantage of high-technology amplification devices.

According to Hull (2001), however, strict methods of lipreading that are presented as a structured sequence of lessons are generally believed to be unsatisfactory for two basic reasons:

1. After the sequence has been completed, patients generally emerge unchanged in their ability to communicate with others. Even though individual patients may thank the audiologist who provided the lipreading sessions by saying, "I surely learned a lot," or "Thank you, your lessons were very interesting," they may have concluded that they did not improve.

2. Those approaches do not lend themselves to a basic need in the process of aural rehabilitation. That is, the programs do not address the specific communicative difficulties that patients face on a daily basis, or help them to communicate in their priority communicative environments with greater efficiency.

The strict approaches described, and others like them, are based on the assumption that if the lessons are adhered to and learned, they will help people with impaired hearing to identify the visual clues of speech. In that regard, then, it was felt that patients would likewise be able to communicate better within their everyday worlds. Although the assumption appeared rational to those who advocated the use of those approaches, it is probably not a valid one.

The Efficiency of Vision in Communication

The early approaches to aural rehabilitation emphasized the use of vision to take the place of, or at least strongly supplement, impaired hearing in communication. How much does vision enhance communication when hearing is impaired? A number of investigators have studied the efficiency of vision in speech reception. The purpose of the majority of those investigations was to study the reciprocal benefits of vision and audition. However, early studies by Berger (1972), Binnie and Barrager (1969), Binnie, Montgomery, and Jackson (1976), Brannon (1961), DiCarlo and Kataja (1951), Erber (1969, 1979), Franks and Kimble (1972), Heider and Heider (1940), Hull and Alpiner (1976b), Hutton (1959), O'Neill (1954), Utley (1946), and Woodward and Barber (1960) have concluded that vision alone can contribute as much as 30 to 50% to speech intelligibility when no auditory information is available.

An early study by Erber (1969), for example, confirmed that for essentially inaudible speech, intelligibility scores in vision-alone conditions remain at about 50%. Hull and Alpiner (1976b) reported that among young adults with normal language function, approximately 50% of linguistically and phonemically balanced words within sentences could be identified by vision alone. They also found that only about 30% of sentences could be identified relative to their content when participants were forced to depend on vision as the only sensory modality.

Whether hearing-impaired adults can, through training, improve in their ability to recognize the phonemes of speech and then transfer that ability to improved understanding of conversational speech continues to be a matter of debate (Walden, Erdman, Montgomery, Schwartz, & Prosek, 1981). Some feel that it is a trait that some possess naturally and others do not. However, early studies on the effect of training on the visual recognition of vowels and consonants (Armstrong, 1974; Black, 1957; Black, O'Reilly, & Peck, 1963; Franks, 1976; Hutton, 1959; Walden, Prosek, Montgomery, Scherr, & Jones, 1977, and others) generally revealed anywhere from subtle to dramatic improvements in phoneme and word recognition. Again, whether vision can be used in speech recognition or whether it varies naturally from person to person continues to be a matter of debate. A lengthy discussion of early research on the complement of vision for the hearing impaired is found in O'Neill and Oyer (1981).

Audition Complements Vision

An early study by Erber (1979), as discussed earlier, demonstrated that vision alone under optimal conditions leads to only about 30 to 50% intelligibility. For children who possess a severe sensorineural hearing loss, vision alone contributed approximately 35 to 41% intelligibility. However, this study, like others, demonstrated the considerable complement of vision to audition and audition to vision. For example, in utilizing a mechanism for systematically manipulating the amount of visual clarity available to subjects (Plexiglas placed at various distances to simulate visual acuity of from 20/20—normal—to 20/400—severe visual deficit), Erber found a 44% advantage when clear visual clues were available and audition was available at a comfortable listening level. This advantage was maintained in spite of a simulated severe high-frequency hearing loss (450 Hz low-pass filter with a 35 dB roll-off per octave). Even with the simulated high-frequency hearing loss, scores increased from 54% intelligibility for single words in the vision-alone mode at 20/20 vision to 98% when a distorted low-pass auditory mode was also introduced, demonstrating the significant complement of vision to low-frequency hearing when there is a high-frequency hearing loss.

In the early study cited above, conducted with severely hearing-impaired children, in which variable distortions of the visual portion were used, results of the identification of content words within sentences indicated that the benefit of the children's dominant sensory modality (vision) is great under optimal conditions (20/20 vision), but still only allows for approximately 33% intelligibility. When their amplified residual hearing was combined with clear vision, youngsters' intelligibility scores increased to 68%. For profoundly hearing-impaired children, the contribution of the auditory modality was found to be only 6%. However, the combined auditory and visual benefit was 47%. When vision was reduced to replicate

a severe loss of vision, scores dropped to 4%. Again, the complement of audition to vision is evident, but only proportionate to the degree of auditory impairment.

The majority of adventitiously hearing-impaired adults are found within the moderate hearing loss categories, where the complement of audition to vision and vice versa is very evident, and the benefits of vision alone are generally minimal. In an early study by Hull and Alpiner (1976a), the reasons for the lack of definitiveness in the visual-only reception of speech are probably that some phonemes look alike; some phonemes are difficult to identify, because they are not visible by observing the lips (only about one third of the phonemes of American English are readily recognizable by observing the face of the speaker). Also, there is a general lack of redundancy of the visemes of speech relative to the comprehension of verbal messages. In the end, audition, even at minimal levels, adds greatly to the synthesis and closure required to comprehend speech.

Other early studies that confirm the complement of audition to vision include those by Binnie et al. (1976), Erber (1971), Hull and Alpiner (1976a), Hutton, Curry, and Armstrong (1969), Miller and Nicely (1955), Montgomery, Walden, Schwartz, and Prosek (1984), O'Neill (1954), Prall (1957), Sumby and Pollack (1954), van Uden (1960), Walden et al. (1977), Walden et al. (1981), among others.

Discussing This Information with Your Patient

Although it is important for patients to recognize the benefits of vision in communication, particularly in adverse listening environments, the efficient use of their residual hearing should also be emphasized during aural rehabilitation. They should be made aware not only of the limitations imposed by their impaired hearing, but also of the amount of residual hearing that is available for use. Both should also be discussed in light of efficient and complementary combined uses of audition and vision in communication.

Current Approaches

Improving Communication Skills through Aural Rehabilitation

Up to this point, the discussion in this chapter has centered on early traditional methods used in attempts at improving hearing impaired persons' ability to communicate in their worlds, including the benefits and limitations of the sensory modalities used in verbal communication. As noted earlier, the approaches to aural rehabilitation for adults that appear to be most effective are those that are holistic in philosophy—that is, they address the specific communicative problems and needs of individual patients. There is more to resolving a communication deficit resulting from an adventitious hearing loss than learning to use one's residual hearing and complementary visual clues. That is not to say, however, that these aspects are not important in the process of enhancing one's ability to communicate with others.

The most critical element in the process of aural rehabilitation is the patient. This is where some of the earlier methods failed. Patient-centered aural rehabilitation services for the adult include those by Alpiner (1987), Alpiner and Garstecki (1996), Alpiner and McCarthy (2000), Binnie (1976), Colton (1977), Fleming, Birkle, Kolman, Miltenberger, and Israel (1973), Giolas (1994),

Hull (1982, 2001), Maurer and Schow (1996), and Tannahill and Smoski (1978). Alpiner (1987) states that the goal of therapy for adults is to provide support, to help patients recognize where their communication problems exist, and to overcome them to the degree possible.

Hull (2001) stresses the importance of addressing the patient's specific communicative needs. Although the majority of the problems hearing-impaired adults encounter revolve around a decreased ability to hear and understand the speech of others especially in adverse listening environments, each patient faces uniquely individual difficulties as a result of his auditory deficit. In order for aural rehabilitation treatment to be appropriate and meaningful for patients, the approach must relate to their specific problems and communicative needs (Hull, 2001, p. 182). It is critical that audiologists adhere to philosophies that address aural rehabilitation as a many-faceted process that goes beyond the earlier procedures that stress primarily speechreading and auditory training.

Approaches to Aural Rehabilitation for Adults

More traditional, early approaches include, for example, those of O'Neill and Oyer (1981). In their discussion of visual training, they refer to a number of avenues to train the hearing-impaired individual to use vision more fully as a means of communication. O'Neill and Oyer suggest that the visual form of training accomplishes two purposes for the patient. Those are, first, the development of visual concentration, and second, the development of synthetic ability.

In the same treatise on aural rehabilitation, O'Neill and Oyer (1981) also present a suggested approach to training patients in the combined use of visual and auditory clues. They state:

> The initial stages of aural rehabilitation involve training without voice so that the hard of hearing person can focus his attention upon the visual aspects of speech. If such an approach is not employed from the beginning, the auditory channel will be used exclusively and the subject will not try to make use of the visual cues. Only because of this initial "sensory" isolation will the individual be alerted to the use of lipreading alone. (pp. 74–75)

Even though their rationale for the visual-only training has merit in some instances for some patients, it behooves audiologists to avoid unisensory approaches.

The O'Neill and Oyer (1981) approach to the combined use of vision and audition includes beginning with practice in environmental noise conditions—in other words, not in an ideal communication situation. The steps advocated by those authors include:

1. Progress from words utilizing lip sounds to words with open articulation (vowel) sounds;
2. Enhance auditory discrimination of isolated sounds;
3. Work with amplified sound, introduced first at threshold, and then gradually increased to make a smooth transfer from vision to combined vision and audition;
4. Associate gestures and facial expression with quality and rate of speech;
5. Use phrases, sentences, and stories;
6. Promote story retention (thought level rather than words or sentences), assessed by multiple-choice tests.

A summary of the first 4 weeks of lessons, as described by O'Neill and Oyer, is as follows:

1st day: Explanation of purpose of program. Discussion of the value of combined practice. Demonstration of contributions of vision alone, audition alone, and vision and audition together.

2nd day: Fifteen minutes of practice on "speech without auditory cues," followed by 15 minutes of practice on "speech without visual cues."

3rd day: Initial listening in noise practice.

4th and 5th days: Thirty minutes of practice understanding individual words against interfering noises. Individual monosyllabic words in contrasting pairs are used in the practice.

6th and 7th days: Practice in listening without auditory cues. Paired words differing only in vowel composition. Fifteen minutes of practice with vowel discrimination against a noise background (recordings of various environmental noises).

8th and 9th days: Review of practice with selected consonants and vowels as incorporated in monosyllabic words.

10th day: Discussion of hearing aids and how they assist in lipreading. Discussion of benefits of hearing aids and effects of auditory "sets", plus discussion of critical listening and viewing.

11th day: Practice in speech discrimination. Sentences and phrases. Viewing alone, auditory alone, and combined. Listening against noise backgrounds using phrases.

12th and 13th days: Intelligibility practice with sentences, without voice, with voice, in noise, and in quiet.

14th and 15th days: Practice in rapid response to sentences.

16th day: Demonstration of "whole" approach with magazine covers. Stress recall of thoughts. Present description of pictures with no voice, low voice, and conversational voice.

17th day: Work on developing tolerance for noise. Discuss that noise has semantic as well as acoustic aspects.

18th day: Practice on colloquial forms using subject areas: newspapers, automobiles, magazines, and cigarettes. Use of intermittent noise backgrounds with combined approach.

19th day: Situation practice. Discussion of people and objects in the clinic. Go over daily newspaper items, short stories from *Reader's Digest* and *The New Yorker*. Use of white noise as background.

20th day: Start incorporating tachistoscopic practice with 5- and 6-digit numbers presented at 1/50 of a second.

Another traditional approach has been presented by Sanders (1993). He believes that what should constitute a tailored management program for adults with impaired hearing can be facilitated by comparing the task to a problem-solving model. His approach involves the following stages:

1. Defining the problem;
2. Assessing the patient's needs;
3. Establishing goals;
4. Determining methods for goal achievement; and
5. Evaluating effectiveness of intervention strategies.

Sanders (1993) states that even though formal approaches to lipreading can be utilized for both adults and children, they "should not detract the teacher from grasping every opportunity to meet the (special) needs . . . both of individual students and of the group" (p. 495). He stresses the importance of viewing aural rehabilitative management from the standpoint of the effects of the disability or handicap that the patient is experiencing as a result of the hearing loss. He emphasizes that one's need for aural rehabilitation services becomes evident when: (a) the patient's communication abilities are no longer adequate to permit the patient to meet the demands encountered in his daily life; (b) the psychological cost of meeting daily demands is judged to be too high; (c) the level of communication abilities, although somewhat adequate, will limit advancement of the adult.

Sanders (1993) advocates the use of a profile questionnaire approach to probe the difficulties that a patient is experiencing, and then to attempt to resolve them to the degree possible. The areas probed include the patient's:

1. Home environment;
2. Work environment; and
3. Social environments.

One must recognize that the relative importance of these areas will differ from patient to patient.

The Committee of Aural Rehabilitation of The American Speech-Language-Hearing Association (ASHA; Freeland et al., 1974), as a result of a historic meeting that resulted in a classic publication on aural rehabilitation, presented an approach that involves more than just a formal approach to the use of visual and auditory clues in communication. Even though it is well over 30 years old, it emphasizes sound methodologies in aural rehabilitation, and includes the following components:

1. Evaluation of peripheral and central auditory disorders;
2. Development or remediation of communication skills through specific training methods;
3. Use of electronic devices to increase sensory input (auditory, vibratory, and others) for speech perception;
4. Counseling regarding the auditory deficit;
5. Periodic reevaluation of auditory function;
6. Assessment of the effectiveness of the procedures used in habilitation.

McCarthy and Culpepper (1987) suggest a "progressive approach" to aural rehabilitation treatment that is based on modifying the patients' behavior and attitudes, the patients' communicative environments, or a combination of both. In modifying the patients' behavior and attitudes, the emphasis is on developing a willingness to:

1. Admit the existence of the hearing loss and its handicapping effects;
2. Admit the hearing loss to others;
3. Take positive action to reduce communication difficulties, for example, by asking others to repeat and speak more clearly and requesting selective seating.

According to these authors, the sequence of their approach involves:

1. Audiologic and hearing aid evaluation;
2. Assessment of communication function;
3. Identification of problem areas due to hearing loss;
4. Verbal discussion in a group or individual basis regarding problems;
5. Admission of hearing loss to self and to others;

6. Modification of behavior, attitudes, and environment;
7. Willingness to utilize amplification in nonthreatening therapy sessions;
8. Reduction of stress in communication situations;
9. Willingness to utilize amplification outside of therapy sessions;
10. More effective communication with normal hearing persons;
11. Termination of therapy (McCarthy & Culpepper, 1987, p. 100).

The McCarthy and Culpepper approach concentrates on the psychological impact of hearing impairment and a patient's response to the deficits experienced in his environment. The philosophy seems appropriate for portions of an aural rehabilitation treatment program, and addresses important areas to be covered. It is to be stressed here, however, that not all audiologists are trained as counselors. Those untrained in counseling should not venture into areas where problems (emotional or otherwise) require help by professionals who are trained to do so.

McCarthy and Culpepper (1987) stress that aural rehabilitation is a comprehensive process composed of interacting components. They state that the purpose of an aural rehabilitation program is to focus on assisting hearing-impaired persons in realizing their optimal potential (Freeland et al., 1974). The important components of an aural rehabilitation program of hearing impaired adults, according to McCarthy and Culpepper (1987), include:

1. Visual training, including speechreading and interpretation of nonspeech stimuli such as gestures and environmental cues;
2. Auditory training, which involves listening training, or developing auditory attending behaviors;
3. Speech conservation; and
4. Counseling.

Giolas (1994) stresses two major components of aural rehabilitation treatment: (a) optimal use of auditory cues and (b) communication strategies. From those, five subcomponents are derived. Those involve (a) a thorough program of hearing aid orientation, (b) the use of visual cues in communication, (c) the conservative uses of lipreading, (d) the manipulation of one's listening environment, and (e) responses to auditory failure and repair strategies.

Hull (2001) presents a holistic approach to aural rehabilitation treatment. It involves (a) counseling, (b) hearing aid orientation, (c) designing a program for increased communicative efficiency that is based on individual patients' prioritized needs, (d) specific treatment procedures that address those prioritized needs, and (e) evaluation of success (or lack of it) in the patient's aural rehabilitation program. This approach lends itself to both younger and older adult patients. Its premises are that, *first*, each patient has special priority needs that revolve around his frequent communicative environments; *second*, most patients can benefit from specific treatment techniques that are based on factors of interactive communication if brought to a higher level of awareness; and *third*, the majority of adults with impaired hearing complain of difficulty communicating in noisy or otherwise distracting environments. Learning about the reasons for difficulty in those environments and practicing strategies of coping or making change in them can be of common benefit to most patients.

Aural Rehabilitation Applications

In the end, specific approaches, alone or in combination, rarely fit the needs of all patients with impaired hearing. It is considered by this author that best practice for audiologists is to develop a holistic or eclectic philosophy regarding aural rehabilitation that will result in services that fit individual patients' specific prioritized communicative needs.

What, then, is aural rehabilitation for adults? A holistic philosophy that would serve audiologists well was written almost 50 years ago by Braceland (1963). He stated that rehabilitation, in its broadest sense, involves a philosophy that a person who possesses an impairment has the right to be helped to become a complete person and, not only to be restored as much as possible to usefulness and dignity, but also to be aided in reaching his own highest potential. That is a far-reaching philosophy that should guide all persons who work in helping professions. In aural rehabilitation, however, such a philosophy should guide the audiologist to serve the needs of individual patients who possess specific communicative needs. Thus, not every adult with impaired hearing should be placed in long-term aural rehabilitation treatment groups, nor do all require extensive hearing aid orientation, nor do all have the same communicative needs.

Such a philosophy suggests that, for some, the process of aural rehabilitation may involve:

1. A session or two to discuss difficult listening situations that they experience in their daily lives and develop strategies for dealing successfully with them;
2. A few sessions of hearing aid orientation to adjust satisfactorily to their hearing aids, those with whom they communicate, and the places where they communicate;
3. A full program of auditory rehabilitation sessions that involve problem solving and the development of communicative strategies either in group or individual sessions. If the difficulties experienced by the patient warrant a full program of

treatment, this author prefers that new patients be involved in individual work at least for several weeks before being introduced into a group setting.

Principles of Aural Rehabilitation

The following are principles that can guide the planning and execution of efficient aural rehabilitation programs for adult patients. However, these principles are not intended to supplant the good judgment of a skilled audiologist. In the absence of an extensive body of knowledge surrounding these topics, however, the following are offered as considerations that have guided this author and were originally discussed in part by Bode and Tweedie (1982), and by Hull (2001, 2007). They further have guided practicing audiologists over the years, as practiced and reported by them.

1. **Aural Rehabilitation treatment should always address the specific needs of the patient.** Although obvious, this principle appears in many instances to have been ignored. If a patient is having difficulty communicating in a specific environment or with a specific person, then it is critically important that the audiologist work with him to develop strategies to address those specific difficulties. The individualized strategies often generalize to other situations as the patient develops the resolve, the self-confidence, and plans of action to overcome the original difficulties.

2. **Because older patients with presbycusis can have both peripheral and central auditory involvement, environmental design strategies can be effective in enhancing speech understanding.** This aspect of aural rehabilitation service not only involves development of listening strategies that accommodate auditory decline in the peripheral and central nervous system of aging patients, but also includes environmental design strategies that can enhance speech understanding. Treatment that enhances cognitive function that can otherwise impair auditory/linguistic processing can also be utilized —including strategies for analysis and synthesis of auditory/linguistic information, speed of auditory processing, accuracy of attending behaviors, and auditory sorting behaviors.

3. **Empowering patients to become more assertive enhances their ability to improve their communication environment, which is an essential component of treatment.** Assertiveness can be an important treatment objective, and should be a goal in patient counseling. The patient can learn to stage-manage communication events and environments to maximize the probability of successful participation. Reducing background noise levels, decreasing the distance from a talker, optimizing lighting for speech-reading cues, requesting that the talker speak with greater clarity or use the microphone (at speaking engagements), and manipulating the design of the environment to one's communicative advantage are examples of how the patient can be a positive catalyst in improving the communication environment.

4. **The clinician should model effective communication.** Clear, articulate speech without unnatural overarticulation should be the norm. Appropriate speech intensity levels for maximum intelligibility in a variety of listening

situations should be sought. Unintentional masking of visible speech by hand or head movements should be noted and avoided. By being an example of a good communicator, the audiologist demonstrates what patients with hearing loss should expect from their most effective communication partners. Further, the patient can teach others about effective communication skills.

5. **The patient and clinician should work together to develop specific auditory training goals and objectives.** Because audiologic rehabilitation is a learning process, the patient must be made aware of his part and responsibility. The patient's active involvement is of paramount importance. Carryover into real-life situations cannot be fully accomplished unless the patient accepts his responsibility in the process.

6. **Individual and group treatment programs should be available to patients.** Group sessions permit the patient to discuss communication problems with peers who may have similar problems, but each patient must be carefully evaluated as to his potential for successful entry into a group environment. Some patients should begin individual treatment before joining a group, either because their communication difficulties may negatively affect their ability to interact in a group environment, or their communication problems are simply not conducive to group discussion. For patients who are a good fit for group work, this type of treatment can be a powerful tool for the development of a more positive attitude about their hearing loss, because others in the group may be able to offer helpful strategies that they found successful. In addition, group problem-solving sessions can be extremely beneficial.

7. **Treatment activities should offer opportunities for successful communication.** Interesting and challenging activities can be planned; social activities for aural rehabilitation groups in which techniques of successful communication can be practiced in a controlled and nurturing environment can be a positive treatment tool. Developing and maintaining motivation are important potential effects of a relationship wherein humor, active involvement, and dynamic interaction are important parts of treatment.

8. **Counseling is essential to the effectiveness of the clinician-patient relationship.** Counseling is one of the most important activities involved in audiologic rehabilitation. In that regard, major attention and effort must be directed toward developing counseling skills in audiology students and clinicians so that they can become effective listeners, provide constructive support, facilitate problem solving, instill confidence, and be a catalyst in the development of strategies to resolve difficult listening and communicative environments.

9. **Patients should be encouraged to maintain a balance between the give-and-take of communication, and to have realistic expectations.** The patient may need counseling to develop skills in how to be assertive and to listen when communicating. Acceptance of realistic expectations also should be addressed. Not every communicative environment can be changed, nor can all speakers be taught how to communicate effectively. The patient may assume too much personal responsibility for specific communicative failures. Further, we must encourage the patient to develop realistic expectations relative to amplification.

No matter what technologic heights hearing aid design has reached, it cannot be expected to match the full range of human hearing, nor can they resolve all of the environments in which the person with impaired hearing finds himself. We live in a world of speakers who are poorer than desired and environments that are not made for communication. Hearing aids cannot correct for those barriers.

10. **Clinicians should assist patients in developing alternative behaviors and responses for specific communication events.** Some patients adopt avoidance or withdrawal behaviors in situations requiring their participation in interactive communication, particularly when they may have previously had frustrating experiences in that place or with that person. Planning for these difficult situations might include activities that involve principles of effective interactive or interpersonal communication that are specific to that environment or with the speaker. These, for example, may include rehearsing their participation in a wedding, as a greeter at a social event, or in conducting a business meeting for an organization.

11. **Incorporating hearing assistive technology can be an effective part of audiologic rehabilitation.** Technology should be introduced, as appropriate, as a part of an aural rehabilitation program, including such items as telephone amplifiers and new commercially available assistive listening devices for specific social or vocational listening situations. New hearing assistive technologies as they become available should be used for instruction and exploration, not to exploit a captive audience for profit.

12. **Innovations to enhance patients' auditory and visual function can be beneficial.** The speed and efficiency with which patients utilize the auditory and visual information derived from communication can be enhanced. For example, *time avenues* for audiologic rehabilitation (compressed speech and interactive laser-video technology) are available and useful. Enhancing central auditory function in older adult patients appears to be an efficient avenue through which speech comprehension can be improved, which can be exciting and helpful for patients. Activities emphasizing speed and accuracy of auditory closure, accuracy of very short-term auditory memory, and speed and accuracy of auditory/visual decision making can also provide benefit to patients.

13. **Patients should be taught a variety of listening strategies appropriate for specific communication situations.** The clinician should explain why certain communicative situations are more difficult than others, and discuss why, in certain noisy situations, an alternative strategy might work better —perhaps turning down a hearing aid and relying more on visual clues through lipreading. The patient will become more confident as he learns that there are usually several ways to overcome difficult communicative environments, and that most people—not just those with hearing loss—at times have difficulty communicating. And in some situations, there may be no solution. Teach patients to recognize and understand these limitations but not fret over them.

14. **Clinicians should create a catalog of possible methodologies to achieve specific objectives and then review this information during planning of individual treatment.** Varying clinical approaches should be gleaned

from the literature. Novel approaches developed by colleagues should be evaluated for future use, and their contributions appropriately cited.

15. **Improving the speech habits of a patient's communication partners can enhance aural rehabilitation treatment.** Clinicians too often focus only on the patient, with little attention given to significant others in the patient's communicative environment. When the most important communication partners improve and refine their speech production and vocal expressiveness—including a decrease in the speed of speech and clearer enunciation without overarticulation—the patient's difficulties in speech understanding can be reduced. This can be an extremely powerful part of treatment, but diplomacy is a critical factor. Providing tactful instruction on speech production to a patient's spouse, children, and other significant communication partners can be a positive addition to aural rehabilitation treatment.

Summary

In this chapter, varying philosophies and approaches to aural rehabilitative treatment have been presented. The theme that the author desired to stress throughout is that clinicians must continually remain vigilant to the special needs of individual patients. Many will require specific strategies to address particular problems in communication that are peculiar to them. Others may benefit from speechreading/lipreading instruction to complement their residual hearing. Whatever the assessed needs of patients, the audiologist must be flexible and knowledgeable in offering those services.

References

Alpiner, J. G. (Ed.). (1978). *Handbook of adult rehabilitative audiology.* Baltimore: Williams & Wilkins.

Alpiner, J. G. (1987). Rehabilitative audiology: An overview. In J. G. Alpiner & P. McCarthy (Eds.), *Rehabilitative audiology: Children and adults* (p. 317). Baltimore: Williams & Wilkins.

Alpiner, J., & Garstecki, D. C. (1996). Aural rehabilitation for adults: Assessment and management. In R. L. Schow & M. A. Nerbonne (Eds.), *Introduction to audiologic rehabilitation* (pp. 316–412). Boston: Allyn and Bacon.

Alpiner, J., & McCarthy, P. (Eds.). (2000). *Rehabilitative audiology: Children and adults* (2nd ed.). Baltimore: Lippincott, Williams & Wilkins.

Armstrong, M. B. S. (1974). *Visual training in aural rehabilitation.* Unpublished doctoral dissertation, University of Illinois, Champaign-Urbana.

Berger, K. (1972). Visemes and homophenous words. *Teacher of the Deaf, 70,* 396–399.

Binnie, C. A. (1976). Relevant aural rehabilitation. In J. L Northern (Ed.), *Hearing disorders* (pp. 213–227). Boston: Little, Brown.

Binnie, C. A., & Barrager, D. C. (1969, November). *Bi-sensory established articulation functions for normal hearing and sensorineural hearing loss patients.* Paper presented at the annual convention of the American Speech and Hearing Association, Chicago.

Binnie, C. A., Montgomery, A. A., & Jackson, P. (1976). Auditory and visual contributions to the perception of selected English consonants. *Journal of Speech and Hearing Disorders, 17,* 619–630.

Black, J. W. (1957). Multiple choice intelligibility tests. *Journal of Speech and Hearing Disorders, 22,* 213–235.

Black, J. W., O'Reilly, P. P., & Peck, L. (1963). Self-administered training in lipreading. *Journal of Speech and Hearing Disorders, 28,* 183–186.

Bode, D., Tweedie, D., & Hull, R. H. (1982). Improving communication through aural rehabilitation. In R. H. Hull (Ed.), *Aural rehabilitation* (pp. 101-115). New York: Grune & Stratton.

Braceland, F. J. (1963, October). *The restoration of man*. Donald Dabelstein Memorial Lecture presented at the annual conference of the National Rehabilitation Association, Chicago.

Brannon, C. (1961). Speechreading of various materials. *Journal of Speech and Hearing Disorders, 26*, 348-354.

Bruhn, M. D. (1949). *The Mueller-Walle method of lip-reading*. Washington, DC: Volta Bureau.

Bunger, A. M. (1944). *Speech reading: Jena method*. Danville, IL: The Interstate Press.

Bunger, A. M. (1961). *Speech reading: Jena method* (2nd ed.). Danville, IL: The Interstate Printers and Publishers.

Colton, J. (1977). Student participation in aural rehabilitation programs. *Journal of the Academy of Rehabilitative Audiology, 10*, 31-35.

Costello, M. R., Freeland, E. E., Hill, M. J., Jeffers, J., Matkin, N. D., Stream, R. W., et al. (1974). The audiologist: Responsibilities in the habilitation of the auditorily handicapped. *Journal of the American Speech and Hearing Association, 16*, 68-70.

DiCarlo, L. M., & Kataja, R. (1951). An analysis of the Utley lipreading test. *Journal of Speech and Hearing Disorders, 16*, 226-240.

Erber, N. P. (1969). Interaction of audition and vision in the recognition of oral speech stimuli. *Journal of Speech and Hearing Research, 12*, 423-425.

Erber, N. P. (1971). Auditory and audiovisual reception of words in low frequency noise by children with normal hearing and by children with impaired hearing. *Journal of Speech and Hearing Research, 14*, 496-512.

Erber, N. P. (1979). Auditory-visual perception of speech with reduced optical clarity. *Journal of Speech and Hearing Research, 22*, 212-223.

Fleming, M., Birkle, L., Kolman, I., Miltenberger, G., & Israel, R. (1973). Development of workable aural rehabilitation programs. *Journal of the Academy of Rehabilitative Audiology, 6*, 35-36.

Franks, J. R. (1976). The relationship of non-linguistic visual perception to lipreading skill. *Journal of the Academy of Rehabilitative Audiology, 9*, 31-37.

Franks, J. R., & Kimble, J. (1972). The confusion of English consonant clusters in lipreading. *Journal of Speech and Hearing Research, 15*, 474-482.

Freeland, E. E., Hill, M. J., Jeffers, J., Matkin, N. D., Stream, R. W., Tobin, H., et al. (1974). The audiologist: Responsibilities in the habilitation of the auditorily handicapped. *Asha, 16*, 68-70.

French-St. George, M., & Stoker, R. (1988). Speechreading: An historical perspective. In C. L. DeFilippo & D. G. Sims (Eds.), New reflections on speechreading. *The Volta Review, 90*, 17-31.

Giolas, T. G. (1994). Aural rehabilitation of adults with hearing impairment. In J. Katz (Ed.), *Handbook of clinical audiology* (pp. 356-423). Baltimore: Williams and Wilkins.

Heider, F. K., & Heider, G. M. (1940). A comparison of sentence structure of deaf and hard of hearing children. *Psychological Monographs, 52*, 42-103.

Hull, R. H. (Ed.). (1982). *Rehabilitative Audiology*. New York: Grune & Stratton.

Hull, R. H. (1997). *Aural rehabilitation* (3rd ed.). San Diego, CA: Singular.

Hull, R. H. (2001). Techniques for aural rehabilitation for aging adults who are hearing impaired. In R. H. Hull, (Ed.), *Aural rehabilitation* (4th ed., pp. 393-424). San Diego, CA: Singular/Thomson Learning.

Hull, R. H. (2007). Fifteen principles of consumer oriented audiologic/aural rehabilitation. *ASHA Leader, 12*, 6-7.

Hull, R. H., & Alpiner, J. G. (1976a). The effect of syntactic word variations on the predictability of sentence content in speechreading. *Journal of the Academy of Rehabilitative Audiology, 9*, 42-56.

Hull, R. H., & Alpiner, J. G. (1976). A linguistic approach to the teaching of speechreading: Theoretical and practical concepts. *Journal of the Academy of Rehabilitative Audiology, 9*, 4-19.

Hutton, C. (1959). Combining auditory and visual stimuli in aural rehabilitation. *The Volta Review, 61*, 316-319.

Hutton, C., Curry, E. T., & Armstrong, M. B. (1969). Semi-diagnostic test materials for aural rehabilitation. *Journal of Speech and Hearing Disorders*, *24*, 318-329.

Kinzie, C. E., & Kinzie, R. (1931). *Lip-reading for the deafened adult*. Philadelphia: John C. Winston.

Maurer, J., & Schow, R. L. (1996). Audiologic rehabilitation for elderly adults: Assessment and management. In R. L. Schow & M. A. Nerbonne (Eds.), *Introduction to audiologic rehabilitation* (pp. 645-684). Boston: Allyn and Bacon.

McCarthy & Alpiner (1978). The remediation process. In Alpiner, J (Ed.), *Handbook of adult rehabilitative audiology* (pp. 88-111). Baltimore: Williams and Wilkins.

McCarthy, P. A., & Culpepper, N. B. (1987). The adult remediation process. In J. Alpiner & P. A. McCarthy (Eds.), *Rehabilitative audiology: Children and adults* (pp. 305-342). Baltimore: Williams & Wilkins.

McCarthy, P. A., & Sapp, J. V. (2000). Rehabilitative needs of the aging population. In J. G. Alpiner & P. A. McCarthy (Eds.), *Rehabilitative audiology* (pp. 402-434). Baltimore: Lippincott Williams and Wilkins.

Miller, G. A., & Nicely, P. E. (1955). An analysis of perceptual confusions among some English consonants. *Journal of the Acoustical Society of America*, *27*, 338-352.

Montgomery, A., Walden, B., Schwartz, D., & Prosek, R. (1984). Training auditory-visual speech recognition in adults with moderate sensorineural hearing loss. *Ear and Hearing*, *5*, 30-36.

Nitchie, E. H. (1950). *New lessons in lip-reading*. Philadelphia: J. B. Lippincott.

O'Neill, J. J. (1954). Contributions of the visual components of oral symbols to speech comprehension. *Journal of Speech and Hearing Disorders*, *19*, 429-439.

O'Neill, J. J., & Oyer, H. J. (1981). *Visual communication for the hard of hearing*. Englewood Cliffs, NJ: Prentice-Hall.

Ordman, K. A., & Ralli, M. P. (1957). *What people say*. Washington, DC: Volta Bureau.

Prall, J. (1957). Lipreading and hearing aids combine for better comprehension. *The Volta Review*, *59*, 64-65.

Sanders, D. A. (1993). *Management of hearing handicap: Infants to elderly* (3rd ed.). Englewood Cliffs, NJ: Prentice-Hall.

Sumby, W. H., & Pollack, I. (1954). Visual contributions to speech intelligibility in noise. *Journal of the Acoustical Society of America*, *26*, 212-215.

Tannahill, J. C., & Smoski, W. J. (1978). Introduction to aural rehabilitation. In J. Katz (Ed.), *Handbook of clinical audiology* (pp. 442-446). Baltimore: Williams & Wilkins.

Utley, J. (1946). Factors involved in the teaching and testing of lipreading through the use of motion pictures. *The Volta Review*, *38*, 657-659.

van Uden, A. (1960). A sound-perceptive method. In A. W. G. Ewing (Ed.), *The modern educational treatment of deafness* (pp. 3-19). Washington, DC: Volta Bureau.

Walden, B., Erdman, S., Montgomery, A., Schwartz, D., & Prosek, R. (1981). Some effects of training on speech perception by hearing-impaired adults. *Journal of Speech and Hearing Research*, *24*, 207-216.

Walden, B., Prosek, R., Montgomery, A., Scherr, C., & Jones, C. (1977). Effects of training on the visual recognition of consonants. *Journal of Speech and Hearing Research*, *20*, 130-145.

Woodward, M. F., & Barber, C. G. (1960). Phoneme perception in lipreading. *Journal of Speech and Hearing Research*, *3*, 212-222.

End of Chapter Examination Questions

Chapter 11

1. Briefly discuss why strict methods of lipreading presented as a structured sequence of lessons are generally felt to be unsatisfactory.

2. In this chapter, the author presents a philosophical statement by Sanders (1993) that describes three indicators of the need for aural rehabilitation. What are those three indicators?
   a.
   b.
   c.

3. According to the author of this chapter, a holistic philosophy for audiologists to follow is in the provision of aural rehabilitation services. What are some of the services that may be provided?

4. Vision alone contributes approximately _____% to speech intelligibility when no auditory information is available.
   a. 20
   b. 50
   c. 31
   d. 70

5. The most critical element in the process of aural rehabilitation is _____
   .
   a. the complement of audition to vision
   b. the degree of auditory impairment
   c. the patient
   d. all of the above

6. McCarthy and Alpiner (1978) suggest a "progressive approach" to aural rehabilitation. It concentrates on the _____ of hearing impairment.
   a. psychological impact
   b. physical impact
   c. economic impact
   d. none of the above

7. Hull (2007) presents a holistic approach to aural rehabilitation. It involves _____. (Please list the components.)

8. (True/False) According to the author of this chapter, "all aural rehabilitation should center only on the degree of hearing impairment of the patient."

9. It is important for patients to recognize the benefits of vision in communication. But that is not all that should be recognized to help in overcoming the handicap of hearing loss. What else should be involved?

10. List four of the early methods of lipreading.
   a.
   b.
   c.
   d.

End of Chapter Answer Sheet

Name _____ Date _____

Chapter 11

1. _____

_____

_____

2. a. _____

b. _____

c. _____

3. _____

_____

_____

4. Which one?   a   b   c   d

5. Which one?   a   b   c   d

6. Which one?   a   b   c   d

7. _____

_____

_____

8. True or False?

9. _____

_____

_____

10. a. _____

b. _____

c. _____

d. _____

12

Counseling Adults Who Possess Impaired Hearing

R. STEVEN ACKLEY

Chapter Outline

Introduction

As stated by Kaplan (2001), the sense of hearing is integrally related to communication and interaction with other people, because people generally relate to others through verbal communication. For the majority of adults who are deaf or hard of hearing, impairment of the sense of hearing means that the ability to interact communicatively with others may also be impaired. The frustrations that arise from misinterpreted verbal messages, or not hearing at all, in a world of verbal communicative exchanges can result in problems for both the adult with impaired hearing and for those with whom she associates who do not possess impaired hearing. For the audiologist, helping people to deal with the problems that are inherent in breakdowns in communication as a result of impaired hearing is an integral part of the process of aural rehabilitation.

Adults Who Are Deaf

Counseling deaf and hard-of-hearing adults involves more than simply understanding issues related to loss of hearing and the psychological impact this loss might impose. In addition, understanding the culture of the Deaf is equally vital to successful counseling management of those who are members of this unique American subculture. The two groups are quite distinct from a counseling perspective. Persons who have lost some hearing or have become profoundly deaf suffer a disability and may be psychologically devastated more so than persons who have incurred a physical disability. Loss of hearing implies loss of communication ability. When the loss is complete, the person is deaf and the learned mode of communication is also completely lost. The deaf person's speech will also be affected. This results in a sense of isolation that no physical disability or other sensory loss, including blindness, can imitate. On the other hand, for those who are born deaf and into a culture of Deafness, there is no loss. Perhaps those who can hear would say the congenitally deaf person adapts to a no-hearing world, whereas Deaf persons would consider themselves privy to a unique and rich culture by virtue of their birthright.

Culturally Deaf persons are those individuals who use American Sign Language (ASL) as their primary means of communication. They identify with and obtain most of their social experiences within the Deaf community. ASL is a complete communication system and no more ambiguous than that of any other well-established and highly evolved linguistic system. As with any modern culture, the language used by the community defines much of the social context, the humor, the tradition, and the cultural nuances that are unique to each culture. But perhaps Deafness is better described as a subculture; just as Italian Americans, African Americans, and Mexican Americans may retain their native culture while participating in the broader American society, so too does Deaf culture in America function within the broad context of American society while maintaining the social and cultural support systems within the Deaf community (Kannapell & Adams, 1984). Social clubs organized by the Deaf bring ASL users together in a recreational way that is of necessity in the same manner that someone who speaks only Spanish may unite with speakers of this language after a week on the job with non-Spanish speakers. Although a culture is often identified by a unique cuisine in addition to its system of communication, this is not the case of the Deaf culture in America. Rather, any and all types of food may be represented in social gatherings. What makes the social context unique among the Deaf is the dependence on ASL communication. Deaf clubs may welcome participants who can hear, but to the extent that these "guests" are fluent in ASL. Children of Deaf adults, or CODAs as they like to be called, often represent a subculture within the Deaf subculture and are afforded the benefit of joining the Deaf community by virtue of their native ASL fluency in addition to their native participation in the broader culture. Bilingualism has distinct advantages beyond the obvious convenience of communication with various peoples. It also offers an entrée into "biculturalism."

It is in the context of the unique culture Deaf people enjoy that counseling issues will need to be considered. Any type of "psychological problem" and the degree to which it is seen varies with every individual's lifestyle and personality and, to some extent, the characteristics of a hearing loss. Although there are individual differences among persons who are hard of hearing or deaf, there are similarities that psychologists identify that are interpreted in a non-hearing loss context. The non-hearing loss attitude is based on a premise that a deficit in hearing is a disability and results in problems that psychologists measure. Congenitally deaf who are in the Deaf culture have no sense of hearing "loss," having no experience to report on what it was like to hear. Persons who are culturally Deaf do not see their condition as a disability that needs to be treated or its psychological consequences as needing to be measured. People who are Deaf see themselves as culturally unique and nothing else. They have no desire to eradicate their highly evolved system of communication or to repair their hearing condition. They do not see ASL as a compensatory communication system any more than we might see spoken language as com-

pensation for our inability to communicate via telepathy. In extreme cases, some Deaf may even defend their right to be Deaf and protest medical efforts that attempt to "cure" deafness, such cochlear implants, as genocide of the Deaf culture.

Adults Who Possess Impaired Hearing

In contrast to the persons described above, adults who are considered to be "hearing impaired" are those who possess a hearing loss of various degrees and configurations, but who possess hearing that is to an extent probably usable for purposes of communication. These persons range from those who require amplification through the use of hearing aids in order to assist them in hearing speech, to those who possess a milder loss of hearing that requires relatively simple changes in their listening environment for purposes of communication with others. Hearing impairment among this population of adults can result in breakdowns in communication that can impact negatively on their occupational, social, educational, and personal lives and can result in depression and withdrawal from situations that require communication. The tendency to withdraw from situations and environments that otherwise involve interactive communication can, in turn, result in personal, social, occupational, and educational problems that can impact on those important aspects of their lives and these can, in turn, have psychological implications.

Counseling provides adults who possess impaired hearing with access to avenues of services that can assist them to learn to cope more efficiently within various aspects of their communicative life in spite of their hearing loss, and an understanding of the causes for the difficulties that are being experienced in hearing and communication. With a better understanding of why the difficulties are being experienced, strategies for overcoming them can be developed.

Hearing loss can result in an extremely frustrating disability in interactive verbal communication, which can, in turn, result in other impairments within environments that require communication. Those include one's job, one's social life, one's personal life. The adjustments that are required can appear overwhelming to an adult who has never had to consider those adjustments before and did not expect to. These individuals require special services that are different from those that are offered adults who are Deaf, as described above, and require different strategies for learning to cope in spite of their hearing loss.

Depression—Feelings of Inadequacy

People who are nonculturally deaf may feel shut off from the world, not only because of difficulty communicating with others, but also because some or all of the subliminal auditory clues that permit one to maintain contact with the hearing world are no longer available. This phenomenon described by Ramsdell (1978) is discussed below. Reaction to this depression may be withdrawing from social situations and from contact with other people. This might be considered a normal response to an acquired condition rather than a typical reaction of someone who is born deaf and into the unique culture of Deafness. Depression is frequently complicated by feelings of inadequacy. People who become deaf and even those who become hard of hearing may feel that they should be able to cope better with a hear-

ing loss and that the inability to do so indicates weakness. In addition, there may be feelings of shame, because of the rationalization that hearing difficulty is associated with abnormalities such as thinking, learning, remembering, or decision-making disabilities. They may apologize for not understanding and assume that the "fault" for communication breakdown is always theirs.

Defense Mechanisms

Denial

In general, threats to self-esteem are handled by one or more defense mechanisms. A common defense mechanism is denial. People with mild to moderate hearing losses may simply not acknowledge they have a hearing loss, because to them acceptance implies abnormality. Those same individuals would probably have no difficulty accepting the reality of a visual problem, because visual problems tend not to be associated with the general adequacy of the person. Denial increases the problem because it makes it more difficult to seek help or accept the need for a hearing aid, because the visibility of the hearing aid would make the hearing impairment apparent to others. It is also a common reaction for the sufferer to assume the communication problems would resolve, if only people would speak plainly.

Hostility and Suspicion

It may be natural again for those who suffer a hearing loss to blame others for their difficulties, accusing them of mumbling or of deliberately excluding them from a conversation. They may become suspicious, accusing others of saying unpleasant things or planning unpleasant situations. Laughter may be misinterpreted as ridicule. They may react negatively to such service providers as a doctor, an audiologist, or a hearing aid dispenser. The service provider may be the messenger of the bad news, and blaming the messenger is common.

It is important for service providers to be aware of the devastating nature of the message they have the power to convey. Discussing an older patient's hearing loss by dismissing it as something that happens when we get old is of little assurance or assistance to the person receiving this information. Although the patient may admit to suspecting hearing loss, it may be no less traumatic than for someone who might suspect cancer, tumor, or terminal illness. Verifying the suspicion may in fact be a devastating blow that is internalized along with a polite chuckle to acknowledge the "getting older" comment. It is vital for the service provider to follow up with the patient immediately and frequently. A call to the patient at home the evening of the visit when the hearing loss was determined will be important to the patient. Discussing something that will make life easier under the circumstances such as a headset or wireless assistive device for the TV may help to sort out the inconvenience of the loss. As follow-up continues, strategies for coping may be introduced along with support groups, on-line services, broader assistive technology, and even communication alternatives. The audiologist is notoriously the "demon" with the Deaf as well as those who lose their hearing. The physician makes the actual diagnosis and so should be classified as "co-demon," but this is typically not the case. The reason is simple: the physician calls the patient at home after the visit. Audiologists usually do not do this. The follow-up call to the patient's home after hours is considered a sign of compassion, outreach, and understanding and unre-lated to the business of hearing, which is conducted during the work day.

Also, it is vital for the service provider to make some effort to communicate visually or manually with Deaf clientele. Learning to fingerspell requires an evening of effort, and this can demonstrate to the member of the ASL-based culture that you not only acknowledge the linguistic system but also support the culture in general. Learning a few signs will go a long way to forming a bond with the Deaf patient. It can instill a sense of trust and help cement the doctor-patient relationship.

Psychological Levels of Hearing

Ramsdell (1978) in his classic treatise on hearing loss has described three psychological levels of hearing for the normal hearing person and the problems associated with loss of hearing at each level. Two are described here for purposes of discussion.

Primitive Level

At the primitive level, sound functions as auditory coupling to the world. Individuals react to the changing background sounds of the world without being aware of it. As Ramsdell (1978) states:

> At this level, we react to such sounds as the tick of a clock, the distant roar of traffic, vague echoes of people moving in other rooms of the house, without being aware that we are hearing them. These incidental noises maintain our feeling of being part of a living world and contribute to our own sense of being alive. (p. 501)

When this primitive function is lost, acute depression may occur. Because the primitive level of hearing is not on a conscious level, the person who is deaf may not be aware of the cause of the depression. Frequently, the depression is attributed to inadequacy in coping with the hearing impairment.

The severity of the depression will be greatest among persons who have a sudden hearing loss, whether it is through trauma, surgery such as acoustic tumor removal, or other causes. Fortunately, hearing loss of sudden onset most frequently affects one ear only, although bilateral losses do occur.

Depression due to the loss of the primitive level will occur in the individual with slowly deteriorating hearing as well. In this case it is more insidious, occurring more slowly, but the resulting depression may be equally great. In some instances, the depression may be more severe because the person may not be aware that hearing is deteriorating. Informing the patient of the true cause of the depression will help alleviate some of the problem, although this knowledge will not eliminate it entirely. Often, properly fitted amplification (hearings aids or cochlear implants) can restore the primitive level, even if speech understanding is not possible. In some cases if amplification is not possible, such as with CN VIII destruction, a vibrotactile device may serve to couple the deaf individual to the world of sound.

The loss of the primitive level is a problem primarily with severe-to-profound adventitious losses. Most adults who are culturally Deaf have never experienced the world of sound and, therefore, are not aware of the absence of subliminal auditory cues.

Warning or Signal Level of Hearing

At the warning level, sounds convey information about objects or events. The doorbell indicates the presence of a visitor. Footsteps indicate that someone is approaching. A siren indicates an emergency vehicle is near. A fire alarm indicates danger. Because warning sounds are frequently intense, loss of the warning level is generally found among persons with severe-to-profound losses. Some warning sounds, however, are of low intensity, and may be missed by persons with less severe hearing losses. These are mainly distant sounds, such as the whistle of an approaching train.

Psychological Impact of Hearing Loss

Insecurity

When the ability to hear warning sounds such as a smoke alarm, a door knock, or a child in another room is lost, feelings of insecurity are understandable. Such problems are found within all segments of the deaf and severely hard-of-hearing population, but to a much less extent among people who are culturally Deaf. A vast array of electronic visual systems has been developed to deal with warning level problems. These systems can monitor a doorbell, a person in another room, a smoke alarm, and any other important sound within the home or office. More complete discussions of alerting device systems can be found in Compton (1993), DiPietro, Williams, and Kaplan (1984), and Kaplan (1987).

Annoyance

Feelings of annoyance are caused by disruption of normal patterns of life due to loss of hearing at the warning level. The person who is deaf or hard of hearing who cannot hear the alarm clock may oversleep in the morning and suffer penalties at work as a result. When the ring of the telephone can no longer be heard, social activities may be affected or business opportunities lost. Visual alerting systems can be very useful in overcoming these problems.

Localization

Localization problems may be considered a special type of warning level difficulty. To predict direction of sound, approximately equal sensitivity is needed in both ears; therefore, the inability to localize sound is a special problem for persons with unilateral losses. What is not always realized, however, is that localization problems also exist for individuals who have bilateral hearing impairment who are aided monaurally.

In addition to alerting device technology, warning level difficulties can be dealt with by training a person who is hard of hearing or deaf to become more visually aware of her environment.

Loss of Esthetic Experiences

For many individuals, music provides an esthetic experience. For some people, the inability to hear the sounds of nature, such as bird calls, may represent significant esthetic loss. Amplification cannot always restore these sounds to the extent that esthetic experiences are restored.

Symbolic Level of Hearing

At the symbolic level, individuals deal with sound as language and a major channel of communication. Nearly all people who are deaf or hard of hearing have difficulty at this level to one degree or another. Many children and adults who have deafness early in childhood experience delayed English language development, which later affects reading and other academic skills. Although adults who are culturally Deaf tend to communicate comfortably in sign language and consider English a second language, they may have difficulties with the vocabulary and structure of English. English language deficits create a variety of communication problems for anyone who needs to function within the mainstream community for any reason.

Although adults who are hard of hearing or deafened do not generally suffer delayed language development, they do face the problem of communicating under conditions of reduced verbal redundancy imposed by impaired auditory reception. Depending on degree, type, and configuration of loss, such individuals lose linguistic cues inherent in a sentence, prosodic cues such as stress and inflection, and phonemic information. The fewer auditory cues that are available, the more likely a person is to misinterpret what is heard, with consequent embarrassment, frustration, and social penalty. This situation is worsened if the communication environment has background noise, competing speech, or other auditory or visual distractions.

At Home

The home can be a source of tension because of communication difficulties for a number of reasons. First, there is more opportunity for interpersonal communication and, consequently, more opportunity for communication breakdown. Second, the person who is hard of hearing or deaf expects the family to be more understanding of the special problems imposed by hearing loss than nonrelatives and is disappointed if that is not the case. Third, households tend to be noisy places. The noise level in a typical kitchen was measured at l00 dB SPL with water running at moderate speed, the refrigerator on, and the radio tuned to a comfortable listening level. Competing noise may give the hard-of-hearing person no usable hearing whatsoever. This fact is puzzling especially to children in the family who may not fully appreciate how the hearing loss can seem to be so selective. How is it that conversation can be at a normal level and without misunderstandings in the quiet living room and yet be impossible in the kitchen? The strain of hearing may also be too great when the sufferer is exhausted at the end of the day. What comes naturally to the family members requires concentration and often great effort by the person with hearing loss. Sorting through a mental catalog of likely utterances that were made in the context leaves the sufferer mentally and physically challenged at the end of a day of this endless activity.

When there are preexisting conflicts within a family, a hearing loss can accentuate them. The hearing impairment can be used as a weapon either by the person who is hard of hearing or by other family members. A supportive family is important to an individual who is deaf or hard of hearing; at the same time, the person with the hearing loss must be willing to assume part of the responsibility for successful communication.

An individual who is culturally Deaf will not have communication difficulties with the family, if the family is willing and able to use sign language as the primary mode of communication. However, the majority of adults who are culturally Deaf grew up in hearing families. Unless the deaf person can communicate orally with the family or the family can sign to the deaf person, limited communication occurs in the home and the stresses are great.

At Work

Work-related problems are common. The extent and nature of a difficulty depend on the nature of the hearing loss, and the type of job the person holds. The greater the amount of oral communication required and the greater the need for precision of understanding, the more difficulty a patient is likely to have. The receptionist who has difficulty understanding speech on the telephone may be in danger of losing her job. The physician who finds it difficult to monitor a patient's heartbeat may find it increasingly difficult to function professionally. Large or small group meetings pose special problems, because of the need to follow rapidly changing conversation, often against background noise or reverberation. If not dealt with, anxiety and frustration created by such demands complicate communication problems caused by the hearing loss.

The majority of individuals who are culturally Deaf work in environments where the communication system is spoken English. To function successfully, they must either develop strategies to communicate comfortably with hearing people or constantly use an interpreter. If communication is limited, the person who is Deaf may be lonely at work and may face limited opportunities for advancement.

The Telephone

A special problem at the symbolic level is inability to use the telephone. The telephone message has become an integral part of our lives, affecting communication at home, work, school, and in social environments. The person who cannot understand speech transmitted by telephone or who cannot hear the telephone ring is affected in every aspect of life. Social contacts are reduced because friends and family cannot be easily contacted. Vocational opportunities are limited to the minority of jobs not requiring telephone use. The inability to use the telephone to summon help is threatening, particularly for an individual who lives alone. However, many of these inconveniences are overcome with text-message capability and e-mail. In fact, the majority of young adults with normal hearing may generally prefer this communication method, and Deaf young adults use it constantly.

Many people who are deaf or hard of hearing can learn to use the telephone more effectively by developing appropriate telephone strategies. Telecommunication devices for the deaf (TDDs) are viable options for those who cannot use the voice telephone, and video phone technology is available to all deaf and hard-of-hearing persons.

At School

The adult or adolescent in school often has special problems. Classrooms are rarely quiet places. Ross (1982) reported that the average noise level in 45 classrooms was 60 dBA; an optimal level for students who are hard of hearing is 35 dBA. At noise levels of 60 dBA or greater, it is often difficult for a normal hearing individual to correctly understand a teacher. The task is immeasurably more difficult for a student who is deaf or hard of hearing, who must function with an auditory system that distorts the incoming speech signal even under favorable conditions.

Not only are many classrooms noisy, but they tend to be reverberant as well, because of large areas of rigid, smooth surface and few absorbent materials such as drapes or carpets. Such room conditions further distort speech and add to the burden of a student who is deaf or hard of hearing who is trying to function with amplification. These conditions interfere with the efficient use of a hearing aid, which amplifies noise, speech, and distortion caused by reverberation with equal effectiveness.

Teachers are not always aware of the special needs of a student who is deaf or hard of hearing and do not always adequately project their voices. Teachers will occasionally speak with their backs to a class while writing at the chalkboard, thus distorting and reducing the intensity of their voices. Speechreading becomes impossible. A barrier to both speechreading and sign language reception in class is the need to take notes; one cannot concentrate on interpreting visual information and write at the same time. All of these problems tend to limit educational opportunities for adults who are hard of hearing or deaf, with consequent vocational limitations. Assistive listening systems to minimize effects of noise and reverberation, note-takers, interpreters, and greater awareness by teachers of the needs of students who are deaf and hard of hearing are needed.

Social Activities

For many adults, sudden or increasing hearing loss results in a restriction of social activities. The difficulty in understanding speech exposes individuals who are deaf or hard of hearing to the danger and embarrassment of misinterpreting what is said. As a result, they may react inappropriately and be exposed to ridicule. It is a rare person who possesses enough ego strength to continually explain the presence of a hearing loss and continually ask people to repeat what has been said. Even well-meaning friends do not always succeed in making a person who is deaf or hard of hearing feel comfortable.

People with normal hearing may feel uncomfortable when they know a listener does not understand what is being said. Often they are at a loss as to how to help the listener understand better, particularly when the person who is deaf or hard of hearing attempts to "bluff" and does it badly. Both partners in the conversation may attempt to deny a hearing loss, but communication is disrupted and speaker and listener are embarrassed.

When the hearing loss is severe or has been present for a long time, speech may deteriorate. In that case, the person who is deaf or hard of hearing may not be clearly understood, adding to the possible social penalties imposed by the hearing loss.

Conversational difficulties increase exponentially in difficult listening situations. Following a conversation alternating between members of a group can be very difficult, particularly with background noise. A dinner party can be extremely anxiety provoking and a cocktail party impossible.

Social activities are further limited when a person who is deaf or hard of hearing can no longer enjoy the theater or lectures. Just as in face-to-face conversation, the person must cope with speakers or actors who may not project adequately, speech that shifts rapidly from one person to another, and poor room acoustics, as well as the loss of sensitivity and distortion imposed by the hearing loss.

More and more, as social activities become restricted, the person who is deaf or hard of hearing becomes isolated and lonely. This condition may ultimately be accepted with resignation, or it may be met with aggression. The individual may deny the reality of the problem and attribute a shrinking social life to the malice of others. Regardless of whether the problem is met with resignation or aggression, the person who is deaf or hard of hearing suffers deterioration in the quality of her lifestyle.

Individuals who are culturally Deaf do not suffer social penalties because of hearing loss so long as their social contacts remain within the Deaf community. That is usually a satisfying and enriching social choice. However, those who wish to socialize outside of the Deaf culture encounter the same barriers as individuals who are hard of hearing and individuals who are not culturally Deaf. Generally, successful cross-cultural friendships occur when a hearing person can sign comfortably and both parties are good communicators.

Other Problems at the Symbolic Level

Every person who is deaf or hard of hearing has had, at one time or another, difficulties in obtaining services. This may involve mailing a package at the post office, purchasing an airline ticket, placing an order at a restaurant, or communicating effectively with a physician. Persons who are deaf or hard of hearing are at a definite disadvantage when dealing with the law. In recognition of this, a legal center for the deaf was established at Gallaudet University. Most hospitals attempt to make special provisions for communicating with patients who are deaf or hard of hearing, but personnel are not always aware of their communication problems. Hearing aids may be removed for safekeeping, effectively destroying any possible communication.

Another problem at the symbolic level is the ability to hear and understand television. Many people who are hard of hearing increase the volume beyond the tolerance level of hearing family members and neighbors, thereby creating a great deal of tension. Many people who are deaf cannot understand the TV signal, regardless of its intensity. The inability to enjoy television is not only a social loss, but eliminates an important source of information. Assistive device technology can make television accessible to almost everyone (Compton, 1993). In addition, many people who are deaf or hard of hearing find the use of closed captioning very useful.

Facilitating Adjustment

The professional faces a twofold task in helping the person who is deaf or hard of hearing adjust to the problems imposed by hearing impairment. First, through educational and personal adjustment counseling (Sanders, 1988), patients must be helped to accept themselves as people who are deaf or hard of hearing and understand the limitations imposed by the hearing loss. Once this is achieved, patients can be helped to manipulate the environment to minimize penalties. Environmental manipulation may involve use of listening aids, modification of communication situations, and education of family, friends, and associates.

Definition of the Problem

To provide meaningful assistance to a patient who is hard of hearing or deaf, it is necessary to obtain information on the specific communicative difficulties encountered in daily activities. Not only is it important to identify specific difficult listening situations, but also to assess coping strategies and attitudes of a patient toward communication and toward herself as a person with a hearing loss.

To one degree or another, the traditional case history explores areas of communicative difficulty and allows the interviewer to assess an individual's motivation to cope with communicative difficulties. However, a case history interview provides only a general overview of a patient's communicative difficulties. It does not provide quantitative information about degree of difficulty in various situations, nor generally does it sufficiently and systematically probe the specific social, vocational, and interpersonal situations creating problems. There are a number of communication scales available to provide more precise evaluation about difficult communication situations, communication strategies used by the patient, and attitudes about hearing loss. This information helps an aural rehabilitation specialist to plan a program of therapy and observe progress as it occurs.

Counseling—The Process

After the specific communicative and attitudinal problems of a patient have been defined, a specific aural rehabilitation program needs to be developed to meet the identified needs. In addition to speechreading, auditory training, and other skill development activities, personal adjustment and informational counseling must be included in the program as needed.

Personal Adjustment Counseling

Although personal adjustment and informational counseling are artificially separated here for purposes of discussion, they are intertwined in an actual rehabilitative program. The personal adjustment counselor functions as a facilitator to help patients modify maladaptive attitudes about themselves as hearing-impaired persons. Kodman (1967) discusses three facilitative conditions that must be present, if the therapist is to be successful.

Accurate Empathy

The first condition is accurate empathy. This is the understanding by a therapist of the true feelings that underlie statements the patient might make. The therapist then responds in such a way that the patient's feelings are reflected back, so that her difficulties can be viewed objectively. For example, a patient might say, "Most people don't speak plainly these days. I'd rather read a book than talk to people." The empathetic clinician might reply, "It must be terribly frustrating not to understand people. Let's talk about some of your experiences." As the patient begins to relate difficult listening experiences, the therapist can continue reflecting back upon the patient's feelings and perhaps, in the process, lead the patient to suggest ways of coping with these situations. This is a nondirective approach. The patient makes decisions based on increased perception of the situation; decisions are not imposed on the patient.

The use of accurate empathy is as important in a group situation as in an individual session. In the group situation, the therapist must reflect the feelings of each member as they are expressed. After a group becomes a cohesive unit, the members may begin to practice accurate empathy toward each other, providing strong positive reinforcement for attitudinal change.

Unconditional Positive Regard

The second condition is unconditional positive regard. This involves acceptance of patients as they are, regardless of any hostility, belligerence, or apparent lack of cooperation. It is sometimes difficult for a novice clinician to accept expressions of negativism from a patient and not to consider such behavior as a personal attack. However, it is important to realize that unpleasant actions or expressions are simply manifestations of a patient's problems. Perspective taking, the ability to take another's point of view (Erdmann, 1993), is a combination of accurate empathy and unconditional positive regard. Patient management is facilitated if an aural rehabilitation specialist can view experiences from the patient's point of view.

Genuineness

A third facilitative condition is genuineness. This condition implies a relaxed, friendly attitude toward a patient, respect for the patient's suggestions, ability to accept criticism, and communication with the patient in a manner she can easily understand. A genuine clinician does not retreat into professional jargon or assume a pose of superiority because of professional stature.

These facilitative conditions are especially important when working with patients who are culturally Deaf. Their language and culture must be understood and respected. ASL is not English; idioms and other figurative language vary from English. ASL tends to be a more direct language, with different pragmatic conventions and far fewer euphemisms than English; expression of ideas tends to be more direct. What may appear to be rudeness may simply reflect differences in the languages. To work effectively with a person who is culturally Deaf, it is important for a clinician to have a working knowledge of the patient's language and be willing to use it. Even if the clinician is not fluent in ASL, she should make every effort to maximize communication with the patient. Most people who are culturally Deaf will meet hearing clinicians halfway communicatively, if convinced of the genuineness of the relationship.

Patients who are culturally Deaf sometimes make decisions from a different cultural base from patients who are not culturally Deaf or are hard of hearing. Some have no desire to mainstream into majority culture; these people enter into therapy with a desire to develop greater communicative independence in those situations where it is advantageous to communicate using English speech or writing. The aural rehabilitation specialist must respect such decisions and work with patients on their own terms.

The qualities of accurate empathy, unconditional positive regard, and genuineness can be developed or enhanced through experience. Audio- or videotaping sessions —with the permission of the patient, of course—and later reviewing the patient-clinician interchange is an excellent way for the novice clinician to improve skills.

Accepting the Reality of the Hearing Loss

One of the most important goals of personal adjustment counseling is to help a patient accept the reality of the hearing loss and the need for help. One must not assume that, because a patient has opted for a clinic evaluation, acceptance of amplification or therapy is a given. The patient may simply be appeasing family or friends or perhaps be taking the first tenuous steps toward seeking help while remaining ambivalent about self-acceptance as a hard-of-hearing person. There is no point in recommending amplification if a patient is not ready to accept it.

It is far better to persuade the individual to enroll in an aural rehabilitation program that includes discussion-counseling to help with acceptance of the reality of the hearing problem. If necessary, the group discussions can be supplemented with individual counseling. It must be made clear that participation in aural rehabilitation is not contingent on hearing aid use. It must be emphasized that the audiologist is ready to assist with selection of a hearing aid if and when a patient becomes ready.

Recognizing a Patient's Fears

When a person feels a loss of self-esteem because of an inability to hear normally, she has a tendency to conceal the hearing loss. The fear is often related to the concern that people will view her as different. To such an individual, a hearing aid is a visible indication that she is an inferior person. Although it may be recognized logically that there is no truth to such fears, a fearful person may not be able to emotionally accept use of a hearing aid. Even when the hearing aid can be completely hidden from view, the problem of acceptance is not solved for some people; they believe that wearing a hearing aid represents tangible evidence of inferiority. These feelings are especially prevalent among adolescents, where peer identification and acceptance are overriding concerns. In addition, many adolescents and adults fear that hearing loss and its visible badge, the hearing aid, will make them less attractive to the opposite sex.

If an individual who is deaf or hard of hearing does succeed in working through the emotional objections to amplification, the usual expectation is that the hearing aid will restore good hearing. If the hearing aid user is not properly prepared for the limitations of amplification and the adjustment necessary to use it well, she will be disappointed during attempts to use the hearing aid. If the hearing aid is discarded, the person who is deaf or hard of hearing may feel even more isolated and depressed, as hopes of solving her communication problem with a mechanical prosthesis have not been fulfilled.

Educational or Informational Counseling

Educational or informational counseling is the provision of information about hearing loss, its effect on communication, and intervention procedures. Although this type of counseling can be accomplished either in an individual or a group situation, the group situation is often more effective, because experiences can be shared and peer reinforcement can occur. However, group participation requires that individuals identify themselves as persons with hearing problems. If a patient is not ready for this level of acceptance, individual therapy is preferable until the goal of ultimate participation in a group can be met.

Topics that should be included in an informational counseling program are:

- The nature of the auditory system and hearing loss, including interpretation of audiograms.
- Effects of hearing loss on communication and impact of background noise and poor listening conditions.
- Importance of visual input, audiovisual integration, and attending behavior.
- Impact of talker differences and social conditions to communication.
- Benefits and limitations of speechreading.
- Benefits and limitations of hearing aids and their use and care.
- Benefits and limitations of assistive devices.
- Use of community resources such as self-help groups.

Identifying Difficult Listening Situations

An important part of informational counseling is identification of difficult communication situations and development of coping strategies that work. The group format is especially effective for identification of and practice with communication strategies, but such training can be incorporated into individual sessions, if necessary.

Assertiveness Training

Assertiveness training can be easily incorporated into aural rehabilitation sessions. It is important for patients who are deaf or hard of hearing to understand that they have a right to understand, that it is acceptable to ask for help in a polite, courteous fashion, and that it is the responsibility of the person with hearing loss to instruct the communication partner in ways of helping. Patients need to learn to distinguish between (a) aggressive, which involves violation of other people's rights; (b) passive, which involves allowing others to violate their rights; and (c) assertive, in which patients protect their rights without violating those of other people.

The aural rehabilitation specialist might pose the problem: "Suppose you meet two friends on a noisy street who are having a conversation. They greet you and try to include you in their conversation, but you are unable to follow what they are saying. What might you do?" The therapist would then try to elicit some of the following examples of assertive behavior:

1. Ask the people to move away from the source of the noise so that you can understand better.
2. Ask one of the two people to briefly summarize what has been said before you entered the conversation.
3. Admit you do not understand and ask for repetition or rephrasing of an idea.
4. Ask the people to speak louder.

The patients would then be asked to give examples of aggressive behavior, such as verbal or physical abuse of the speakers, and of passive behavior, such as saying nothing about the lack of understanding. Table 12-1 and Table 12-2 have further suggestions for coping with difficult listening situations.

Role playing can be incorporated into assertiveness training sessions very effec-tively to help patients define appropriate behaviors. Homework assignments involv-ing the use of these behaviors in actual life situations can follow the role playing and be followed up by discussions during sub-sequent classes.

TABLE 12–1. How to Cope with Difficult Listening Situations

- Ask the speaker to speak in a good light and to face the listener, so that speechreading skills can be used.

- Ask the speaker to speak clearly and naturally, but not to shout or exaggerate articulatory movements.

- If you do not understand what a speaker is saying, ask the speaker to repeat or rephrase the statement.

- If entering a group in the middle of a conversation, ask one person to sum up the gist of the conversation.

- If someone is speaking at a distance, that person should be asked to stand closer.

- If the speaker turns her head away, ask her to face you to permit optimal speechreading and listening.

- If you are attempting to understand speech in the presence of noise, try to move yourself and the speaker away from the source of the noise.

- When in a communication situation requiring exact information, such as asking directions or obtaining schedules for a trip, request that the speaker write the crucial information.

- If the speaker is talking while eating, smoking, or chewing, request that she not do so, because it makes speechreading difficult.

- A person who has a unilateral loss should be sure to keep the good ear facing the speaker at all times.

- If possible, avoid rooms with poor acoustics. If meetings are held in such rooms, request that they be transferred to rooms with less reverberation.

- If a speaker at a meeting cannot be heard, request that she use a microphone.

- Arrive early for meetings, so that you can sit close to the speaker. Avoid taking a seat near a wall to minimize the possibility of reverberation. This is particularly important for those who use hearing aids.

- If you are going to a movie or to the theater, read the reviews in advance to familiarize yourself with the plot.

- In an extremely noisy situation, limit conversation to before the noise has started or after the noise has subsided. Normal hearing people do this all the time. For example, if a plane goes overhead and a conversation is going on, most people will halt their conversations and wait until the plane has passed.

TABLE 12–2. Helping Students Who Are Deaf or Hard of Hearing

- Preferential seating is important for anyone with a hearing problem. The adult who is deaf or hard of hearing will usually know which place in a classroom is best. However, as the focus of attention may change during a lecture, the student should be assured that any change of seat will not be considered disruptive.

- The teacher should be careful to speak only when a student who is deaf or hard of hearing can see her lips. The following situations should be avoided if possible:
  - Talking with one's back to the class, as when writing on the chalkboard.
  - Standing in front of a window or a bright light. The light should be shining on the speaker's face, not in the student's eyes.
  - Teaching from the back of the room, where the student cannot see.
  - Walking around the classroom while talking.

- The teacher should:
  - Speak in a careful yet natural manner. Avoid exaggerated lip movements.
  - Restate or rephrase statements when the student fails to understand.
  - Not cover the face with a hand or a book while reading.
  - Not stand too close to a student who must lipread. She might have to tilt her head back to see the speaker's face, causing unnecessary strain and fatigue.

- Students who are deaf or hard of hearing rely heavily on written material to obtain information. It is helpful to inform them in advance what material will be covered on a particular day, so that pertinent material can be read in advance.

- It is not possible for a student who is deaf or hard of hearing to use visual cues in class and take notes simultaneously. The teacher can either prepare special lecture notes or request that a fellow student share notes with a student who is deaf or hard of hearing.

- The teacher should use the chalkboard or the overhead projector as much as possible. If the written material must be copied by the student, lecturing should not occur at the same time.

- Oral tests should never be given to a student who is deaf or hard of hearing.

- The teacher should be available for extra tutoring. A student who is deaf or hard of hearing should be encouraged to meet with the teacher after class for explanation of material not understood.

Once patients are able to function assertively, they are ready to learn the many behaviors that facilitate communication. There are two broad categories of communication strategies: anticipation and repair.

Anticipatory Strategies

Anticipatory strategies involve thinking about a communication situation in advance and figuring out ways to minimize difficulties. They include such things as educating speakers to keep their faces visible, coming early to a meeting to get a seat close to the speaker, identifying tables in restaurants that provide optimal lighting and minimal noise and making advance reservations to secure those tables, arranging for note-takers or interpreters in classes or meetings, and obtaining assistive devices. An excellent anticipatory strategy involves predicting vocabulary or dialogue that is likely to occur in a particular situation and practicing such language in advance. Patients need to learn how to use such strategies and when they are appropriate. Detailed discussion of communication strategies and exercises for practice can be found in Kaplan, Bally, and Garretson (1987), Tye-Murray (1991, 1993), and Tye-Murray, Purdy, and Woodworth (1992).

It is important to realize that it is difficult for many people who deaf or hard of hearing to be assertive, particularly as they are often rebuffed. Coping with difficult listening situations in the manner suggested requires practice and development of a "thick skin." Clinicians should be sure to make their patients understand that they are aware of the difficulties involved in implementing these suggestions.

Educating Significant Others

Because communication involves not only the person who is deaf or hard of hearing but also family members, friends, and others, educational counseling of these people is important to the adjustment of the patient. Family members or associates must understand the nature of a patient's hearing problem and the specific ways in which communication is affected. After testing it is highly desirable to include spouses, children, parents, or friends in the counseling session for the initial explanation of the hearing loss.

The limitations imposed by some types of hearing loss are baffling to the layperson who finds it difficult to understand why some things can be heard easily and other conversations are handled poorly. The effect of a high-frequency hearing loss on speech perception, the practical effects of a word recognition problem, and the devastating effects of competing noise or competing speech on speech understanding must be carefully explained. For complete understanding, several explanations at different times may be necessary for both a patient and significant others. For that reason, normal hearing family members or friends should be encouraged to enter a rehabilitation group with a patient.

Summary

The psychological impact of hearing impairment or deafness on adults is real and can be severe. The avenues available to those who serve these persons can be employed in constructive and meaningful ways to restore feelings of self-worth and to assist patients in adjusting to the demands of their world. Only audiologists who are willing to enter into a close working relationship with these adults with hearing impairment should become a part of the process of facilitative counseling.

Acknowledgment. The content of this chapter was first prepared by Harriet Kaplan, PhD, for a chapter on counseling on behalf of persons with impaired hearing in the fourth edition of Hull's *Aural Rehabilitation*. The author wishes to thank her for her contributions to the content of the current chapter.

References

Castle, D. L. (1980). *Telephone training for the deaf.* Rochester, NY: National Technical Institute for the Deaf.

Compton, C. L. (1989). Assistive devices. *Seminars in Hearing, 10,* 66–77.

Compton, C. L. (1993). Assistive technology for deaf and hard-of-hearing people. In J. G.

Alpiner & P. A. McCarthy (Eds.), *Rehabilitative audiology: Children and adults* (2nd ed., pp. 440–468). Baltimore: Williams & Wilkins.

DiPietro, L., Williams, P., & Kaplan, H. (1984). *Alerting and communication devices for hearing impaired people: What's available now.* Washington, DC: National Information Center on Deafness, Gallaudet University.

Erber, N. P. (1985). *Telephone communication and hearing impairment.* San Diego, CA: College Hill Press.

Erdmann, S. A. (1993). Counseling hearing-impaired adults. In J. G. Alpiner & P. A. McCarthy (Eds.), *Rehabilitative audiology: Children and adults* (2nd ed., pp. 374–413). Baltimore: Williams & Wilkins.

Kannapell, B., & Adams, P. (1984). *An orientation to deafness: A handbook and resource guide.* Washington, DC: Gallaudet University Press.

Kaplan, H. (1987). Assistive devices. In H. G. Mueller & V. C. Geoffrey (Eds.), *Communication disorders in aging* (pp. 464–493). Washington, DC: Gallaudet University Press.

Kaplan (2001). In Hull R., (2001). *Aural rehabilitation* (4th ed.). San Diego, CA: Singular.

Kaplan, H., Bally, S. J., & Garretson, C. (1987). *Speechreading, a way to improve understanding.* Washington, DC: Gallaudet University Press.

Kodman, F. (1967). *Techniques for counseling the hearing aid client. Maico audiological library series* (Vol. 8, Reports 23–25). Minneapolis, MN: Maico Hearing Instruments.

Lamb, S. H., Owens, E., & Schubert, E. D. (1983). The revised form of the Hearing Performance Inventory. *Ear and Hearing, 4,* 152–159.

Ramsdell, D. A. (1978). The psychology of the hard-of-hearing and the deafened adult. In H. Davis & S. R. Silverman (Eds.), *Hearing and deafness* (pp. 502–523). New York: Holt, Rinehart, and Winston.

Ross, M. (1982). *Hard-of-hearing children in regular schools.* Englewood Cliffs, NJ: Prentice-Hall.

Rupp, R. R., Higgins, J., & Maurer, J. F. (1977). A feasibility scale for predicting hearing aid use (FSPHAU) with older individuals. *Journal of the Academy of Rehabilitative Audiology, 10,* 81–91.

Sanders, D. A. (1988). Hearing aid orientation and counseling. In M. C. Pollack (Ed.), *Amplification for the hearing impaired* (pp. 343–389). New York: Grune and Stratton.

Tye-Murray, N. (1991). Repair strategy usage by hearing-impaired adults and changes following communication therapy. *Journal of Speech and Hearing Research, 34,* 921–928.

Tye-Murray, N. (1993). Aural rehabilitation and patient management. In R. S. Tyler (Ed.), *Cochlear implants: Audiological foundations* (pp. 323–345). San Diego, CA: Singular.

Tye-Murray, N., Purdy, S. C., & Woodworth, G. G. (1992). Reported use of communication strategies by SHHH members: Client, talker, and situational variables. *Journal of Speech and Hearing Research, 35,* 708–717.

End of Chapter Examination Questions

Chapter 12

1. Compare and contrast the terms *nonculturally deaf* and *culturally Deaf.*

2. According to the author, in contrast with persons who possess normal hearing, adults who have hearing impairment generally have feelings of inadequacy and assume that the "fault" for communication breakdowns is always _____.

3. Name and describe the three psychological levels of hearing presented in this chapter.
    a.
    b.
    c.

4. According to the author, _____ is one of the most important goals of personal adjustment counseling for those with hearing impairment.

5. When persons feel a loss of self-esteem because of an inability to hear normally, they:
    a. are usually open about their disability and discuss their problems without hesitation.
    b. have a tendency to conceal their hearing loss from others.
    c. seek professional help to work through their problems without referral.

6. The term *educational or informational counseling* refers to:
    a. the provision of information about hearing loss.
    b. the effect of a hearing loss on communication.
    c. discussions of intervention procedures.
    d. all of the above.

7. List three coping strategies that can assist hearing-impaired adults, as described by the author.
    a.
    b.
    c.

8. **What steps should teachers take to assist students who have sufficient hearing loss to be able to function with greater efficiency in the classroom? List four.**

    a.

    b.

    c.

    d.

9. **According to the author of this chapter, the home of a deaf or hearing-impaired person is:**

    a. Their "safe place" where they stay a majority of the time.

    b. A quiet place for them to return to after being out in the "real world."

    c. A place for interpersonal communication and consequently more opportunity for communication breakdowns.

End of Chapter Answer Sheet

Name _____ Date _____

Chapter 12

1. Culturally Deaf

_____

_____

Nonculturally deaf

_____

_____

2. _____

3. a. _____

  b. _____

  c. _____

4. _____

5. Which one(s)?   a   b   c

6. Which one(s)?   a   b   c   d

7. Which one(s)?   a   b   c

8. a. _____

  b. _____

  c. _____

  d. _____

9. Which one(s)?   a   b   c

13

Hearing Aid Orientation for Adults Who Possess Impaired Hearing

RAYMOND H. HULL

Chapter Outline

Introduction

One of the important areas of expertise for audiologists is the fitting and dispensing of hearing aids and non-hearing aid assistive listening devices. This has become such an integral component of the scope of practice of audiologists that "audiology" and "dispensing of prosthetic listening devices" go hand-in-hand both in the preparation of future professionals in audiology, and in the practice of audiology. Other than the accurate fitting of the most appropriate hearing aid(s) for individual patients, probably the other single most important element in the successful fitting and dispensing of hearing aids and other assistive listening devices is effective hearing aid orientation and hearing aid counseling. This chapter provides a historical and practical look at considerations in the orientation to and uses of hearing aids by adults who possess impaired hearing.

Considerations for Hearing Aid Orientation for Adults

No matter what type of hearing aid has been fit for adult patients, audiologists confirm the need for hearing aid orientation (HAO) services, and most claim they are offering them. Problems, however, have occurred in effective and efficient provision of those services. The American Speech-Language-Hearing Association's (ASHA's) early "Guidelines on the Responsibilities of Audiologists in the Rehabilitation of the Auditorily Handicapped" (Freeland et al., 1974) emphasized that hearing aid users and their families should be provided with information about the use of amplification. These guidelines also mentioned the need for periodic reassessment

of an amplification device and a patient's adjustment to it. These admonishments by ASHA and the American Academy of Audiology have continued and are assumed to be critical in the fitting and dispensing of hearing aids. Guidelines by AHSA (1998) stress essentially the same elements, but recognize the audiologist as the primary dispenser of the instruments. The elements in these guidelines stress the topics recommended to be included in hearing aid orientation on behalf of adults. Those are:

1. Battery management and safety
2. Instrument features and landmarks
3. Use and routine maintenance
4. Working knowledge of hearing aid components
5. Insertion and removal of the instruments

According to those 1998 ASHA guidelines, the process of assessment through orientation should involve six major stages that constitute the hearing aid fitting process embedded in the rehabilitation plan: assessment, treatment planning, selection, verification, orientation, and validation.

The *assessment* stage is essential to determine the type and magnitude of hearing loss. This is also when intervention is planned and candidacy for amplification is determined. At the *treatment planning* stage, the audiologist, patient, and family or caregivers review the findings of the assessment stage and identify areas of difficulty and need. During the *selection* stage, the physical and electroacoustic characteristics of the desired hearing aids are defined. During the *verification* stage, the audiologist determines that the hearing aids meet a set of standardized measures that include basic electroacoustics, cosmetic appeal, comfortable fit, and real-ear electroacoustic performance. During the *orientation* stage, the audiologist counsels the patient on the use and care of the hearing aids, fosters the patient's realistic expectations of performance from the hearing aids, and explores the candidacy for assistive listening devices and audiologic rehabilitation assessment and treatment. During the *validation* stage, the audiologist determines the impact of the intervention on the perceived disability attributable to the hearing loss.

These guidelines are not intended to precisely dictate how hearing aids should be fitted. Rather, they are intended to suggest several strategies that audiologists may choose from to maximize the probability of user satisfaction with and perceived benefit from amplification. Audiologists should exercise professional judgment in choosing which segments of the guidelines are appropriate to their clinical environment and individual patients. Although the emphasis of the guidelines is on the technical aspects involved in fitting hearing aids, audiologists are reminded that fitting hearing aids is an ongoing process that requires joint participation of the audiologist, patient, and family or caregivers.

It is assumed that most hearing aid users need hearing aid orientation or, at least, more comprehensive and realistic orientation services than some apparently receive. In a review of 377 Army patients, Scherr, Schwartz, and Montgomery (1983) found 32.6% of them required some follow-up orientation in the use of their hearing aid(s). These patients were experiencing minor problems, such as feedback and earmold discomfort, and most needed at least some counseling on using amplification.

According to Eggen (1988), the major complaints of hearing aid users reported by 60 Michigan audiologists and hearing aid dealers were:

1. Background noise;
2. Sound quality of patient's voice;
3. Insertion of the hearing aid;
4. Feeling of a fullness in the ear;
5. Sounds too loud;
6. Adjusting the volume control; and
7. Comfort of the hearing aid.

All of these complaints can be addressed through ongoing hearing aid orientation.

Madell, Pfeffer, Ross, and Chellappa (1991) surveyed 92 patients who had returned dispensed hearing aids at the New York League for the Hard of Hearing. The most frequent reasons for returning hearing aids were (a) less benefit than expected, (b) discomfort, and (c) problems hearing in noise. Such surveys substantiate the need for effective hearing aid orientation before and after hearing aid fitting, although with advances in hearing aid technology, elements of the process of hearing aid orientation will differ in relation to the type of instruments and their components.

Although post-hearing aid fitting orientation has been found to be important in a patient's adjustment to hearing aids, the prefitting expectation of the patient regarding the benefits and uses of hearing aids along with the patient's acceptance of his hearing loss and an understanding of the elements involved in impaired hearing appear to be critical to a patient's success in wearing hearing aids. According to a study by Jerram and Purdy (2001), subjects in their study of 225 adults with impaired hearing who were measured as having better prefitting expectations of hearing aids and better personal adjustment to hearing loss were more successful in wearing their hearing aids, wore them more, and positively influenced their use in both easy and difficult listening situation. So it appears that precounseling regarding hearing aid use can also be important in successful hearing aid use. In fact, in the mind of this author, it can be equally important, although follow-up instruction on the use of a patient's hearing aids and positive reinforcement on their uses are also important aspects of successful hearing aid use.

Hearing Aid Orientation in Retrospect

Hearing aid orientation has been an extensive and integral part of aural rehabilitation, even during the early years of the audiology profession. For example, Carhart (1946) described an elaborate hearing aid selection procedure used with military personnel during World War II that included activities designed to familiarize adults with hearing aid use. These activities were all carried out prior to the final selection of an individual's hearing aid. The major emphasis on HAO in that hearing aid selection program is apparent when reviewing the military's three goals to (a) obtain a hearing aid with optimal efficiency in everyday situations for each patient; (b) provide each patient with an understanding of hearing aids, establish habits of efficient use, and initiate hearing training; and (c) help the person foster a full psychological acceptance of hearing aids (Carhart, 1946). The hearing aid orientation process proposed by Raymond Carhart was quite elaborate. In-depth HAO in those days was particularly critical because in those early years hearing aids were not only cumbersome to wear, but were also difficult to use and maintain. Many persons did not want to wear them because of their size and general amplification characteristics. They were definitely not comparable to the miniaturized digital forms of amplification that we have available to us today!

Preliminary to the actual hearing aid selection in Carhart's early protocol, orien-

tation activities included an explanation about the person's hearing impairment and handicapping conditions, what to expect and what not to expect from wearing a hearing aid, any special problems that might occur, along with group instructions about hearing aid selection procedures. As a part of Carhart's protocol (1946), in an effort to select hearing aids from the total available stock of about 200 instruments, the hearing aid selection began with an informal trial of instruments during an interview. Audiometric and case history information also was used in narrowing the selection to 7 to 10 hearing aids. Certainly, this trial also served as an orientation to hearing aids.

The second stage of the Carhart (1946) comprehensive process involved a 24-hour trial of each preselected aid with a listening hour following every trial. Frequently, 25 to 30 persons participated in a single listening hour. Individuals rated 13 different kinds of controlled sounds on a 5-point rating scale for each of the preselected hearing aids. The sounds included six musical, three speech, and five environmental selections. A similar rating was done for each person's ability to localize sound, listen on the telephone, and experience a 24-hour trial. Finally, a sound discrimination test was administered. Prospective hearing aid users were allowed to adjust their aids for comfort during all of these listening experiences. These ratings, with a weighted score for the discrimination test, were combined and used in eliminating all but three aids for potential selection. The final selection was made from the three remaining hearing aids, based on controlled comparisons of these instruments for speech reception threshold, speech discrimination, tolerance, comfort level, and signal-to-noise ratio tests.

Granted, comprehensive HAO activities in the Carhart process were possible with these prospective hearing aid users because they were a "captive audience" in a Veterans Administration hospital environment. This was because their full-time assignment was to be rehabilitated for a return to civilian life or active duty. Further, the elaborate selection process was important because hearing aids at that time were certainly not prescription instruments. Moreover, the cost of such a program in its entirety for full-time employed civilians might be prohibitive. Despite these limitations for the general adult population, many aspects of this early HAO program were adapted for use by others in the field in familiarizing prospective adult hearing aid users to wearable amplification (Hardick, 1977; Hawkins, 1985). These early orientation procedures were as comprehensive (and lengthy) as they were novel.

Essential Hearing Aid Orientation Services

Some HOA services are essential to all hearing aid orientation programs. The user should receive:

1. Understanding of the function of the component parts and adjustments of hearing aids;
2. Practice in fitting, adjusting, and maintaining amplification;
3. Understanding of the limitations of amplification;
4. Knowledge of why the particular aid was selected;
5. How to begin using a newly selected hearing aid;
6. How to troubleshoot hearing aid problems; and
7. How to exercise a hearing aid user's legal rights.

According to Schow (2001), also found in Mueller, Johnson, and Carter (2007), the elements of an effective hearing aid orientation should include the following, initialed HIO Basics:

1. Hearing expectations: The patient needs to know the benefits and limitations of hearing aids.
2. Instrument operation: It is imperative that the patient know how to operate the hearing aids.
3. Occlusion effect: Test for and eliminate the occlusion effect to the degree possible if it exists.
4. Batteries: The patient needs to know which batteries his hearing aids use, how to insert and remove them, how to obtain them, and their approximate lifespan.
5. Acoustic feedback: It is important for the patient to be aware of what acoustic feedback sounds like, what causes it, and what to do if it persists.
6. System troubleshooting: The patient should be provided a troubleshooting chart to assess problems. Table 13–1 is an example of a hearing aid troubleshooting chart.
7. Insertion and removal: Insertion and removal of the hearing aids should be demonstrated, and the patient should have the opportunity to practice those basics and become proficient before leaving the office.
8. Cleaning and maintenance: The basics of hearing aid cleaning, prevention of moisture damage, implications of hairspray, excessive heat, and others must be discussed.
9. Service: The warranty and repair policies must be discussed and handed to the patient in written form, including how repairs are handled.

TABLE 13–1. Example of a Hearing Aid Orientation Chart

HEARING AID ORIENTATION AND ISSUE

Client: _____ Date: _____

Make & Model: _____ Serial #: LE _____

Serial #: RE _____

Style: BTE ITE ITC CIC

Hearing aid use and maintenance:

_____ Hearing aid components (microphone, receiver, battery door, volume control, earmold)

_____ Battery insertion and removal

_____ Battery size: 675 13 312 10

_____ Battery safety—National Button Battery Hotline (202) 625-3333 (call collect)

_____ Volume adjustment/on-off control

_____ Telephone use/switch

_____ Memory button; Programs 1. _____, 2. _____, 3. _____

_____ Hearing aid insertion and removal

_____ Daily maintenance and cleaning

_____ What to do if the hearing aid gets wet; avoid moisture, extreme temperatures, dropping the aid

_____ Hearing aid storage (soft case vs. hard case, away from pets, room temperature)

Service:

_____ Warranty: _____ year(s) repair and one-time loss and damage. There is a deductible for hearing aid replacement of $_____ per hearing aid.

_____ Follow-up visits

_____ Repairs (drop off aid at clinic, come on-call or call for appointment 978-3289)

_____ On-call—Wednesday 1:30–4:00 p.m., no appointment necessary, but always call to ensure service is available (978-3289)

_____ Battery program

_____ Manufacturer's manual

_____ Trial period/return policy ($_____ return fee per hearing aid). Trial period end date: _____

_____ Medical clearance/medical waiver

TABLE 13–1. *continued*

Notes: _____

_____

_____

_____

_____

_____

_____

The above information has been discussed with me and I have been provided a copy of this form.

Client's Signature	Date	Dispensing Audiologist	Date

Note. Adapted with permission of the WSU Audiology Clinic.

Hearing aid orientation need not be restricted to a limited time frame following the selection and fitting of hearing aids. Orientation may continue for several weeks or many months until a person achieves his fullest understanding of hearing aid use and maximum potential performance in operating and communicating through amplifying devices. Certain aspects of HAO, such as explaining the component parts and adjustments of hearing aids and the anticipated limitations and benefits to be derived from amplification, might be presented before performing a hearing aid selection. Miller and Schein (1987) subscribe to providing HAO before fitting hearing aids. Thus, this chapter's author suggests that HAO not be limited to any specific aspect of rehabilitative services or time frame. Moreover, some aspects of HAO can be presented efficiently in a group and the sharing of common experiences can result in valuable rehabilitation.

Understanding the Component Parts and Controls of Hearing Aids

It is disheartening to evaluate an intelligent adult who purchased a hearing aid a year earlier, but is unable to tell the audiologist the location of the hearing aid microphone or the purpose of the hearing aid components. Adult hearing aid users should be able to name, locate, and describe the functions of the major hearing aid components, including the microphone, battery, receiver, tubing (if it is a behind-the-ear [BTE]), ear hook or "goose neck" (if it is a BTE hearing aid), and earmold (if it is not an in-the-canal [ITC] hearing aid). Similarly, hearing aid users should be able to locate and explain the function of the controls on their hearing aids, such as the gain-control and on-off, tone, and telephone switches if their hearing aids possess those components.

An effective HAO must go beyond providing information, however. It must assess user understanding and performance to see if goals in these areas are accomplished. This author suggests employing a user performance checklist or rating scale to record whether users can satisfactorily can name, locate, and describe the functions of the component parts and controls of their hearing aids (Byrne, Porbinson al Nerval, 1991). Objectives, as always, will have to be tailored to individual needs and capabilities.

Videotapes have been prepared by service facilities and can be purchased commercially (Orton, 1989) to illustrate the component parts of hearing aids and how to fit, adjust, and maintain different models of hearing aids. Some hearing aid manufacturers have DVDs available on hearing aid use and maintenance. These tapes and DVDs can be shown to individuals or used efficiently with groups of individuals who have hearing impairment and their family members and/or friends or given to the patient as part of the fitting process. They should be shown to family members and friends while the patient is present.

Practice in Fitting, Adjusting, and Maintaining Amplification

A hearing aid user, particularly a new user, needs more than a description and demonstration of how to fit, operate, and maintain a newly selected hearing aid. To determine if orientation has been successful, an assessment of a user's ability to perform these tasks is essential. Preferably, this assessment should be done when the aid is fitted and repeated at a follow-up appointment within a month. A simple user-performance checklist or rating scale can be used to record a user's ability to perform the many fitting, adjustment, and maintenance functions

associated with the user's hearing aid. For example, audiologists should rate a hearing aid user's ability to insert and remove the earmold or ITE hearing aid from the ear, operate the hearing aid controls, and change the battery, and also make certain that all aspects of the hearing aid fitting and orientation have taken place. This performance-based check should be used for all hearing aid fittings to make sure that all has been accomplished that is to be accomplished before the patient leaves his appointment. Do not assume a person is adequately oriented to hearing aid use just because he has previously worn a hearing aid, or assume that you, the audiologist, have completed all aspects of the fitting and orientation. An example of a performance-based checklist is presented in Table 13–2, adapted from Sandlin (2000).

The hearing aid user should be given a list of maintenance suggestions and be provided an opportunity to demonstrate basic maintenance skills. The following suggestions are some examples of what might be included on a maintenance list:

Hearing Aid Maintenance List

■ Protect hearing aids against exposure to excessive heat from sources such as hair dryers, radiators, heaters, and closed cars on a hot sunny day.

■ Avoid exposing hearing aids to excessive humidity of rain, saunas, steam baths, or placing aids in a pants pocket and sent to the laundry.

■ Place hearing aids in a container with silica gel at night to remove any moisture, particularly for persons who perspire excessively or are involved in sports or yard work.

■ Prevent hairsprays, insecticides, and other sprays from being directed at the instruments.

TABLE 13–2. Example of a Hearing Aid Fitting Checklist.

HEARING AID FITTING CHECKLIST

Patient Name _____ Address _____

Phone _____

Date of Hearing Aid Fitting_____

Company _____ Serial No(s) _____

Battery Size _____.

Dispensing Checklist

_____ Medical Clearance and Release of Information on file.

_____ Explained steps for care and maintenance of hearing aid(s).

_____ Is able to insert batteries and check for hearing aid function.

_____ Provided card with battery size specified.

_____ Provided extra batteries and battery mailing card.

_____ Provided cleaning tools and instructions.

_____ Patient understands Return Policy.

Comments _____

_____

_____ Warranty and Warranty Expiration _____

_____ Explained Warranty Coverage _____

_____ Special Instruction to Patient _____

_____

_____ Date and Method of Payment _____ Amount Paid _____

Balance Due _____

_____   _____
Patient Signature   Date   Audiologist Signature   Date

License No. _____

Note. From Audiology Services of Central Kansas, 22 Center St., Eden, Kansas. Reprinted by permission.

- Clean earmolds and tubing periodically with mild soap and water or commercially available cleaning solutions.
- Keep hearing aids away from dogs and small children when not wearing them.
- Remove hearing aids from the ear and handle them over a soft surface, so, if dropped, potential damage is reduced.

Limitations of Amplification

Prospective hearing aid users, as well as their family members and friends, frequently have unrealistic expectations about the benefits of wearable amplification (Kricos, Lesner, & Sandridge, 1991). These expectations range from total lack of benefit to the expectation of "normal" hearing. These perceptions must be explored if audiologists hope to successfully acquaint hearing aid users and the persons with whom they communicate with amplification. A very positive, although straightforward, approach will be required with an acquaintance or family member who is extremely skeptical about the benefits of amplification. Conversely, a realistic approach is needed for an individual who expects a hearing aid to resolve all hearing problems, especially if speech discrimination ability is significantly reduced. Two other potential limitations include restricted dynamic range and tolerance problems and monaural fitting when binaural hearing aids were appropriate (Hurley, 1993).

Why Was a Particular Hearing Aid Selected?

Hearing aid users should be told why:

1. A particular type of hearing aid, such as an in-the-ear or BTE instrument, was selected,
2. The aid is a particular make,
3. A monaural aid for the right or left ear or binaural instruments were chosen,

4. The particular external controls were chosen and how they should be set,
5. The type of earmold was selected, and
6. Special features were selected.

Adjustments to Newly Selected and Fit Hearing Aids

The length of time necessary for satisfactory adjustment to newly selected hearing aids will vary substantially from person to person depending on the amount and type of impairment, whether amplification has been used previously, the extent of concomitant handicapping conditions such as mental impairment, muscular coordination, or visual impairment, the age of onset and progression of hearing impairment, and the person's daily activities. An intelligent, long-time successful hearing aid user who has just procured a replacement instrument might immediately begin wearing the new hearing aid during all of his waking hours without needing any formalized HAO beyond an explanation of any new or different hearing aid controls or maintenance instructions. Conversely, a developmentally disabled adult who has a long-standing hearing impairment and has never tried amplification may require ongoing HAO along with involvement of family or those who provide services on his behalf. New hearing aid users generally are encouraged to begin employing their aids in easy listening situations and then progress to more difficult listening experiences. An easy listening situation would involve listening:

1. To a single known speaker,
2. In a non-noisy environment,
3. To familiar topics,
4. While watching the speaker,
5. With good lighting on the speaker's face, and
6. With minimal visual or auditory distractions.

After new users adjust to easy listening situations, they will be encouraged to enter other less optimal environments. HAO is not complete until patients have adjusted to using their new hearing aids in a variety of daily listening activities, particularly in those situations where they want and need to communicate for social, vocational, or educational purposes.

How to Troubleshoot Hearing Aid Problems

If hearing aid users sufficiently understand the functions of the component parts and controls of hearing aids, they intuitively may be able to solve most of their own hearing aid problems. However, troubleshooting ability should not be left to chance; quite the contrary—hearing aid users should be told about possible problems that can occur, how to locate the problems, and how to seek a resolution. A set of used hearing aids with a variety of problems is very helpful in demonstrating troubleshooting techniques. Moreover, a chart listing problems, possible causes, and remedies should be provided to hearing aid users. The clinician can ask users to study their charts and be prepared to answer questions about malfunctioning aids. At a later appointment patients should be able to demonstrate their understanding of the material by locating problems and remedying them with a stock of used aids. Hearing aid users should be encouraged to keep the troubleshooting chart with important papers for immediate reference, if hearing aid problems arise. The chart might cover these problems:

1. Squealing (whistling)
2. No amplification
3. Reduced amplification
4. Intermittent amplification or scratchy, frying, crashing sound
5. Sharp sound (as though through a barrel)
6. "Tinny" or "thin" sound
7. Sound too noisy
8. Reduced clarity of speech
9. Ear canal hurts
10. Problem not describable, but change noticed

Additionally, the chart should list possible causes, how to locate the problems, and the remedies. The chart should indicate clearly which causes can be remedied by the user and which ones should be fixed by a hearing aid dispenser. The hearing aid user should be encouraged to call the audiologist who selected the hearing instrument, if problems arise that the user is unable to resolve. The audiologist's address and phone number should be printed prominently on the chart.

These charts are available commercially through a variety of sources. Hearing aid manufacturers frequently include these charts in the User Instructional Brochure that is required to accompany hearing aids by the U.S. Food and Drug Administration (U.S. Food and Drug Administration [FDA], 1994a).

Consumer Rights of Hearing Aid Users

Individuals should be informed of their legal rights and options as owners or users of wearable amplification. The cost of aids and most expenses associated with hearing impairment, for example, are allowed as medical expenses in computing federal income tax. Many prospective purchasers of hearing aids may qualify for public or private funds to cover the cost, such as funds available through Medicaid, Rehabilitation

Services Administration, Veterans Administration, or employee health benefits. They should also be informed of their legal rights and restrictions under the Labeling and Conditions for Sale Regulation promulgated by the FDA. Certain information must be provided to prospective hearing aid users in the form of a User Instructional Brochure, as mandated by the FDA. Although many hearing aid manufacturers provided brochures with their instruments prior to this regulation, the extent and uniformity of information varied substantially. This was particularly true concerning electroacoustic characteristics of hearing aids.

Since as early as August 15, 1977, the effective date of the FDA regulation, all hearing aids are to be accompanied by a user instructional brochure containing the following categories of information:

1. Illustration of the hearing aid showing controls, adjustments, and battery compartment.
2. Printed material on the operation of all controls designed for user adjustment.
3. Description of possible accompanying accessories.
4. Instructions on how to use, maintain, and care for as well as replace or recharge batteries.
5. How to and where to procure repair services.
6. Conditions to be avoided in preventing damage to hearing aids, such as dropping or exposing to excessive heat or humidity.
7. Warning to seek medical advice when encountering any side effects such as skin irritation or increased accumulation of cerumen.
8. Statement that a hearing aid will not restore normal hearing or prevent or improve a hearing impairment caused by organic conditions.
9. Statement that with most persons, infrequent use of wearable amplification will not allow them to attain full benefit from hearing aid use.
10. Statement that hearing aid use is only one aspect of hearing rehabilitation and may need to be augmented by auditory training and lipreading instruction.
11. Warning statement to hearing aid dispensers to advise prospective hearing aid users to see a licensed physician before dispensing hearing aids if any of eight medical conditions exist (see any User Instructional Brochure for these conditions).
12. Notice to prospective hearing aid users indicating, among other things, that hearing aids cannot be sold to individuals until they have obtained a medical evaluation from a licensed physician (preferably one who specializes in diseases of the ear); however, a fully informed adult may waive the medical evaluation.
13. Electroacoustical data obtained in accordance with the American National Standards Institute (1996) Standard for Specification of Hearing Aid Characteristics (this information may be included on separate labeling that accompanies the hearing aids).

Other information may be included in the User Instructional Brochure if it is not false, misleading, or prohibited by this regulation or by Federal Trade Commission (FTC) regulations. Audiologists, hearing aid sales personnel, and physicians specializing in diseases of the ear should have a reference copy of this important FDA regulation. In addition to the services discussed in this chapter, an individualized rehabilitation plan for a patient might require counseling, auditory training, situational training, speechreading, motivational training, and speech production training. Although some or all of these additional five rehabilitative services might be required, they are not essential for all patients. Moreover, these latter services are discussed in more detail in other chapters of this textbook.

Summary

Because of the limited survey and research data on adult HAO services, the author challenges all specialists working with adults who possess impaired hearing to provide hearing aid orientation services that are tailored to each patient, and to be aware of the HAO needs of each patient even though those will vary greatly among patients. The prospects for improvement in hearing and related communication function are great if patients are successfully oriented to their hearing aids and their function. The hearing aids will become an important part of their life as their use becomes a natural part of it.

References

Alpiner, J. (1987). Evaluation of adult communication function. In J. Alpiner & P. McCarthy (Eds.), *Rehabilitative audiology: Children and adults* (pp. 44-114). Baltimore: Williams & Wilkins.

American National Standards Institute. (1996). *Specification of hearing aid characteristics*. ANSI A 3.22-1996. New York: American National Standards Institute.

American Speech-Language-Hearing Association. (1984). Position statement: Definition of competencies for aural rehabilitation. *Asha, 26*, 37-41.

American Speech-Language-Hearing Association. (1990). Scope of practice, speech-language pathology and audiology. *ASHA, 32*, 1-2.

American Speech-Language-Hearing Association. (1998). Guidelines for hearing aid fitting for adults. Available at http://www.asha.org/policy GL1998_00012

Armbruster, J., & Miller, M. (1986). *How to get the most out of your hearing aid*. Washington, DC: Alexander Graham Bell Association for the Deaf.

Carhart, R. (1946). Selection of hearing aids. *Archives of Otolaryngology, 44*, 1-18.

Castle, W. E. (Ed.). (1967). A conference on hearing aid evaluation procedures. *ASHA Reports, 2*, 21-38.

Chmiel, R., & Jerger, J. (1993). Some factors affecting assessment of hearing handicap in the elderly. *Journal of the American Academy of Audiology, 4*, 249-257.

Cox, R. M., Gilmore, C., & Alexander, G. C. (1991). Comparison of two questionnaires for patient-assessed hearing aid benefit. *Journal of the American Academy of Audiology, 2*, 134-145.

Cox, R. M., & Rivera, I. M. (1992). Predictability and reliability of hearing aid benefit measured using the PHAB. *Journal of the American Academy of Audiology, 3*, 242-254.

Demorest, M., & Erdman, S. (1987). Development of the communication profile for the hearing impaired. *Journal of Speech and Hearing Disorders, 52*, 129-143.

Eggen, R. E. (1988). *A survey of hearing aid orientation process in the state of Michigan*. Unpublished master's independent study, Central Michigan University, Mount Pleasant.

Freeland, E. E., Hill, M. J., Jeffers, J., Matkin, N. D., Stream, R. W., Tobin, H., et al. (1974). The audiologist: Responsibilities in the habilitation of the auditorily handicapped. *Journal of the American Speech and Hearing Association, 16*, 68-70.

Gatehouse, S. (1993). Role of perceptual acclimatization in the selection of frequency response for hearing aids. *Journal of the American Academy of Audiology, 4*, 296-306.

Gauger, J. S. (1978). *Orientation to hearing aids*. Rochester, NY: National Technical Institute for the Deaf.

Gendel, J. (1984). *Questions most often asked about earmolds*. New York: New York League for the Hard of Hearing.

Hardick, E. J. (1977). Aural rehabilitation programs for the aged can be successful. *Journal of the Academy of Rehabilitative Audiology, 10*, 51-67.

Harless, E. L., & McConnell, F. (1982). Effects of hearing aid use on self concept in older persons. *Journal of Speech and Hearing Disorders, 47*, 305-309.

Hawkins, D. B. (1985). Reflections on amplification: Validation of performance. *Journal of the Academy of Rehabilitative Audiology, 18*, 42-54.

Hurley, R. M. (1993). Monaural hearing aid effect: Case presentations. *Journal of the American Academy of Audiology, 4*, 285-294.

Jerram, J. C. K., & Purdy, S. (2001). Technology, expectations, and adjustment to hearing loss: Predictors of hearing aid outcome. *Journal of the American Academy of Audiology, 12*, 64-79.

Krames Communications. (1987). *Hearing aids: A guide to their wear and care.* Daly City, CA: Author.

Kricos, P. B., Lesner, S. A., & Sandridge, S. A. (1991). Expectations of older adults regarding the use of hearing aids. *Journal of the American Academy of Audiology, 2*, 129-133.

Lamb, S., Owens, E., & Schubert, E. (1983). The revised form of the Hearing Performance Inventory. *Ear and Hearing, 4*, 152-157.

Lesner, S. A., Lynn, J. M., & Brainard, J. (1988). Feasibility of using a single-subject design for continuous discourse tracking measurement. *Journal of the Academy of Rehabilitative Audiology, 21*, 83-89.

Madell, J. (1986). *You and your hearing aid.* New York: New York League for the Hard of Hearing.

Madell, J., Pfeffer, E., Ross, M., & Chellappa, M. (1991). Hearing aid returns at a community hearing and speech agency. *The Hearing Journal, 44*, 18-23.

Mahon, W. J. (1989). A close look at hearing aid repair. *The Hearing Aid Journal, 42*, 9-12.

Mahon, W. J. (1989). 1989 U.S. hearing aid sale summary. *The Hearing Aid Journal, 42*, 9-14.

Martin, F. N., & Morris, L. J. (1989). Current audiologic practices in the United States. *The Hearing Aid Journal, 42*, 25-44.

McReynolds, L. V., & Thompson, C. K. (1986). Flexibility of single-subject experimental designs. Part I: Review of the basics of single-subject designs. *Journal of Speech and Hearing Disorders, 51*, 194-203.

Miller, M. H., & Schein, J. D. (1987). Improving consumer acceptance of hearing aids. *The Hearing Journal, 40*, 25-30.

Mueller, H. G., Johnson, E. E., & Carter, A. S. (2007). Hearing aids and assistive devices. In R. L. Schow & M. A. Nerbonne (Eds.), *Introduction to audiologic rehabilitation* (pp. 31-76). Boston: Allyn and Bacon.

Newman, C. W., Jacobson, G. P., Hug, G. A., Weinstein, B. E., & Malinoff, R. L. (1991). Practical method for quantifying hearing aid benefit in older adults. *Journal of the American Academy of Audiology, 2*, 70-75.

Orton, C. (1989). *Help with your hearing aids* [Videotape]. Stinson Beach, CA: Orton-Palmer & Associates.

Palmer, C. V. (1992). Assistive devices in the audiology practice. *American Journal of Audiology, 1*, 37-57.

Sanders, D. A. (1993). Profile questionnaire for rating communicative performance in a home environment, occupational environment, social environment. In M. Pollack (Ed.), *Amplification for the hearing impaired* (pp. 385-395). Orlando, FL: Grune & Stratton.

Sandlin, R. E. (2000). *Textbook of hearing aid amplification.* San Diego, CA: Singular.

Scherr, C. K., Schwartz, D. M., & Montgomery, A. A. (1983). Follow-up survey of new hearing aid users. *Journal of Academy of Rehabilitative Audiology, 1*, 202-209.

Schow, R. L. (2001). A standardized AR battery for dispensers is proposed. *The Hearing Journal, 54*, 10-20.

Schow, R. L., Balsara, N. R., Smedley, T. C., & Whitcomb, C. J. (1993). Aural rehabilitation by ASHA audiologists: 1980-1990. *American Journal of Audiology, 2*, 28-37.

Self-Help for Hard of Hearing People. (1986). *I think I have a problem. What do I do?* Bethesda, MD: Author.

Self-Help for Hard of Hearing People. (1987). *ABCs of hearing aids.* Bethesda, MD: Author.

Sinclair, J. S., & Goldstein, J. L. (1991). Long-term benefit, satisfaction, and use of amplification among military retirees. *Journal of the Academy of Rehabilitative Audiology, 24*, 55-64.

Smaldino, S. E., & Smaldino, J. J. (1988). The influence of aural rehabilitation and cognitive style disclosure on the perception of hearing handicap. *Journal of the Academy of Rehabilitative Audiology*, *21*, 57–64.

Tyler, R. S. (1994). The use of speech-perception tests in audiological rehabilitation: Current and future research needs. *Journal of the Academy of Rehabilitative Audiology*, *27*, 67–92.

U.S. Food and Drug Administration. (1994, Sept/Oct). FDA Holds Hearings on Hearing Aid Performance Claims. *Audiology Today*, *26*, 203–206.

U.S. Food and Drug Administration. (1994). Hearing aid devices, professional and patient labeling and conditions for sale. *Federal Register*, *42*, 9286–9296.

U.S. Office of Education, Bureau of Education for Handicapped Children. (1977). Implementation of Part B of the Education of the Handicapped Act. *Federal Register*, *42*, 42474–42518.

Walden, B., Demorest, M., & Hepler, E. (1984). Self-report approach to assessing benefit derived from amplification. *Journal of Speech and Hearing Research*, *27*, 49–56.

Williams, P., & Jacobs-Condit, L. (1985). *Hearing aids, what are they?* Washington, DC: National Information Center on Deafness, Gallaudet University.

End of Chapter Examination Questions

Chapter 13

1. Hearing aid users may complain about certain aspects of hearing aid use. Name at least four of the seven major complaints of hearing aid users.
   a.
   b.
   c.
   d.

2. According to the author, what are the most frequent reasons for hearing aid returns?

3. What are some of the reasons that hearing aid orientation (HAO) programs may have to be modified to fit the needs of individual patients?

4. Why is it important to involve family members and friends of hearing aid users in HAO programs?

5. Hearing aid orientation must be an extensive and integral part of the _____ program.

6. All hearing aid orientation programs should contain the same basic elements. List five of the most essential elements of hearing aid orientation.
   a.
   b.
   c.
   d.
   e.

7. New hearing aid users generally are encouraged to begin using their hearing aids in easy listening situations and then progress to more difficult listening experiences. An easy listening situation would involve listening to:
   a. flute playing
   b. a group of people at a party
   c. a single speaker who is known to the listener
   d. a familiar radio station

8. The most common hearing aid problem that may arise is:
   a. a dead battery
   b. acoustic feedback
   c. uncomfortable earmold
   d. all of the above

9. **In addition to the seven hearing aid orientation services discussed in this chapter, _____ is always welcomed by a hearing-impaired patient.**
   a. a follow-up call by the audiologist
   b. a grant for funds
   c. rescheduling of appointments
   d. an individualized rehabilitation plan

End of Chapter Answer Sheet

Name _____ Date _____

Chapter 13

1. a. _____

    b. _____

    c. _____

    d. _____

2. _____

_____

_____

3. _____

_____

_____

4. _____

_____

_____

5. _____

6. a. _____

    b. _____

    c. _____

    d. _____

    e. _____

7. Which one(s)?   a   b   c   d

8. Which one(s)?   a   b   c   d

9. Which one(s)?   a   b   c   d

Non-Hearing Aid Assistive Hearing Technology for Adults with Impaired Hearing

JOSEPH J. SMALDINO

Chapter Outline

Introduction

Montgomery and Houston (2000) describe the management of communication deficits of hearing impaired adults in statistical terms. In this conceptualization the goal of a management program is to increase the probability that successful communication will occur in an ever-changing verbal and acoustic environment. In order to increase the odds of success under these changing conditions, rehabilitative goals and interventions are developed based on individual needs and individual capabilities. Because of the hearing loss, suitable fitting of a hearing aid is an important element used to increase chances of successful management with hearing impaired adults. Recent technological advances in hearing aid capabilities have provided solutions to many communication problems, but hearing aids cannot be relied upon to solve every patient's communication deficits. In these instances, when hearing aids are not enough, a plethora of auditory (assistive listening device) and nonauditory (assistive device) technologies can be recruited to be used in conjunction with the hearing aid or in place of the hearing aid in especially difficult communication situations. Unfortunately, hearing assistance technology is often given low priority during the development of management plans for hearing impaired adults (Ross, 2004). When it is considered that these technologies can further enhance the chances of successful communication over the hearing aid alone, the low priority can significantly reduce the effectiveness of the rehabilitative plan and overall communication success.

The purpose of this chapter is to (a) provide a framework for hearing assistance technology candidacy and selection and (b) review various types of hearing assistance technologies.

Listener and Talker Rights

Many adults with hearing loss can communicate effectively in person-to-person communication when the communication partners are close to one another and when there is a satisfactory acoustic environment (low levels of background noise and reverberation). It is well established, however, that communication is significantly degraded for the same individuals (with or without a hearing aid) when the acoustic environment is undesirable (high levels of background noise and room echoes [reverberation] and when communicating in groups or at a distance; Crandell, Smaldino, & Flexer, 2005). Under these circumstances, the hearing impaired person is prevented from participating on equal terms with normal hearing people. In recognition of the need for equal participation in communication environments, the Americans with Disabilities Act of 1990 (ADA, 1990) requires access to assistive listening devices in employment, state and government services, public accommodations and commercial facilities, and in telecommunications. Overall, the right as well as the need of both listeners and talkers to participate in interpersonal communication is an important theme to keep in mind.

Compton (1995) developed a scheme that emphasizes the central role that assistive technology plays in the overall management of the hearing impaired adult. An adapted version of her "continuum of audiological" care is shown in Figure 14–1. Several important aspects should be noted in the scheme: (a) Assistive technology evaluation and deployment is an integral part of the management plan; it is not considered an "add-on" or "afterthought." (b) Assistive technology bridges the gap between the

Overall Hearing Management Plan

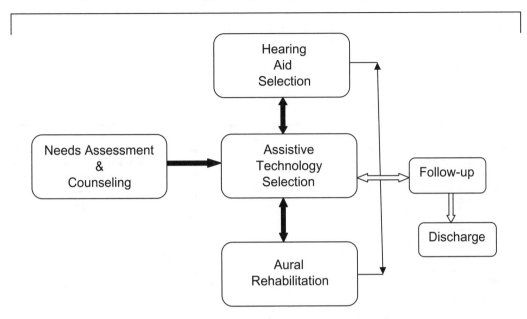

Figure 14–1. Continuum of audiological care showing the central position of assistive technology in overall hearing management plan. *Note.* Adapted from "Selecting What's Best for the Individual," by C. Compton, 1995, in Tyler, R. & Schum, D. (Eds.), *Assistive Devices for Persons with Hearing Impairment* (p. 225), Boston: Allyn & Bacon.

hearing aid and the aural rehabilitation procedures, and as such often permits the maximum benefit from both the hearing aid and the therapeutic interventions. (c) The professional must be conversant with available assistive technology in order to effectively incorporate them into a comprehensive management plan.

Hearing Assistance Technology Needs Assessment

A thorough needs assessment is pivotal to the effective selection and fitting of a hearing aid, effective design of rehabilitative therapeutic services, and the effective selection of assistive technology (see Figure 14-1). Much has been written about techniques for evaluating the therapeutic needs of an individual and selection of hearing aid characteristics (Alpiner & Schow, 2000; Palmer & Mueller, 2000). Less has been written about the selection of assistive technologies for the hearing impaired adult. One of the most comprehensive hearing assistance technology (HAT) communication needs assessment questionnaires has been developed by Compton (2000) and is an ideal starting point for identifying assistive technology needs. A shorter checklist assessment developed by Vaughn and Lightfoot (1996) is shown in Table 14-1. Once a need is determined, then affordability, reliability/ durability, operability, portability, compatibility, and cosmetic factors must be considered

TABLE 14–1. Short Communication Needs Assessment Checklist

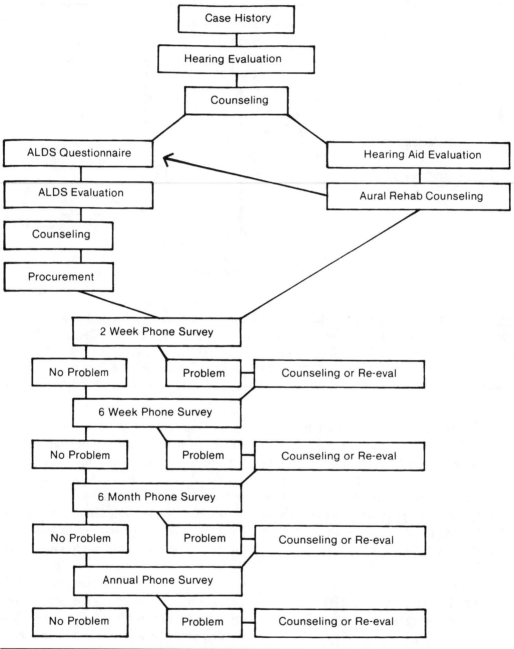

Note. From Vaughn, G. R., & Lightfoot, R. K. (1989). Resource materials. In R. L. Schow & M. A. Nerbonne (Eds.), *Introduction to aural rehabilitation* (pp. 586–605). Austin, TX: Pro-Ed.

(Compton, 1995). When selecting a personal hearing aid for a patient, audiologists consider the patient's degree of loss and her acceptance of amplification. When dispensing HAT, audiologists must follow the same selection protocol. In addition, however, they need to make a careful analysis of the patient's lifestyle. The successful selection of a HAT depends not only on the satisfaction of the listener, but also that of the talkers who wish to communicate with her.

When Assistive Technology Can Help

In an attempt to systematize HAT selection, Compton (1995) suggested that assistive technology can be used to address one or more of four communication needs. She suggests that most people face the following four needs: (a) face-to-face communication, (b) broadcast and other electronic media, (c) telephone conversations, and (d) important warning or environmental sounds. The major technologies described in the decision circles, which assists in making decisions regarding which technology is most appropriate (found in Figure 14-2), will be overviewed in the following section.

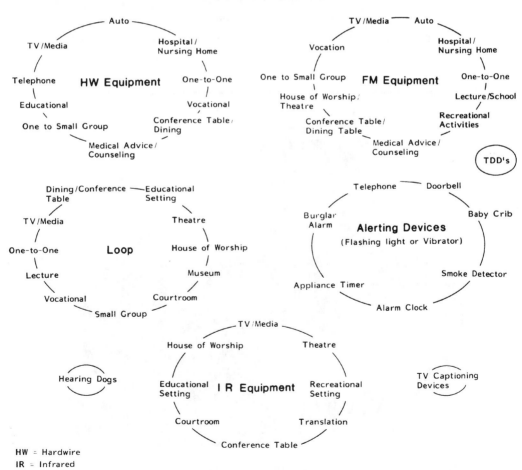

Figure 14–2. Decision circles for use of assistive technologies.

Categories of Hearing Assistance Technology

Hearing assistance technology can be generally categorized as follows:

1. Hardwire
2. Infrared
3. Frequency modulation (FM)
4. Audio induction loop

Television and telephone aids are found across these categories.

Hardwire Devices

Hardwire devices are extremely popular because they are readily available, amplify the sound level, use simple and familiar technology, are easy to operate, and, most of all, are inexpensive. The basic components of a hardwire HAT are: (a) an amplifier, (b) a microphone, (c) possibly a tone control, and (d) an earphone or insert ear plugs (Figure 14–3 is an example). They resemble other kinds of portable audio devices such as an iPod and MP3 player but are typically larger. Because they are not marketed as hearing aids per se, they are not required to have Food and Drug Administration approval or oversight. Some are capable of high output levels so care must be taken to avoid unsafe listening levels. Additional components may be purchased to accommodate such special needs as television or telephone listening. The listener usually puts the hardwire amplifier in a pocket so that the volume control and on/

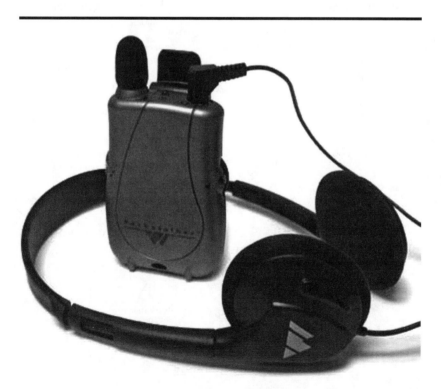

Figure 14–3. Basic hardwire hearing assistance technology (HAT).

off switch are accessible. She puts the earphones on her ears and places the microphone on or near the desired sound source. For television viewing, for example, the microphone might be attached to an extension cord and placed in close proximity to the television speaker.

Other accessories might include an induction loop for use with a hearing aid telecoil and rechargeable battery. In some environments, such as nursing homes, these devices can serve as the primary amplification device for residents unable or unwilling to use hearing aids. They can also be used as a temporary listening device when hearing aids malfunction, are sent out for repair, or are lost. In medical environments, such as a doctor's office, the devices are useful when communicating with hearing impaired patients who need hearing aids but do not have them. In noisy environments, such as in a vehicle, a hardwired system microphone can be passed around during a conversation, affording the hearing impaired passenger an effective means to be involved in the communications (Ross, January, 1999).

Infrared Listening Systems

Infrared light technology is widely used in the field of electronics. Televisions, stereos, and DVD recorder/players employ the use of infrared light for operation of their remote controls. Infrared light beams are now used to carry audio signals from the special light emitting diodes (LEDs) of the transmitters to the infrared receivers worn by normally hearing listeners and listeners who have hearing impairment. Although varying amounts of infrared light are in all sources of light, technology has reduced the problems of infrared interference from incandescent and fluorescent lighting. The natural infrared light from the sun is so great that the use of

an infrared system is typically confined to indoor environments. Depending on specific needs, various sizes and signal strengths are available for home, small meeting areas, or large areas such as auditoriums and churches. Infrared systems are line-of-sight devices, meaning that the receiver must be in line-of-sight with the transmitter. It is possible, however, for the receiver to respond to a signal that has bounced off of a surface such as a smooth ceiling or wall, tile floor, glossy painted wall, or other reflective surface. When considering the placement of transmitters in a facility, care must be taken that the signal is not obstructed by supporting structures or by the heads of the persons who are seated or standing between the listeners and the transmitter.

One great advantage of infrared light transmission is that it does not pass through walls or curtains; thus, infrared HATs provide transmission privacy. Some of the locations in which this privacy is desirable include courtrooms, boardrooms, or theaters. Infrared prevents the illegal recording of a performance outside places such as those listed above, or listening in to proceedings in a courtroom. A second advantage of an infrared HAT is that it is usually not affected by radio frequency transmissions or by electromagnetic interference.

Infrared listening systems have been installed in many theaters and churches for patrons who have hearing impairment, as well as for normally hearing persons who enjoy the high audio quality of infrared reception.

Infrared listening systems are appropriate for all situations in which a listener is in a fixed position. These situations include the large area infrared transmitter systems for houses of worship, theaters, or concert halls. The entire listening area must be saturated with infrared light, so large and or numerous LEDs must be employed.

For small area usage, such as home television viewing or small group meetings, a smaller transmitter provides adequate infrared light coverage. Figure 14–4 illustrates a small infrared system.

Reception of any infrared signal can be accomplished by several means. The most common is by the use of an "under-the-chin" receiver that receives the infrared signal, converts it to acoustic energy, and delivers it to the ear of the listener. Figure 14–5 shows a person using an infrared receiver. Note the volume control pictured on the left and the "eye" shown on the right. A second type of receiver is a body receiver that is worn with a cord that delivers the signal electronically to (a) an earplug or earphone, (b) a magnetic induction silhouette worn behind

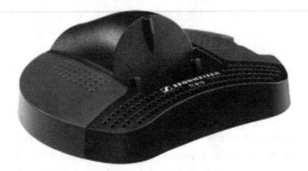

Figure 14–4. An example of an infrared transmitter. (Courtesy of Sennheiser.)

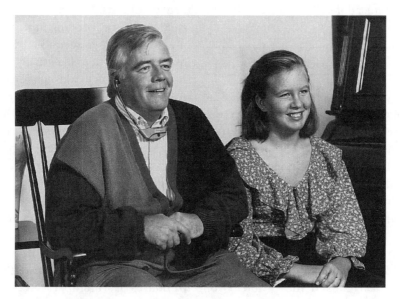

Figure 14–5. Person wearing an infrared receiver. (Courtesy of Sennheiser.)

the ear or against the T-coil of a hearing aid, (c) a magnetic neck loop, or (d) a personal hearing aid with direct audio input. Most recently, infrared (IR) technology has been used in the classroom setting and is referred to as sound-field amplification. An IR transmitting microphone is worn by the teacher. The IR receiver is connected to a public address amplifier, which in turn is connected to loudspeakers distributed throughout the listening area. Figure 14–6 shows an IR sound-field system. Students benefit from a louder signal that is less distorted by background noise, distance, and room echoes. Portable sound-field systems are being used by adults in small group settings and in places where excessive background noise impedes communication.

Frequency Modulation Devices

Frequency modulation (FM) systems employ frequency modulated radio waves to transmit a signal from the talker or sound source to listeners. The FM transmitter may be thought of as a miniature radio station that transmits to FM receivers, similar in concept to the radios used by the general pub-

lic. The FM transmitter sends the signal at a specific frequency and the receiver must be tuned to the same frequency in order to receive the transmission. The transmitted signal is often signal processed and then amplified or delivered to a primary amplification device such as a hearing aid or cochlear implant.

FM systems are commonly used in educational settings and can be described as a personal FM auditory trainer or as sound-field amplification. When used as a personal FM system, the teacher wears an FM transmitting microphone that sends an FM radio signal to a student wearing a receiver. Sometimes the receiver is connected to the student's hearing aid via a direct audio input connection (Figure 14–7) or connected to an induction coil neck loop and input to the hearing aid via the aid's telecoil. Most recently, some hearing aids have FM receivers integrated into the hearing aid itself and so require no external connections to the receiver whatsoever (Figure 14–8). When used as a sound-field amplification system, the configuration is similar to the IR sound-field system. The main differences between the two types of sound-field systems is that the FM transmitter radio signal is not confined

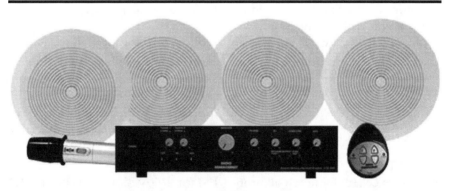

Figure 14–6. Example of an infrared soundfield amplification system. (Courtesy of Audio Enhancement.)

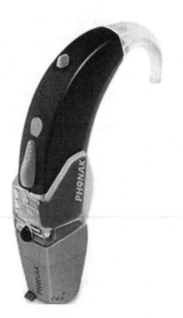

Figure 14–7. Hearing aid with external FM receiver attached. (Courtesy of Phonak.)

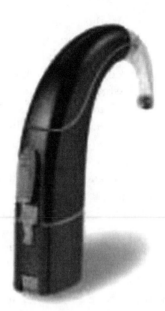

Figure 14–8. Hearing aid with integrated FM receiver attached. (Courtesy of Phonak.)

like the IR signal and so each classroom must have a separate designated frequency in order to prevent unintended FM signals from being received by the students.

The Federal Communications Commission (FCC) has assigned two separate FM frequency ranges for assistive listening systems. The established 72–76 MHz range is somewhat prone to interference from emergency vehicles and is slowly being phased out. The newer 216–217 MHz range is assigned exclusively for low-power assistive listening devices and is not as susceptible to interference.

FM HATS and Special Needs

FM for One-To-One Communication. FM systems are excellent for nearly all problem listening environments. In one-to-one communication, the microphone and transmitter can be handheld by the talker or they can be permanently positioned on the corner of a desk or table for interviewing and counseling situations.

FM for Automobiles. For use in automobiles or other transportation modes, the microphone of an FM transmitter can be clipped to the front or back of a car seat to be as close to as many talkers as possible.

FM for Restaurants. Restaurant noise can be overcome by placing an FM microphone as close to the sound source as possible by (a) clipping it to the talker's lapel, (b) placing it in the center of the table, or (c) hanging it from the ceiling or light fixture above the table.

FM for Television and Radio. Television and radio reception can be improved by positioning a microphone in front of the internal speaker of the television or radio.

The volume level on the set should be adjusted so that it is at a listening level that is comfortable for the normally hearing listeners in the area.

FM and Glass Barriers. One of the most difficult situations for persons who have hearing impairment is caused by the glass barriers used at bank teller windows and in office reception areas. If there is an opening in the glass barrier, the microphone can be passed through the opening for the best speech signal.

Large Area FM Applications. The problems encountered in large area listening can be overcome by giving the microphone to the talker or by placing it at the sound source. FM transmission is highly satisfactory for activities such as religious gatherings, lectures, group meetings, classrooms, or even movie theaters. As a courtesy, permission should be given by the talker or the management of a facility prior to the placement of a transmitter. This will avoid any misunderstanding about the legality of the recording.

FM and Outdoor Activities. Outdoor instructional activities such as horseback riding, bicycling, snow skiing, and golfing can be enhanced by FM technology.

FM and Mobility Training for the Blind. Rehabilitation specialists for the blind have included FM devices as an important tool for mobility training and other activities in which the blind person is at a distance from the instructor.

Audio Induction Loop Systems

The audio induction loop system is one of the oldest assistive listening devices. In Europe, loops have been used widely in conjunction with personal hearing aids. They are found in most public buildings. In several countries, the law requires the installation of this technology in churches and other public areas. The popularity of this system in Europe resulted from the widespread use of hearing aid telecoil (T-coils). The use of loops spread to the United States in the 1950s. The basic components of an audio loop system include: (a) a microphone, (b) an amplifier, and (c) a coil of wire that is looped around a room or a personal listening area. Sound is converted to an electrical signal by the microphone and fed to the amplifier. The amplifier is connected to the long loop of wire, which produces a fluctuating electromagnetic field around the wire. If a hearing aid telecoil is in proximity to the fluctuating magnetic field, a current is induced in the telecoil that is an electrical replica of the original signal. This signal is fed into the hearing aid circuitry, amplified and processed, and delivered to the hearing impaired listener. Although the size of the loop can vary, it is best suited for medium and small listening areas.

The loop has a number of applications: (a) it can be placed around a group of chairs in an auditorium, (b) it can encircle a single chair in a living room for television viewing, (c) it can be worn around the neck, or (d) it can take the form of a small silhouette induction loop that can be placed next to the hearing aid T-coil. A major disadvantage of loop technology is the interference caused by stray electromagnetic fields from electric wiring, fluorescent lights, and transformers. Distance from the loop and improper head positioning can cause a reduction in the signal. Consumers report the greatest advantage to loop technology is that no special receiver is required for users who have personal hearing aids with working T-coils. Loop systems are easy to install and the technology is relatively simple and easily understood.

In the late 1970s and early 1980s, a major movement by consumer groups and health care professionals interested in the improvement of T-coil technology for personal hearing aids resulted in more efficient and sensitive T-coils in hearing aids. As a result, there has been an expanded application of induction loop HAT in the United States.

Alerting and Signaling Devices

Nearly all the sounds used by normal hearing people for signaling or warning purposes can be converted into visual or vibratory stimuli so that they can benefit the deaf or hearing impaired individual. There are a huge number of devices available, so the following is a snippet to give the reader a feel for the range of devices available. Figure 14-9 shows examples of a variety of devices.

1. Alarm clocks can be found that have visual or vibratory alerting modes (see Figure 14-9(a).
2. Door knock lights can be activated by the sound of the knock or be hardwired and turned on to alert the hard of hearing person that a person is knocking on the door (see Figure 14-9(b).
3. Phone ringer enhancers change the pitch or volume of the phone ring or flash a light when there is an incoming call (see Figure 14-9(e).
4. Smoke alarms with especially loud horns, flashing lights, vibration, or combination of alerts (see Figure 14-9(d). Sound/movement activated lights go on when there is sound or movement detected. These are especially helpful when the hearing impaired person is not wearing a hearing aid or when

remote alerting such as baby monitoring is needed.
5. Vibratory paging alerts the hearing impaired person to important information.
6. Text messaging via cell phones or other text message device provides weather alerts and the like.

Hotels are required by the ADA (1990) to provide guests signaling and warning devices upon request (Figure 14-10 is an example of an ADA compliance signage). Typically, these ADA compliance kits include a text telephone; a multifunction alerting system that provides alerts for the telephone, the doorbell, the alarm clock, and a general purpose sound monitor; a telephone handset amplifier; and a flashing light smoke detector.

Service Delivery

In spite of the well-documented benefits of HATs, actual delivery of these technologies is hampered by a variety of barriers: (a) professionals perceive that the time needed to select and dispense hearing aids leaves little time to discuss HATs with patients; (b) given the huge diversity of HATs, limited space is often cited as an impediment; and (c) relatively low profit margins of HAT are viewed as a bad investment of time compared to hearing aids (Bankaitis, 2008). Ross (2004) suggests that the barriers can be mitigated by thinking of HAT as necessities, not luxuries—necessities that can significantly improve a hearing impaired person's quality of life and increase the chances of effective communication. If given the priority they deserve in the communication management plan for hearing impairment, HAT will be better integrated into our service delivery models and more hearing impaired individuals will benefit from these technologies.

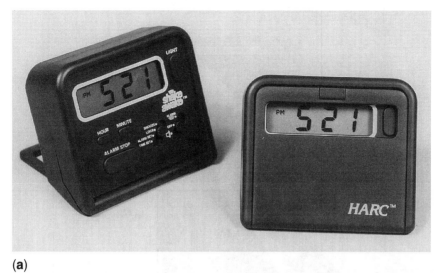

(a)

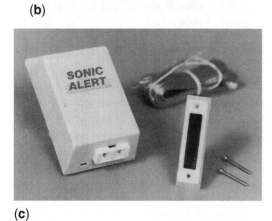

(b)

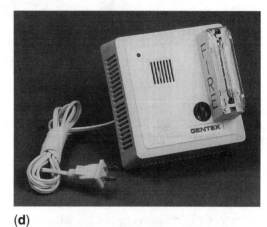

(d)

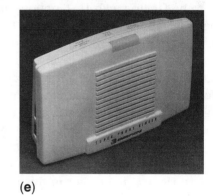

(e)

(c)

Figure 14–9. Examples of alerting/signaling devices. (**a**) Amplified alarm clock. (**b**) Alerting door knock light flasher. (**c**) Sonic Alert (Courtesy of Hal Hen). (**d**) Amplified smoke alarm (Courtesy of Hal Hen). (**e**) Amplified telephone ringer (Courtesy of Hal Hen).

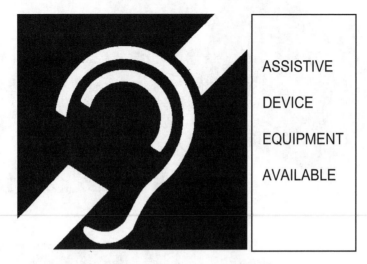

Figure 14–10. Example of ADA compliance signage.

Summary

If quality care involving HAT is to be made available, audiologists, hearing aid dispensers, speech-language pathologists, and other members of the hearing health care team need to be familiar with HAT options and recognize the value that they provide. They should also be familiar with the philosophy and practical considerations involved in the selection and utilization of these devices. Professionals, persons who have hearing impairment, and significant others can refer to the assistive listening devices and systems (HAT) decision circles for examples of how the various types of HAT can be used (see Figure 14-3 earlier in this chapter for the decision circles). The examples in the decision circles are not all-inclusive, but provide a sampling of the most popular applications. When patients are counseled about their special needs for hearing help, professionals can use the decision circles to narrow the selection. Sometimes a single piece of equipment is sufficient; but sometimes a lifestyle demands a "hearing help plan" that involves the future procurement of additional HAT.

References

Alpiner, G., & Schow, R. (2000). Rehabilitative evaluation of hearing-impaired adults. In G. Alpiner & P. McCarthy (Eds.), *Rehabilitative audiology* (pp. 305-331). New York: Lippincott Williams & Wilkins.

Americans with Disabilities Act of 1990. 42 USC 12101. (1990).

Bankaitis, A. (2008). Hearing assistance technology. In M. Valente, H. Hosford-Dunn, & R. Roeser (Eds.), *Audiology treatment* (pp. 400-417). New York: Thieme.

Compton, C. (1995). Selecting what's best for the individual. In R. Tyler & D. Schum (Eds.), *Assistive devices for persons with hearing impairment* (pp. 224-249). Boston: Allyn & Bacon.

Compton, C. (2000). Assistive technology for enhancement of receptive communication. In G. Alpiner & P. McCarthy (Eds.), *Rehabilita-*

tive audiology (pp. 501-554). New York: Lippincott Williams & Wilkins.

Crandell C. C., Smaldino, J. J., & Flexer, C. (2005). *Sound field amplification: Applications to speech perception and classroom acoustics.* Clifton Park, NY: Thompson Delmar Learning.

Federal Communications Commission. (1991). 47 CFR Parts 0 and 64. *Federal Register, 56* (148, August), 36729-36733.

Martin, F. N. (1994). Management of hearing impairment. In F. N. Martin (Ed.), *Introduction to audiology* (pp. 443-444). Englewood Cliffs, NJ: Prentice Hall.

Montgomery, A., & Houston, T. (2000). The hearing impaired adult: Management of communication deficits and tinnitus. In G. Alpiner & P. McCarthy (Eds.), *Rehabilitative audiology* (pp. 377-401). New York: Lippincott Williams & Wilkins.

Palmer, C., & Mueller, G. (2000). Hearing aid selection and assessment. In G. Alpiner & P. McCarthy (Eds.), *Rehabilitative audiology* (pp. 332-376). New York: Lippincott Williams & Wilkins.

Ross, M. (2004). Hearing assistance technology: Making a world of difference. *The Hearing Journal, 57,* 11-17.

Ross, M. (1999). *Beyond hearing aids: Hearing assistance technologies.* Retrieved July 7, 2008, from http://www.hearingresearch.org/Dr.Ross/beyond_hearing_aids.htm

Vaughn, G. R. (1986). Bill of rights for listeners and talkers. *Hearing Instruments, 37,* 8.

Vaughn, G. R., & Lightfoot, R. K. (1983). Lifestyles and assistive listening devices and systems. *Hearing Instruments, 3,* 128-134.

Vaughn, G. R., & Lightfoot, R. K. (1989). Resource materials. In R. L. Schow & M. A. Nerbonne (Eds.), *Introduction to aural rehabilitation* (pp. 586-605). Austin, TX: Pro-Ed.

Vaughn, G. R., Lightfoot, R. K., & Teter, D. L. (1988). Assistive listening devices and systems (HATS) enhance the lifestyles of hearing-impaired persons. *American Journal of Otology, 9,* 101-106.

End of Chapter Examination Questions

Chapter 14

1. **The probability that successful communication will occur with the selection and use of appropriate HAT:**
   a. is decreased.
   b. is increased.
   c. stays the same.
   d. is not a factor.

2. **(True/False) According to public law, it is the responsibility of the person who is hearing impaired to provide her own HAT for use in public places.**

3. **According to Compton, assistive technology can be used to address these four communication needs:**
   a.
   b.
   c.
   d.

4. **(True/False) Hardwire devices are generally the most difficult devices for people with dexterity problems to operate.**

5. **The acoustic conditions of a listening environment in which a HAT may be most helpful includes:**
   a. high levels of background noise.
   b. high levels of room echoes (reverberation).
   c. low levels of background noise.
   d. low levels of room echoes (reverberation).

6. **(True/False) FM HAT includes personal and sound-field.**

7. **Once a need for HAT is determined, which of the following factors should be considered?**
   a. affordability
   b. reliability/durability
   c. operability
   d. portability
   e. compatibility
   f. cosmetics

8. (True/False) Nearly all the sounds used by normal hearing people for signaling or warning purposes can be converted into visual or vibratory stimuli so that they can benefit the deaf or hearing impaired individual.

9. What are the three basic components of a loop listening system?
    a.
    b.
    c.

10. The main reasons given as barriers to HATs in service delivery models for hearing impairment include:
    a. time
    b. space
    c. low profit margins
    d. appreciation of their value to patients

End of Chapter Answer Sheet

Name _____ Date _____

Chapter 14

1. Which one(s)?   a   b   c   d

2. Circle one: True   False

3. a. _____

   b. _____

   c. _____

   d. _____

4. (Circle one)   True   False

5. Which one(s)?   a   b   c   d

6. (Circle one)   True   False

7. Which one(s)?   a   b   c   d   e   f

8. (Circle one)   True   False

9. a. _____

   b. _____

   c. _____

10. Which one(s)?   a   b   c   d

PART IV

Considerations for Older Adults with Impaired Hearing

15

Influences of Aging on Older Adults

JUDAH L. RONCH AND MICHAEL NOVOTNY

Chapter Outline

Introduction

In working with speech, language, and hearing problems, older persons may constitute a sizeable portion of the patients seen, depending upon the service environment. As ours is a youth-oriented society in which myths, stereotypes, and half-truths about aging abound, practitioners must confront and overcome any personal biases about aging. Not to do so dilutes the strength of the therapeutic endeavor and disempowers older patients.

This chapter is presented to help service providers appreciate the realities of aging—both positive and negative and to thereby better understand and serve older persons with the problems discussed elsewhere in this book. Answers to the question, "Who are these aging persons?" often are based on idealizations, personal experiences, or ignorance of the realities of aging. Attitudes toward the aged can be discerned from the words people use to designate this segment of society and by the psychological devices younger persons use to differentiate and distance themselves from "them."

For many years, the "old" have occupied a position of respect, and throughout history society's vocabulary has reflected this attitude. Terms such as senator, alderman, guru, presbyter, and veteran all have their roots in the words of various languages for *old* and denote a position of honor and privilege by the aged. The current public vocabulary about aging includes expressions such as *golden age* and *senior citizen*, but the aged often are referred to in private by words denoting negative attitudes about being old and fears about aging. Older people are often seen as—and easily can feel—obsolete in a rapidly changing, youth-oriented technological society. Thirty-three years ago Butler (1975) termed aging people "the neglected stepchildren in the human life-cycle." Despite more social awareness about the anticipated cohort of aging "baby boomers," to be old is still too frequently a status that is more feared than appreciated.

Currently, the aged constitute about 15% of the U.S. population, or about 1 in every 8 Americans. The percentage of people 65 and older has tripled since 1900, with the largest gains being made in the number of people beyond the age of 85. Americans beyond the age of 65 numbered almost 40 million in 1996. By the year 2031, when the baby boom population peak reaches age 70, there will be about 76 million older persons in the United States.

To answer the question implied by this chapter's title, emphasis is placed on integrating data about aging with examples of the diverse people who make up the aged group. The author hopes that those who work with the aged may begin to develop a realistic understanding of the diverse nature of the aging process, in general, as well as appreciate the diversity of aged persons as individuals. As the coming "age wave" (Dychtwald & Flower, 1989) leads to greater numbers and heterogeneity of older persons, service providers will have to keep finding new, more accurate answers to the question, "Who are these aging persons?"

Dimensions of Aging: Is There a Typical Aging Person?

There are as many experiences of aging as there are aged persons. However, some characteristics of the aging population merit attention, so that the overall circumstances of the aged may be better understood.

Gerontologists have found it useful to divide the aged into the *young-old* (ages 65–74), the *old-old* (ages 75–84), and the *oldest-old* (people more than 85 years of age; Moody, 2006). There are significant differences in the life tasks, abilities, resources, health, and other factors between 50- or 55-year-olds and people age 85 and a greater likelihood (although not a certainty) of similarities among a cohort of 65-year-olds. Still, all persons of the same age do not experience aging in the same way, and physiological, psychological, and social changes do not unfold solely according to chronological age.

Biological aging refers to the length of life in years, psychological aging to the adaptation capacity of the organism, and social aging to the performance of a person relative to his culture and social group (Hoyer & Roodin, 2003). Rather than looking solely at a person's chronological age to explain what we see, greater insight can be derived by looking at the multiple spheres in which a person grows, develops, and gains experience and satisfaction. People of the same biological age are quite diverse in their adaptational capacity and social accomplishments. It is, therefore, important to realize that each aged person must be appreciated in terms of both his similarity to other elders and the lifelong patterns of individuality brought into the later stage of life.

The Interdisciplinary Perspective

Because an elderly person is really a complex organism attempting to interact with an equally complicated environment in a dynamic, mutually demanding way, it is necessary to understand the many factors that make up the world of an older adult. It has been said that no single discipline, whether it be psychiatry, sociology, biology, or economics, can claim to offer a comprehensive explanation of how aged people act, think, and feel or what the multiple determinants of their behavior are (Busse & Pfeiffer, 1977).

If a practitioner is to obtain maximum understanding of the whys and hows of behavior in the aged, knowledge must be gathered and integrated into an interdisciplinary perspective to develop the most accurate, parsimonious, and factually powerful explanation available. In this light, it becomes apparent why a psychologist must know that depression in an elderly woman who barely survives on a monthly Social Security check cannot be alleviated by psychotherapy alone. Treatment of the woman's social and economic realities takes primacy over delving into her childhood experiences. The process also means that psychotic behavior in an elderly man may appropriately be alleviated by having a physician adjust his insulin dose rather than give him an antipsychotic drug or write him off as "senile." Similarly, professionals who are trained along the traditional lines of disciplinary focus must be willing and able to understand the need to know as much as possible about all of the factors outside of their primary discipline that must be in harmony, and how lifestyle can influence functional adaptation, if an aged patient is to function well and enjoy life (Vickers, 2003).

Quality of Life Issues: Stress and Its Sources

Older age is a stage of life in which people have multiple stresses, often with a previously unknown (positive and negative) variety of internal and external resources available to reduce the stress and promote comfort. Eisdorfer and Wilkie (1977) in their early writings defined a stressful stimulus as one that is "perceived in some way as potentially harmful, threatening, damaging, unpleasant, or overwhelming to the organism's adaptive capacity" (p. 252). Different events will be variably stressful, depending on the time of life they are experienced (Neugarten, 1973) and the experience of the person with such stimuli and how they appraise the stress. Many sources of stress can be consequences of the objective reality of the aging process and the biological, psychological, and social changes that may occur (Lawton, 1977). These changes may induce further stress, depending on an individual's personality and characteristic response to change and resultant success, helplessness, or loss of control. The period of life beginning in the fifth decade and continuing for the rest of one's life is a time when many aspects of a person's world undergo change. The experience of older individuals may vary widely but many older persons encounter significant, stressful changes in these areas (among others):

- The family of origin: parents, brothers, and sisters become ill or die and children relocate or die.
- Marital relationship: death or illness of spouse, estrangement due to empty-nest syndrome, pressures caused by retirement.
- Peer group: friends die or become separated by geographical relocation for health, family, or retirement.
- Occupation: retirement and loss of work-role identity.
- Recreation: opportunities may become scarce because of physical limitations or unavailability from lack of interest or opportunity or few resources.

- Economic: income reduced by retirement; limited income tapped by inflation or medical costs not covered by insurance.
- Physical condition: loss of youth with concomitant biological decline of body function, causing risk of poor health and its emotional consequences.
- Emotional/sexual life: loss of significant others through death, separation, and reduction in sexual activity because of societal expectations, personal preference, or death of partners.

Degree of Stress

Old age can be a difficult and stressful time because two things occur in a complementary and simultaneous manner. The various domains of life, as suggested previously, are prone to stresses in greater numbers. At the same time, each domain is the source of a greater degree of stress than in the past. When experienced in combination with the all-too-often limited biological, psychological, and societal resources available to alleviate stress quickly and efficiently, the organism's ability to adapt is compromised. In other words, older persons may experience more stress in increasing domains of life (with fewer internal and societal supports available to them to promote a comfortable readaptation) and they are likely to become disorganized and feel incapable of coping. It then becomes imperative that stress be reduced as much as possible, if an older person is to successfully negotiate a potentially treacherous old age using their retained strengths and continue to derive pleasure from living.

If treatment is to be appropriate, effective, and dignified, it must be borne in mind that rarely can a person of any age (and surely not an aging person) benefit from a helping relationship that does not recognize the total life situation of the patient. It is only when the total person is addressed and understood that discrete problems may be most beneficially remediated and stress effectively reduced.

The Psychological Experiences of Aging

Aging is a biopsychosocial experience and, as such, requires an understanding of aging as a series of mutually interactive processes rather than as discrete events (Cohen, 1988). The changes of physical aging, for example, produce both a discrete decrement in organ efficiency (e.g., heart output, visual ability, hearing acuity, gastrointestinal motility) and a subjective emotional reaction to the resulting functional losses. Thus, it is not how much physical, psychological, or social loss a person experiences, but what that particular loss means to that individual that is the key to understanding the personal, subjective impact of the loss. An avid reader whose vision is failing from macular degeneration, a social gadabout who cannot hear well, and a housekeeper who can no longer dust when she gets anxious because she fractured a hip and cannot walk are three of the many possible individual examples of persons at risk for strong emotional reactions, including anxiety and depression.

The many physical changes that accompany aging have a psychosocial impact not only on a person's subjective sense of well-being and self-esteem (i.e., they must potentially confront the evidence of their "agedness"), but on service providers as well. The service providers' usual techniques, common habits, style of helping, and ability to provide services in their usual settings may have to be modified to assist some older persons. This may prompt providers to think about (consciously or unconsciously) their feelings about aging and youth, control and power, emotions about aging persons they care about, and other psychosocial issues relevant to the providers' personal experiences.

Psychological Changes: Myths and Realities

The myth that cognitive and emotional regression are inevitable with advancing years still persists with surprising tenacity, despite a growing body of evidence to the contrary. Sadly, many health care professionals and the lay public adamantly hold on to the old stereotypes about "normal senility" and a "second childhood" characterized by selfishness, childlike dependency and stubbornness, or passivity in older persons. These nihilistic notions not only lower the self-esteem of older persons who believe these to be the cause—rather than the result—of psychosocial and/or physical problems, but often contribute to the exclusion of older persons from sources of potential help for their difficulties.

Cognitive Abilities

Measures of cognitive performance used to investigate age differences in memory, learning, and intelligence are complicated by the intervening effects of sociocultural factors, for example, educational experience, ethnicity, test motivation, and overall physical health of individuals participating in the studies. Changes in learning capacity, intelligence (as reflected on a standardized test performance), or memory ability that are purely a function of chronological aging alone have been difficult to demonstrate. It is even less clear how any changes found by investigations reflect actual changes in everyday functional abilities experienced by older persons in the general population. Recent research demonstrates that cognitive functioning can be acquired by engaging in creative activity (Cohen, 2005).

Anyone working with an older person would probably find it beneficial to ascertain each older patient's ability to attend to, remember, and integrate new information in an appropriate and consistent way as they work together. A patient's sensory difficulties, comfort about being in a helping relationship, fear of failure, embarrassment at receiving assistance or having a problem, or personality variables (see the following paragraphs) will frequently have a more profound effect on his ability to change behavioral patterns than will any change in cognitive ability. A factor such as cognitive style (how one attempts to understand, analyze, and solve problems) is usually an important dimension that has more relevance to how older persons adapt to new demands than do intelligence, memory capacity, or learning ability in a cognitively intact older person.

Emotions and Aging

The emotional life of older persons is the outcome of how lifelong personality traits and tendencies are affected by the experiences one has while aging. Longitudinal stability of personality, interests, sources of emotional gratification, comfort with emotional expression, and characteristic defenses used against anxiety appear to be consistent over time (see Britton & Britton, 1972; Butler & Lewis, 1982; Neugarten, 1973). Thus, the myth that older people develop rigid, cantankerous, infantile, or controlling personalities because they have grown old is

not substantiated, and it may reflect observations of older people who are unhappy, powerless, ill, debilitated, or responding emotionally to their life circumstances.

Rather than aging leading to a personality change, negativities are more likely either an exacerbation of lifelong personality traits or a response to stress and helplessness not exclusive to later life in any particular older person or the aging population as a whole (how many times do younger persons react similarly when angry, depressed, helpless, or sick?). People at any age will react to unpleasant or upsetting circumstances in their own characteristic fashion. It is negative stereotyping of the aged to conclude that because a particular response is seen in an older person that it is a universal, age-related reaction.

Oberleder (1966) observed many years ago that emotional characteristics of older persons seem to fall into four basic categories:

1. The psychological characteristics that result from societal expectations about old age, to which the aged adhere to expedite conformity and acceptance (social aging).
2. The psychological reactions to the losses and deficits incurred as a result of the aging process.
3. Those characteristics that are independent of age and arise from poor health.
4. The psychological characteristics that are basic to an elderly person and have been so throughout the individual's life span.

Later life is like other phases of the life span, in that a person has much developmental work to do to attain a sense of well-being. According to Butler and Lewis (1982), some developmental tasks of later life include:

1. The desire to leave a legacy and develop a feeling of continuity (through money, land, ideas, children, or students).

2. The need to serve an "elder" function and to share their knowledge and experience (a task made difficult by the information explosion and rapid obsolescence of old knowledge by new technology).

3. An attachment to familiar objects (as in the case of Mr. W., who wanted to leave his awful rooming house, but feared losing his books, clothes, and other treasured possessions if he couldn't find a new room of adequate size).

4. A change in the sense of time, resulting in a sense of immediacy, with emphasis on the "here and now" and willingness to try new experiences (Cohen, 2005).

5. A sense of the finite life cycle and a need for completion, resulting in a renewed emphasis on spirituality, religion, and culture. (In Japan, old men frequently begin to write poetry as a way of expressing their relationship to life.)

6. A sense of consummation and fulfillment, described by Erikson (1959) as the drive toward ego-integrity. Some authors (Butler & Lewis, 1982; Lieberman & Tobin, 1983) have observed that it is common for the elderly to seek to escape their identities through the continuous process by which people "create the self" (Scheibe, 1989), using distortion and other devices that help a person look better in his own eyes.

The continuity of emotional development in later life has been described as occurring along multiple lines of development rather than on a unitary dimension (Colarusso & Nemiroff, 1981). This provides a more accurate notion of the complexity of emotional issues faced by aging persons and allows clinicians to help patients focus on specific issues that, either alone or interactively, are producing emotional distress. Domains such as (a) intimacy, love, and sex; (b) the body; (c) time and death; (d) relationship to children; (e) relationship to parents; (f) work; (g) finances; and (h) play are dimensions that are operative throughout the adult years. These require a person's ongoing psychological work, if he is to attain mastery and well-being. An individual's ability to meet the many, often taxing demands made by the realities of aging are central in determining an older person's emotional satisfaction and personal development.

Affectional and Sexual Needs

It is widely believed that sexuality in the aged is (or ought to be) nonexistent and that if it does exist, it is surely a sign of aberrant, senile, second childhood regression. This belief is based on many subjective feelings, such as that old people are physically unattractive or that any sexuality in older persons is wrong and shameful (a notion probably rooted in the anxieties young people have about the sexual activity of their parents).

Actually, sex is a matter of great concern in later life and is the source of many satisfactions, as well as emotional problems. For example, Masters and Johnson as early as 1966 (Masters & Johnson, 1966) found that sexual response in old age diminished in speed and activity, but not in the capacity to achieve orgasm. They also found that like most aspects of the behavior of older persons, levels of sexual activity tended to be stable over a person's lifetime. Consistent with the cultural values of this cohort, older men may be more active sexually than are women. However, the preponderance of women and the lack of sexual partners among the older population, as well as older people's belief in their asexuality, are strong influences working against sexual satisfaction in the aged. Suffice it to say that sexual activity can become increasingly more desired and acceptable in people as they age, and society appears to have realized that this has both emotional and commercial benefits.

Psychological Dysfunction in Later Life

It is noteworthy that although generalizations about aging may become more accurate as a result of recent methodologically sophisticated research, there is no universal aging experience. Although psychological problems are not inevitable or universal in older persons, there are certain realities that predispose older persons to being particularly vulnerable to mental dysfunction. Notable among these is the likelihood that physical problems influence mental functioning and vice versa in a dynamic fashion. Cohen (1988) illustrates four paradigms of effect:

1. Severe psychological stress leads to compromised physical health. For example, depression can lead to dehydration, which can cause electrolyte imbalance, and a resulting dementia may be misdiagnosed as Alzheimer's disease.
2. Physical disorders can lead to psychiatric disturbance. For example, hearing loss can lead to apparent mental confusions (and possibly late-life paraphrenia).
3. Coexisting mental and physical disorders develop a mutual, dynamic influence on the clinical course of each. For example, congestive heart failure can lead to depression, with indirect suicidal behavior, leading to failure to take medications properly. Further deterioration of cardiac status may result in deepened depression.

4. Psychosocial factors affect the course of physical health problems. For example, elderly persons with diabetes living in isolation are at risk for complications as a result of inadequate monitoring of diet and medication. Physical sequelae (e.g., infection of an extremity) may result, exposing the patient to the risk of amputation and further functional dependence.

Thus, it becomes prudent to consider a "multifactorial basis" for emotional and physical disorders in the elderly (Cohen, 1988), and to engage in coordinated interdisciplinary treatment modalities and procedures when emotional difficulties surface. Older persons faced with psychosocial, physical, economic, existential, and other stressors are at risk of developing anxiety disorders, depression, and other serious but treatable psychological disturbances.

Drugs and Older Persons

As more medications are used by the elderly than by any other age group (U.S. Food and Drug Administration, 1997), it is likely that service providers who treat the older person will frequently encounter potential or actual negative side effects of the many drugs older people take. Medication for cardiovascular problems and psychotropic prescriptions are the most frequently prescribed and have a high potential for harmful side effects in older persons (Salzman, 2001). Psychotropics include antidepressants, antianxiety drugs, antipsychotics (neuroleptics), and sleeping medications.

The dynamics of drug action in an older person's body mean that psychotropic drugs are particularly likely to take longer to work, stay in the body for a longer period of time, and be more potent than they would be in a younger person's body (Cohen, 1988).

Older persons are also at risk for drug-drug and drug-food interactions. With the great numbers and variety of drugs used by older persons, it is not rare that an older person experiences confusion, depression, and other changes in psychological functioning because of the mind-altering effects of medication mixtures. This picture is further compounded when older persons use drugs differently from how they are prescribed. Sensory problems (a person is unable to read the small print on the bottle), difficult-to-open "child-proof" containers, "informal" prescriptions given out by neighbors, self-medication (if the doctor says one pill works, two will work more quickly), and other factors lead to medication usage errors that have been found to be rather significant in older persons (Vestal, 1985).

The risk-to-benefit ratio of using each drug must be considered. Drugs will not erase the effects of aging. They will not make a person suddenly pleasant or amiable or get him to change lifelong personality traits. And they will most certainly not make aging free of discomfort and travail.

Social Pathologies: Isolation, Poverty, Homelessness

Social isolation may be the most significant cause of mental illness in the aged. It may occur as a result of multiple friend and family losses and from the lack of opportunity to form new relationships. This problem is especially severe for women beyond the age of 65, nearly half of whom are widows, and who, by the age of 75, outnumber men nearly 2 to 1. Both men and women frequently sense the loss of their role in society, their sense of being needed, and consequently their self-esteem.

Contrary to popular opinion, the aged usually are not abandoned by family and friends. In 2000, approximately 22 million (or 63%) of older adults lived in family homes (U.S. Census Bureau, 2001a). These living arrangements, however, may be undesirable and family conflicts may arise under the pressure of new stresses or unresolved family issues. As the number of frail elderly in our society increases, so can the strain on family relationships, health, and resources.

Economic conditions under which the majority of aged must survive further compound the stresses of old age. The major source of income for older families continues to be Social Security, which does not compensate for present increases in the cost of living. According to the U.S. Census Bureau , in 1999 the median income for full-time, year-round workers over the age of 65 was $31,600 for men and $22,500 for women (U.S. Census Bureau, 2004). About 3.5 million elderly persons were below the poverty level. Nevertheless, Hoyer and Roodin (2003, p. 37) caution that the number of elderly poor fails to include the "near poor" (those caught between the poverty level and 125% of the poverty level) and the "hidden poor" (individuals who meet the requirements of poverty as based on their incomes, but are supported by relatives who are not poor). Poverty brings with it an increased risk of chronic disease, dental problems, poor vision, and hearing impairments, along with poorer medical care.

Thus, isolation, poverty, and other social pathologies may contribute significantly to psychological dysfunction in later life. For half of America's older persons, poverty does not become reality until after they reach age 65. Although each cohort of aged persons is coming to later life with more financial resources, better education, increased longevity, and better prospects for a longer and healthier retirement, many older persons find that retirement and the accompanying loss of income (about 50%) exposes them to the harrowing effects of poverty or near-poverty conditions.

Retirement

The primary factor in producing a drastic change in economic status for the aged is retirement. Although this is an event that is sometimes eagerly sought, it is more regarded as an achievement in principle but dreaded as a crisis when it actually occurs. There are many reasons for this, particularly in our work-oriented society. One is that retirement is actually a two-pronged process, wherein a person "retires" both economically and socially and loses a work role, a source of identification, and frequently the social contacts and relationships the work situation provides (Back, 1977). In addition, retirement in a society like that in the United States involves withdrawal from productive activities and the transfer of control over resources to others. With the latter, power is yielded to the next generation, and the formerly powerful must cope with a new degree of powerlessness.

The newer, more youthful cohorts of older persons increasingly have discovered that one must retire to something, be it leisure or a second career or third (often lasting 20 years). Not all people feel that unstructured leisure time is satisfying. With increased longevity, growth in numbers, and rising pension incomes, more middle- and working-class elders are finding that they retain a greater proportion of their power than did the generations before them. Thus, older persons are increasingly better prepared for an active retirement phase of life by virtue of improved economic, political, and educational opportunities. Economic boom times throughout recent decades have

not distributed our nation's wealth equally throughout all social classes, however, and the number of older people retiring with limited means is not declining, despite prosperity for some.

The average retirement age of American men has continued to drop during the past few decades. Nevertheless, a large portion of the working population is working longer. Since 1986, mandatory retirement provisions have been eliminated for the vast majority of workers. Although there are numerous factors that ultimately influence the decision to retire, Social Security (or a lack thereof) is the driving factor. Among its other refinements, the Social Security amendments of 1977 and 1983 helped implement raised FICA taxes and an increase in full retirement age. Similarly, penalties for early retirement and positive incentives for delayed retirement have made working in later life a more attractive option. The encompassing effect of increased longevity, burgeoning federal and personal debt, and unfunded liabilities of entitlements has distinguished retirement as a process of transition where older adults will continue to work.

Ethnicity and Aging

To be old and poor is bad enough. To be old, poor, and a member of a racial or ethnic minority (particularly if one is a woman) places the aged person in "multiple jeopardy" (Butler, 1975). African Americans, Latinos, Native Americans, Asians, and other minority groups are overrepresented among the old poor and underrepresented among the nation's elderly. African Americans, for example, compose 13% of the population but only 9% of the elderly population and they are disproportionately represented among the poor aged, especially if they are women (Moody, 2006).

The situation is worse for elderly Latinos who compose only 5% of the total Latino population in the United States (U.S. Census Bureau, 2001b). There are about 7 million elderly Latinos in the continental United States, including persons of Cuban, Mexican, Puerto Rican, and South American origin, and this number does not include the millions of undocumented aliens of Latin origin. Further, Native Americans get to be old much less frequently than any other group in the United States. And the few Native Americans who do grow old may be left impoverished and cut off from traditional family supports (Butler & Lewis, 1982).

Ethnicity

African Americans, Asians, Latinos, Native Americans, and other minorities continue to be outnumbered by White elderly, but the minority population has been growing and by the year 2030 it is expected to compose over one quarter of the elderly population (Administration on Aging, 2005). Assistance with health care costs is of special concern to minority elderly, because of social discrimination that has resulted in poverty, malnutrition, and resulting health problems. Cultural and language differences, as well as lack of cultural sensitivity among health care providers, often keep the minority elderly from using available public programs. Quality of life for these elderly is, therefore, bleak because of lack of educational opportunities, low level of employment with few health benefits and small pensions, and poor health care.

Many minority elderly speak English as their second language. As they age, they may find it difficult to adjust to the differences in language and culture between themselves and the rest of society. For many, English fluency may decrease as they begin to experience difficulty in the way that their central nervous system processes their second language. This can be compounded in persons with hearing loss or dementia, whose anxiety approaches panic and terror as they are less and less able to understand what they hear and increasingly revert to their native language in an attempt to make order out of linguistic-cognitive chaos.

The Aged and the Family

The family life of older persons does not escape change as people age and, as in other aspects of life, there is a high likelihood of loss. Stresses may take their toll on marital relationships, for example, when one spouse becomes ill and thereby creates a "disequilibrium" in the marriage and the inherent caregiving balance of old role relationships. Whether it is a physical or emotional illness that is the problem, the "patient" can come to be resented for all of the demands for care (realistic or exaggerated) he makes on the healthier spouse. The latter, in turn, may become depressed and angry and also develop physical or psychiatric symptoms. Typically, the woman becomes the one "in charge" and is confronted with her own feelings about being a caregiver and decision maker. In some relationships, however, men play this role, or two friends of the same sex who share a household may assign roles based on the realities of need and not gender. Thankfully, there is an increasing recognition of the opportunities for personal growth available when someone becomes a caregiver (e.g., to give back, to have one's nurturing side emerge), and caregiving is no longer seen only as a burden.

When a spouse is not available or capable of providing needed supports, the next most sought after resource is a child. Four fifths of older persons have living children (Butler & Lewis, 1982), and about 83% of these aged live less than an hour's distance away from one child (Sussman, 1986). Similarly, a small percentage of elderly (less than 5%) are socially isolated (Moody, 2006). Generally, it is a daughter to whom older persons turn in times of crisis (Brody, 1981), a choice usually based on longstanding family dynamics and gender role expectations. The one chosen may be the one who lives closest, is the wealthiest, was the most or least favored as a child, wishes to increase his favor with the parents, or historically could be prevailed on by the siblings to do almost anything. The AARP Public Policy Institute estimates the care provided by family caregivers at approximately $350 billion a year (Gibson & Houser, 2007). Despite the value of their contributions, and in spite of their staggering numbers, family caregivers continue to be the most neglected group in the health and long-term care system. Without attention to this situation, the billions in unpaid supportive services provided by informal caregivers might be jeopardized as these same caregivers suffer from physical, emotional, and financial hardships. Carol Levine (2000) provides a more qualitative description of the impact of caregiving on the physical and mental well-being of the caregiver.

Many older persons are now developing alternative living arrangements, which involve cohabitation of unmarried men and women (because either their children or Social Security regulations discourage marriage), moving in with a friend of the same sex to allow for companionship and reduced expenses, or entering communal residences where tasks are shared by all residents. The advent of assisted living has revolutionized elder care and created a viable but not yet universally affordable option.

Relationships between aged parents and their children (who are usually in middle age, that is, caught in the middle of their parents and their children) do not necessarily deteriorate, nor do all marriages. Although some

families are able to be involved positively and happily with each other no matter what stresses arise, others may be fraught with tension, guilt, anxiety, and multigenerational unhappiness. In most cases, the outcome is influenced significantly by the nature of the family relationship as it had been for years and not as a result of the aging process of some of its members.

Feelings of Caregivers about Aging Persons

Butler (1975) in his early writings coined the term *ageism* to denote the "systematic stereotyping of and discrimination against people because they are old, just as racism and sexism accomplish this with skin color and gender" (p. 12). Much of this bigotry functions to provide a temporary distance between younger generations and their own eventual aging, although long-lived ageists stand to become objects of their own prejudice (Butler & Lewis, 1982).

Professionals in many fields have been found to have definite prejudices against treating elderly patients (Butler & Lewis, 1982). An early classic study of this disturbing phenomenon (Group for the Advancement of Psychiatry, 1971) found that some of the reasons for this may be that the aged stimulate the anxiety and conflicts professionals have about their own aging and aging relatives, and the belief that old people cannot be helped. They may feel that their professional expertise and time is wasted on "senile" or soon-to-be-dead patients, that it is a waste of their good training, or that they are uncomfortable giving to an emotionally demanding older person in what is unconsciously perceived as an incongruous role reversal.

On a realistic level, many professionals find it difficult to give as much of themselves as the aged patient demands of their nurturing or social interaction. An older person often will want to talk about his children, retell old stories, or do anything to hold the attention of the often overworked professional. When one does not have an audience or a responsive and regular conversation partner, the "ticket of admission" often can be a physical complaint. This may be evident as hypochondriasis, a depressive equivalent, but the complaint of physical illness or other symptom really can be understood as a safe way of saying, "I want to be taken care of" (Pfeiffer, 1973). These complaints usually are about a physical problem, as psychological or emotional problems are stigmatic or too threatening to talk about.

Just as all older persons are not sick or needy, it is equally unrealistic to perceive aged persons as all being "lovely," "wonderful," and otherwise without human faults. Such stereotyping usually hides fears about one's own aging and an inability to see older persons as people first. The tendency to idealize and romanticize aging and aged persons projects a wish for one's own future and thoughts about how lovely it would be to be treated as faultless and ideal. It is essentially demeaning and infantilizing—hence, dehumanizing.

Summary

An aged person, although undergoing changes in almost every aspect of life, is fundamentally no less like himself than in the earlier part of life. In the later stages of life, as in every other life stage, individual differences are maintained, with no reduction in the dimensions or magnitude of variation. Despite myths, stereotypes, and prejudicial distortions to the contrary, people retain their essential personalities and continue to manifest most of their essential abilities to adapt

and change as they become old. Major sources of inability to cope or adequately adapt come mainly from the severe stresses and limited resources that the elderly experience in a variety of ways, depending on genetics, life experiences, past and present environment, and traditional ways of dealing with life.

Knowing older persons as people who possess characteristic individuality and a lifetime of experience enables the most productive possible relationship with them. In addition, it aids in establishing fertile ground for the development of their trust and thus encourages them to assume an optimistic, strength-based, growth-oriented approach toward treatment as well as toward life. Nothing is worse than for older persons to perceive the negative, impatient attitude of those who purport to help them but who have, in fact, given up hope of providing appropriate aid simply because the person in need is old. In many cases, calming reassurance and objective listening do wonders in reducing anxiety and encouraging older persons to mobilize their own resources to help produce improved functioning.

Who, then, are these aging persons? The question might be rephrased to ask not only who, but what are they like, and why are they so? The answers are crucial not only to the achievement of a full understanding of the aged, but on a most personal level, to ourselves, for we are all ultimately aging persons.

References

Administration on Aging. (2005). *A profile of older Americans: 2004.* Retrieved February 15, 2008, from http://www.aoa.gov

Back, K. W. (1977). The ambiguity of retirement. In E. W. Busse & E. Pfeiffer (Eds.), *Behavior and adaptation in later life* (pp. 78–98). Boston: Little, Brown.

Britton, J. H., & Britton, J. O. (1972). *Personality changes in aging*. New York: Springer.

Brody, E. (1981). "Women in the middle" and family help to older people. *The Gerontologist, 21*, 471–480.

Busse, E. W., & Pfeiffer, E. (1977). Functional psychiatric disorders in old age. In E. W. Busse & E. Pfeiffer (Eds.), *Behavior and adaptation in later life* (pp. 158–211). Boston: Little, Brown.

Butler, R. N. (1975). *Why survive? Being old in America*. New York: Harper & Row.

Butler, R. N., & Lewis, M. (1982). *Aging and mental health* (3rd ed.). St. Louis, MO: C.V. Mosby.

Cohen, G. (1988). *The brain and human aging*. New York: Springer.

Cohen, G. (2005). *The mature mind: The positive power of the aging brain*. New York: Basic Books.

Colarusso, C., & Nemiroff, R. (1981). *Adult development*. New York: Plenum.

Dychtwald, K., & Flower, J. (1989). *Age wave*. Los Angeles: Jeremy P. Tarcher.

Eisdorfer, C., & Wilkie, F. (1977). Stress, disease, aging and behavior. In J. E. Birren & K. W. Schaie (Eds.), *Handbook of the psychology of aging* (pp. 251–275). New York: Van Nostrand Reinhold.

Erikson, E. (1959). The problem of age identity. *Psychological Issues, 1*, 101–164.

Gibson, M. J., & Houser, A. N. (2007). *Valuing the invaluable: A new look at the economic value of family caregiving*. Retrieved May 1, 2008, from http://www.aarp.org/research/ housing-mobility/caregiving/ib82_caregiving .html

Group for the Advancement of Psychiatry. (1971). *Aging and mental health: A guide to program development* (Vol. 8). New York: Author.

Hoyer, W. J., & Roodin, P. A. (2003). *Adult development and aging* (5th ed.). New York: McGraw-Hill.

Lawton, M. P. (1977). Impact of the environment on aging and behavior. In J. E. Birren & K. W. Schaie (Eds.), *Handbook of the psychology of aging* (pp. 276–301). New York: Van Nostrand Reinhold.

Levine, C. (2000). *Always on call: When illness turns families into caregivers*. New York: United Hospital Fund.

Lieberman, M., & Tobin, S. (1983). *The experience of old age*. New York: Basic Books.

Masters, W. H., & Johnson, V. E. (1966). *Human sexual response*. Boston: Little, Brown.

Moody, H. R. (2006). *Aging: Concepts and controversies* (5th ed.). Thousand Oaks, CA: Pine Forge Press.

Neugarten, B. L. (1973). Personality changes in late life: A developmental perspective. In C. Eisdorfer & M. P. Lawton (Eds.), *The psychology of adult development and aging* (pp. 311–335). Washington, DC: American Psychological Association.

Oberleder, M. (1966, November). *Psychological characteristics of old age*. Paper presented at the U.S. Department of Public Health Geriatric Training Conference, Philadelphia.

Pfeiffer, E. (1973). Interacting with older patients. In E. W. Busse & E. Pfeiffer (Eds.), *Mental illness in later life* (pp. 5–18). Boston: Little, Brown.

Salzman, C. (Ed.). (2001). *Psychiatric medications for older adults*. New York: The Guilford Press.

Scheibe, K. (1989). Memory: Identity, history and the understanding of dementia. In L. E. Thomas (Ed.), *Research on adulthood and aging: The human science approach* (pp. 456–501). Albany, NY: SUNY Press.

Sussman, M. B (1986). The family life of old people. In R. Binstock, & E. Shanas, (Eds.), *Handbook of aging and the social sciences* (pp. 229–252). New York: Van Nostrand Reinhold.

U.S. Census Bureau. (2001). *The 65 years and over population: 2000*. Washington, DC: Author.

U.S. Census Bureau. (2001). *The Hispanic population in the United States: 2000*. Retrieved February 10, 2008, from http://www.census .gov/prod/2001pubs/p20-535.pdf

U.S. Census Bureau. (2004). *We the people: Aging in the United States: 2000*. Retrieved February 15, 2008, from http://www.census.gov/ prod/2004pubs/censr-19.pdf

U.S. Census Bureau. (2005). *65+ in the United States: 2005*. Retrieved March 1, 2008, from http://www.census.gov/prod/2006pubs/p23 -209.pdf

U.S. Food and Drug Administration. (1997, October). Medications and older people. *FDA Consumer Magazine*. Retrieved May 4, 2008, from http://www.fda.gov/FDAC/features/ 1997/697_old.html

Vestal, R. (1985). Clinical pharmacology. In R. Andres, E. Bierman, & W. R. Hazzard (Eds.), *Principles of geriatric medicine* (pp. 85–109). New York: McGraw-Hill.

Vickers, R. (2003). Strengths-based health care: Self advocacy and wellness in aging. In J. Ronch & J. Goldfield (Eds.), *Mental wellness in aging: Strength-based approaches* (pp. 33–84). Baltimore: Health Professions Press.

End of Chapter Examination Questions

Chapter 15

1. Currently, the aged constitute _____% of the United States population, and by the year 2031, there will be about _____ million older persons in the United States.

2. Describe and explain the difference between biological aging and social aging.

3. List five different life events that might be stressful to an elderly person.
   a.
   b.
   c.
   d.
   e.

4. Who are the young-old, the old-old, and the oldest-old?

5. Oberleder, as presented by the author, describes four categories of emotional characteristics of older persons. What are they?
   a.
   b.
   c.
   d.

6. Explain the four realities listed by the author that predispose older persons to being particularly vulnerable to mental dysfunction.
   a.
   b.
   c.
   d.

7. What are *two* risk factors involved with older persons taking drugs or medications?
   a.
   b.

8. What are two prejudices that some professionals are found to possess that may negatively influence their treatment on behalf of older adults?
   a.
   b.

End of Chapter Answer Sheet

Name _____ Date _____

Chapter 15

1. _____ percent   _____ million

2. _____

_____

_____

3. a. _____

b. _____

c. _____

d. _____

e. _____

4. young-old _____

old-old   _____

oldest-old _____

5. a. _____

b. _____

c. _____

d. _____

6. a. _____

b. _____

c. _____

d. _____

7. a. _____

   b. _____

8. a. _____

   b. _____

16

Auditory and Nonauditory Barriers to Communication in Older Adults

DAWN KONRAD-MARTIN AND GABRIELLE SAUNDERS

Chapter Outline

Introduction: Presbycusis—The Problem and Its Impact

Many older adults describe living in a noisy world where everyone mumbles and talks too fast. This distorted speech is difficult to comprehend with any degree of confidence and to do so takes great effort. We call this problem presbycusis. Presbycusis can be defined more formally as hearing loss due to the many physical changes in the ear and brain that occur with age, and includes any exposures that damage these systems over time. As human beings, there are emotional and practical reasons why we need to connect with other people through communication. Hearing is our primary source of communication with others. An inability to hear has the effect of isolating an individual from her family, friends and society.

Impact of Hearing Loss on Aging Adults

Why do older adults commonly report that they can hear, but have trouble understanding speech? The main reason is that speech understanding in the elderly is indeed often poorer than hearing sensitivity would suggest, because of impaired retrocochlear and/or central auditory function. Thus the impression that those around her are mumbling is justifiable. Unfortunately, the friends and family of the hearing-impaired person may assume she is being inattentive or not listening properly. In fact, hearing loss has been referred to as the "invisible handicap" because it tends to be overlooked by both the sufferer and by her friends and family. The onset of presbycusis is gradual, so often the individual is unaware she has a hearing problem. An unfortunate consequence of this is the

use of maladaptive coping strategies, such as dominating the conversation and bluffing to avoid the need to hear others, or simply withdrawing from conversing altogether.

The impacts of hearing loss are far-reaching, ranging from feelings of depression, paranoia, insecurity, and anxiety to loss of confidence at work, decreased participation in social activities, and stress on intimate relationships (Kochkin & Rogin, 2000). Individuals with hearing loss are less likely to access and use health care services (Ebert & Heckerling, 1995) and may have higher rates of comorbid conditions and death (Barnett & Franks, 1999; Gates, Cobb, D'Agostino, & Wolf, 1993). The family of hearing impaired persons is also impacted by presbycusis. They report feeling irritation at having to act as an interpreter, stress and anxiety at not being able to rely on their partner, isolated in their social life, and ill at ease in public with their hearing impaired spouse (Hetu, Jones, & Getty, 1993).

Incidence of Hearing Loss in Older Adulthood

It is clear that hearing loss is a high-burden disorder that directly impacts both the sufferer and the family. The incidence of hearing loss among the elderly is considerable. Figure 16–1 shows data collected from almost 6000 individuals aged 20 to 69 who took part in the National Health and Nutrition Examination Survey (Agrawal, Platz, & Niparko, 2008). The figure shows the percentage of the population for each cohort that has hearing loss, defined either as having pure-tone average (PTA) of ≥ 25 dB HL for frequencies of 0.5, 1, and 2 kHz (light bars) or a PTA of ≥ 25 dB HL for frequencies of 3, 4, and 6 kHz (dark bars). Another study shows that over age 69, the incidence of hearing loss continues to rise so that 59.9%

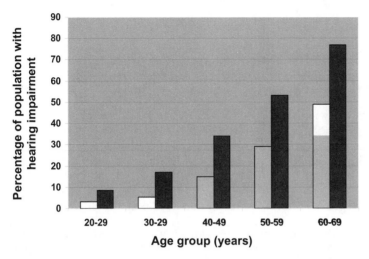

Figure 16–1. Hearing loss incidence defined using a 0.5, 1, and 2 kHz pure-tone average (PTA) and a 3, 4, and 6 kHz PTA. Data from the 1994 to 2004 National Health and Nutrition Examination Survey. *Note.* Data from "Prevalence of Hearing Loss and Differences by Demographic Characteristics among U.S. Adults," by Y. Agrawal, E. Platz, and J. Niparko, 2008, *Archives of Internal Medicine, 168*(14), pp. 1522–1530. Reprinted with permission.

of people aged 73 to 84 had hearing loss as defined by a PTA of ≥ 25 dB HL for frequencies of 0.5, 1, and 2 kHz, with the incidence as high as 76.9% when the definition of hearing loss consists of 2, 4, and 8 kHz (Helzner et al., 2005).

Longitudinal studies in older adults also document the decline of hearing with age. The rate at which hearing loss progresses throughout a lifetime is related to age, gender, and initial threshold values. In one large study, threshold shifts averaged across age groups and gender for adults aged 60 and over were as follows: 0.7 dB per year at 0.25 kHz, increasing to 1.2 dB per year at 8 kHz and 1.23 dB per year at 12 kHz (Lee, Matthews, Dubno, & Mills, 2005). As is seen in Figure 16-2, the decline in men is greater in the higher frequencies up to age 80 years. Lower frequency thresholds (0.5-2 kHz) changed at a lesser rate than the higher frequency thresholds for both sexes (Congdon et al., 2004). An important implication of

this data is that hearing sensitivity at *all* frequencies is typically abnormal in the later decades of life. These sensitivity changes almost certainly disrupt speech understanding, and thus the need for auditory rehabilitation in the later decades of life is the norm.

The U.S. Census Bureau suggests there are currently almost 40 million people over age 65, with almost 6 million of these being over age 85 years. This translates to at least 31 million with hearing loss (Kochkin, 2005). It is projected that by 2050 there will be 88.5 million people over age 65 and 19 million over age 85 (U.S. Census Bureau, 2008). Although there do not appear to be any estimates of the economic cost of presbycusis, it is known that the average lifetime societal costs of severe–to–profound hearing loss in the United States are $297,000 per hearing impaired individual (Mohr et al., 2000); thus, as the prevalence of presbycusis increases, so will its economic and social burden on society.

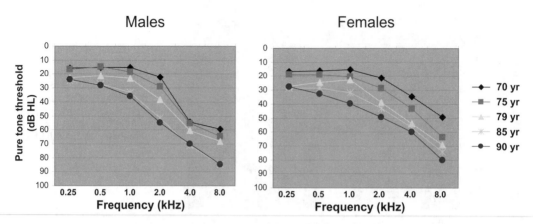

Figure 16–2. Progression of hearing loss with age. Data from the Gerontological and Geriatric Study, 1971, Gotteborg, Sweden. *Note.* From "Hearing in Advanced Age. A Study of Presbycusis in 85-, 88-, and 90-Year Old People," by R. Jonsson, and U. Rosenthall, 1998, *Audiology, 37*(4), pp. 207–218. Reprinted with permission.

Effects of Age on Hearing Abilities

Presbycusis involves deficits at multiple sites within the auditory pathway. Contributions to presbycusis from specific peripheral and central auditory stages of processing are difficult to distinguish clinically, but it is important to do so as far as is possible because the techniques appropriate for addressing cochlear dysfunction are substantially different from those appropriate for addressing temporal processing or cognitive deficits. Table 16–1 provides an overview of changes in hearing abilities that accompany aging. Also listed are the underlying types of processing, and the sites of lesion that these changes may implicate. The rationale for visualizing the auditory system in this way is to provide a systematic approach to clinical intervention.

Aging and Peripheral Auditory Function

Age-related changes in outer and middle ear function are apparent from changes in the appearance of the outer ear and the frequent observation of an air-bone gap at 4 kHz in older adults (Glorig & Davis, 1961). Effects of age are shown through measures of wide-band energy reflectance and impedance, and include a decrease in reflectance from 800 to 2000 Hz as well as a substantial increase near 4000 Hz (Feeney & Sanford, 2004). These age-related changes are consistent with a decrease in middle ear stiffness caused by changes in the elasticity of tissues (reviewed by Zafar, 1994). Outer and middle ear contributions to age-related sensitivity loss are considered relatively minor, but a common related problem is collapse of the ear canal during testing when using supra-aural headphones. This problem yields inaccurate thresholds and can be prevented by the use of appropriately calibrated insert earphones.

Age-related changes in the peripheral auditory system have been extensively studied, but it remains a challenge to separate effects of the normal aging process from exposures to external sources of damage in humans. Changes to inner ear and auditory nerve function are thought to underlie the

TABLE 16–1. Hearing Ability Deficit, Associated Type of Processing, and Lesion Sites

Deficit in Hearing Ability	Type of Processing	Lesion Sites
Sounds are not audible	Auditory acuity and signal detection	External ear, middle ear, and inner ear
Small operating range between sounds that can just be detected and those that are intolerably loud	Auditory acuity and signal detection	Inner ear
Frequency contrasts not detectable		
Rapid changes in sound or complex acoustic features of signal not detectable	Neural processing and transmission	Auditory nerve, brain
Trouble storing and retrieving information	Working memory and attention	Brain
Trouble coding, organizing, associating information	Integration with existing linguistic and other mental constructs	

shifts in hearing sensitivity that accompany aging. In a series of famous studies (e.g., Schucknecht, 1974; Schucknecht & Gacek, 1993), Schucknecht outlined four types of inner ear presbycusis that he had identified:

1. *Sensory presbycusis.* This profile was associated with atrophy and degeneration of the cochlear hair cells and supporting cells. Damage was greatest toward the basal, high-frequency coding end of the cochlea. Originally considered the most common of the four types, Schucknecht later deemphasized this type as a major cause of presbycusis.
2. *Neural presbycusis.* Reduced size and number of spiral ganglion cells and auditory nerve fibers was found. This type was considered a common form of age-related damage.
3. *Metabolic or strial presbycusis.* Degeneration of the cochlear lateral wall and

particularly of the stria vascularis was observed. This type was considered a major cause of presbycusis.

4. *Mechanical presbycusis.* Changes in physical properties of the cochlea were proposed to alter basilar membrane mechanics. This type was deemphasized in later studies.

Schucknecht described a specific audiometric configuration for each of the four types of presbycusis he defined. However, according to the Working Group on Speech Understanding and Aging of the Committee on Hearing Bioacoustics and Biomechanics (1988), age-related hearing loss configurations reflective of the four categories has not been substantiated in humans, except for the sensory category. There is also evidence for the metabolic type, which appears to be genetically determined (Gates, Couropmitree, & Myers, 1999). Pure neural types are infrequently observed, with the mechanical form still considered hypothetical.

Animals reared in quiet provide a way to examine the effects of age in the absence of exposures to noise or other damaging agents. In animal models, aging is associated with a wide range of threshold variability, but variability is less among littermates, consistent with a genetic component to age-related hearing loss (Hellstrom & Schmiedt, 1990). Cochlear hair cell damage does not appear to be a major component of age-related hearing loss in quiet-aged gerbils, though limited outer hair cell damage and loss is part of the emerging picture (Tarnowski, Schmiedt, Hellstrom, Lee, & Adams, 1991). In contrast, atrophy of the stria vascularis is a common feature (Suryadevara, Schulte, Schmiedt, & Slepecky, 2001). In addition, spiral ganglion cells were reduced in number in all frequency regions and the size of remaining neurons was decreased in old gerbils and rats reared in quiet (Keithley & Feldman, 1979; Schulte, Gratton & Smythe, 1996). Given that there was a normal complement of inner hair cells in these animals, this suggests there is an age-related primary degeneration of the auditory nerve. Consistent with these anatomical results, studies have shown evidence for a loss of temporal precision in the action potentials of groups of auditory nerve fibers in the peripheral auditory systems of old gerbils (Hellstrom & Schmiedt, 1996).

Hearing sensitivity is important to consider in that it influences the audibility of speech. However, hearing sensitivity is also important in that it is intimately linked to other hearing abilities that impact speech understanding. Specifically, the outer hair cell system provides frequency-specific amplification to low-level sound input. This nonlinear amplification is responsible for low pure-tone thresholds, but also affects hearing acuity by affording fine frequency tuning and the ability to detect a wide range of stimulus intensities. Lack of frequency tuning reduces frequency contrasts within the speech signal, and so acts as a source of signal distortion. Abnormal growth of loudness is a limiting factor for hearing aid fitting. Abnormal auditory nerve function could reduce the ability to follow rapid changes in the speech signal over time, so that the input signal is degraded, and the ability to process temporal cues (i.e., temporal processing ability) is reduced.

Aging, Central Auditory Function, and Cognition

In 1972, Jerger published the findings of a study comparing the performance of young normal hearing listeners, young hearing impaired listeners, and old hearing impaired listeners on four measures of speech understanding (Jerger, 1972). He found that the normal hearing listeners performed better than the two hearing impaired groups, but that the older hearing impaired listeners performed more poorly than the young listeners with the same degree of hearing impairment. In other words, the older listeners performed more poorly than their hearing sensitivity would suggest they should. Since that time, other studies have shown that, as compared to younger listeners, the elderly have poorer performance on tests of temporal processing (Gordon-Salant & Fitzgibbons, 2001), speech in noise (Plomp & Mimpen, 1979), and higher level linguistic processing (Wingfield, McCoy, Peelle, Tun, & Cox, 2006). The presence of auditory processing deficits combined with elevated thresholds means the individual must use greater perceptual effort to process incoming sensory signals than normal, which likely explains why even mild-to-moderate hearing impairment affects memory (McCoy et al., 2005).

There are pronounced effects of age on neural structures, neural processing, and signal transmission within the central auditory system, which likely contribute to a decline in the ability to discriminate complex acoustic features of a sound. Studies in post-mortem human brains show an age-related reduction in the number and size of neurons in the brainstem (Briner & Willot, 1989; Kirikae, Sato, & Shitara, 1964) and auditory cortex (Brody, 1955). Evidence for changes in brain neurochemistry has also been found, including a reduction in the putative inhibitory neurotransmitter gamma-aminobutyric acid (GABA) within the inferior colliculus (Caspary, Raza, Lawhorn-Armour, Pippin, & Arneric, 1990). Reduced inhibition is likely to affect the neural encoding of timing cues. Deficits in the timing of firings of groups of neurons in the auditory pathway would be expected to affect the use of timing cues to detect sound sources in space, and to discriminate temporally varying signals in noise, such as speech. Thus, these age-related changes in the central auditory system may contribute to temporal processing and speech understanding deficits in the elderly.

Brain imaging studies suggest that even when performance is matched between groups of older and younger adult subjects, older brains behave differently for a range of tasks, including tasks that assess verbal and spatial working memory. Interestingly, some studies show activity in regions of the brain that are not activated by the same task in younger adults (Grady & Craik, 2000; Reuter-Lorenz, 2002; Reuter-Lorenz et al., 2000). These studies describe a relative over-activation that is often found in prefrontal locations, which has led to the hypothesis that overactivity is related to older adult brains "working harder" to make up for deficits due to reduced processing efficiency or degraded input. Studies have also shown activation in a similar region, but in the opposite cerebral hemisphere in older compared with younger adults. Evidence from studies specific to the auditory modality suggests deprivation due to hearing loss leads to the rewiring of the central nervous system (Willott, 1991), which complements the brain imaging studies. The many changes that accompany aging suggest that each older patient will be unique in terms of particular abilities, limitations, and rehabilitative needs.

Nonauditory Barriers to Communication

Normal aging is accompanied by changes in all organs and systems of the body: eyes, hearing, taste, muscles, skin, brain, heart, and so on. The relevance here is that some of these changes directly affect communication and auditory rehabilitation.

Aging, Vision Loss, and Communication

Vision loss is almost as common as hearing loss among the aging population. It is estimated that more than three million people aged 65 and older have some form of uncorrectable visual impairment. Like hearing loss the numbers increase dramatically with age (see Figure 16–3).

Vision loss disrupts interpersonal communication in at least two ways. First, without speech reading cues from the lips and tongue, it is much more difficult to understand speech, especially speech in noise. One study showed that an elderly group of people scored about 43% when listening to sentences presented in noise. Their scores increased to over 90% when visual cues were

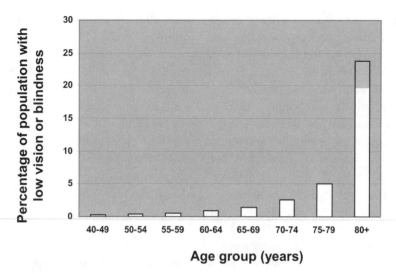

Figure 16–3. Percentage of population with uncorrectable visual impairment by age group. *Note.* Data from "Causes and Prevalence of Visual Impairment among Adults in the United States," by N. Congdon et al., 2004, *Archives of Ophthalmology, 122*(4), pp. 477–485. Reprinted with permission.

added (Walden, Busacco, & Montgomery, 1993). Second, the loss of non-verbal visual cues, like gestures, facial expressions, posture, and eye contact, means that the listener misses information about the speaker's mood and intent, which can result in misunderstandings and miscommunication.

Aging, Cognition, and Communication

The auditory processing and cognitive processing deficits associated with aging that were described above have a variety of implications for interpersonal communication, particularly for the communication that takes place between clinical providers and their elderly patients. Elderly patients have a difficult time understanding speech, especially if it is spoken quickly or there is back-

ground noise present. As a result of the extra effort required to decode the incoming sensory input, there is less brain capacity left for the information to be transferred into memory, and consequently recall of information is poor. Also, because processing the sensory input is effortful, the patient will tire more quickly.

Nonauditory Barriers to Auditory Rehabilitation

Typically, auditory rehabilitation consists of three visits to the audiologist. At the initial visit the patient's hearing is evaluated, needs are discussed, a rehabilitation plan is devised, and assistive technology (usually hearing aids) ordered. At the second visit the hearing aids are fitted, information about their use and upkeep is provided, and communication strategies are discussed. At the third visit, the audiologist assesses whether the patient is successfully using the hearing aids, and the hearing output is fine-tuned as necessary based on patient reports. Some audiologists provide additional visits in the form of group auditory rehabilitation counseling sessions at which additional communication strategies and problems are discussed. Clearly, with so much taking place in short encounters, it is critical the audiologist optimizes communication with the patient, and that the audiologist and patient work closely together to select the auditory rehabilitation most likely to lead to success in terms of effectiveness and patient satisfaction. How can this be best achieved and what are the key points to consider? Below we discuss some of these.

Communication Needs

The lifestyles and needs of the elderly population are varied, ranging from those individuals who maintain a job and an active social life and are involved with their community, to those with poor health whose communication needs are limited to a caregiver, the telephone, and the television. The assistive technology provided should reflect the patient's communication needs, which might mean selecting a high-end hearing aid and personal FM system for the active individual or a personal amplifier for the television and an in-line telephone amplifier for the individual whose life is limited to home. There are questionnaires, such as the Client Oriented Scale of Improvement (Dillon, James, & Ginis, 1997) and the Glasgow Hearing Aid Benefit Profile (Gatehouse, 1999), that have patients specify the listening situations of most importance to them.

These questionnaires take only a few minutes to complete, and provide an easy way for the audiologist to ensure they are addressing at least some of the patient's needs.

Hearing Aids

Although hearing aids do not restore the ability to detect frequency cues or address other age-related changes associated with presbycusis that diminish the clarity of speech, they can address poor hearing sensitivity by amplifying inaudible sounds. Studies show hearing aids to be a successful form of intervention. For example, the National Counsel on the Aging (Kochkin & Rogin, 2000) study of over 2000 hearing impaired individuals found that hearing instruments resulted in improved interpersonal relationships, reduced anger and frustration, reduced depression, depressive symptoms, and anxiety, enhanced emotional stability, increased earning power, decreased social phobias and self-criticism, enhanced group social activity, and improved cognitive function.

Hearing aids come in different shapes and sizes, with many different bells and whistles. The needs and lifestyle of the user, her ability to manipulate a hearing aid, and her visual ability all impact the choices that should be made. More specifically, an individual with good fine motor skills, good visual acuity and an active lifestyle might be best suited to a hearing aid with sophisticated signal processing. On the other hand, someone with peripheral neuropathy or a degenerative disease like Parkinson will encounter difficulties inserting a hearing aid, changing the batteries, and using manual hearing aid controls. Similarly, severe vision loss might make it impossible to see tiny hearing aid switches and batteries. It is the audiologist's responsibility to ensure that patients select hearing aids with features they need and with controls they can handle and see.

1. *Hearing aid style:* One consideration is the style of the hearing aid selected. The current choices are behind-the-ear (BTE), in-the-ear (ITE), in-the-canal (ITC), completely-in-the-canal (CIC), and mini-BTEs. These styles each have their pros and cons associated with the output the hearing aid can provide before feedback, its size, the possible features that can be incorporated, and its visibility. Research shows that ITE hearing aids are easiest to handle, and CIC aids are most difficult. Discussion of the pros and cons of each can help the patient and audiologist together select the style most appropriate for a specific individual.

2. *Automatic versus manual controls:* Another consideration is the extent to which the hearing aid is automated, which today can be almost entirely so if the user wishes. However, some individuals prefer to maintain manual control over certain features. For instance, compression algorithms generally ensure the hearing aid output remains within the user's dynamic range; thus, a volume control wheel is no longer critical. However, many people, particularly experienced hearing aid users who have always had volume control, prefer one. Similarly, many hearing aids these days have *automatic directionality*, which means that the polar pattern of the microphones changes automatically, based on the surrounding signal and noise and the algorithm in the hearing aid. Many people like automated directionality because this removes the burden of making decisions during conversation. However, with automatic directionality,

changes are made based on a signal processing algorithm, which may or may not reflect what the user considers preferable; therefore, manual control might justifiably be preferred.

Patient-Provider Communication

Good communication between the patient and the audiologist is essential to successful outcome. As outline above, hearing loss, vision loss, and the effects of cognitive aging can all compromise successful interactions. There are a number of relatively simple ways to improve communication with the older patient. They can be divided into those associated with optimizing the physical environment and those associated with behavioral changes during communication, as seen below:

1. *Environmental accommodations*
   a. Face the patient to increase likelihood of her being able to see your face and lips.
   b. Keep the office space bright. Use incandescent lighting.
   c. Do not sit in front of a window because backlighting makes your face more difficult to see.
   d. Make sure there are no moving distractions nearby, such as a window that looks out onto a busy reception area, or a TV screen.
   e. Have a magnifying glass available for showing patients small objects or written materials.
2. *Behavioral accommodations*
   a. Get the patient's attention *and* establish eye contact before beginning any discussion.

b. Speak slowly and clearly but do not exaggerate sounds and do not shout. Shouting distorts the auditory signal and exaggeration distorts transitions between phonemes, making them more difficult to understand.

c. Repeat and emphasize key points, but avoid providing unnecessary information.

d. Inform the patient when the topic of discussion is going to change. For example, "Now that you have told me about your hearing loss, we are going to move on to talking about some possible ways to help you."

e. Suggest to patients that they have a family member or friend accompany them to their visit. The more people listening, the more likely it is that someone will recall the information provided.

f. Provide written materials summarizing the key points discussed during the visit to reinforce the information. The patient can take these home to read in a nonstressful environment. Some guidance based on a publication from the Centers for Disease Control and Prevention and Agency for Toxic Substances and Disease Registry (1999) for developing readable materials is provided in Table 16–2.

TABLE 16–2. Developing Readable Materials for Use in the Treatment of Older Adults

Content	Formatting	Printing
Include only critical information	Use 14-point font or larger	Print on nonglossy paper
Avoid long lists	Put key information at the start and end of the brochure	Use contrasting colors, e.g., black on white
Make concrete statements		
Use short sentences	Use informative headings to chunk the information	Keep pictures simple; annotate them with bold arrows to explain the point of each
Use positive statements, e.g., "Keep your hearing aid dry," as opposed to "Do not get your hearing aid wet."	Use bullets, not ongoing text	
	Do not justify the right margin	Use a simple font; avoid big curlicues, etc.
State up front the purpose of the material, e.g., "This booklet tells you how to look after your hearing aids."		Leave lots of white space between text and pictures
	Use columns of about 40–50 characters	
Use vocabulary and sentence structure of grade 8 and below		

Note. From *Simply Put. Tips for Creating Easy-to-Read Print Materials Your Audience Will Want to Read and Use*, by Centers for Disease Control and Prevention and the Agency for Toxic Substances and Disease Registry, 1999, retrieved October 8, 2008, from http://www.cdc.gov/od/oc/simpput.pdf

Summary

When one considers the numbers of older adults with hearing impairment, the physical changes that accompany age, and the impacts communication deficits have on daily function and quality of life, it should become clear that recognition and management of hearing impairment is critical. It is especially critical in the United States at this time, because the population is aging and thus the number of people with hearing impairment is increasing, placing yet greater burden upon society and on the medical community. Individual differences among older patients should be addressed with regard to potential impacts on auditory rehabilitation. For instance, peripheral impairments could be corrected through sophisticated signal processing approaches in hearing aids, central and cognitive processing impairments could be best addressed though FM devices and some form of auditory training, whereas behavioral and comorbid conditions need to be addressed through counseling and wise choices on the part of the clinician. Current research in presbycusis places greater focus on the ways in which age affects the processing of sound in general and of speech in particular. Current and new studies should consider not only changes of the peripheral auditory system, but also changes in the aging brain.

References

Agrawal, Y., Platz, E., & Niparko, J. (2008). Prevalence of hearing loss and differences by demographic characteristics among U.S. adults. *Archives of Internal Medicine, 168*(14), 1522–1530.

Barnett, S., & Franks, P (1999). Deafness and mortality: Analysis of linked data from National Health Interview Survey and National Death Index. *Public Health Report, 114*(4), 330–336.

Briner, W., & Willott, J. F. (1989). Ultrastructural features of neurons in the C57BL/6J mouse anteroventral cochlear nucleus: Young mice versus old mice with chronic presbycusis. *Neurobiology of Aging, 10*, 259–303.

Brody, H. (1955). Organization of the cerebral cortex: III. A study of aging in the human cerebral cortex. *Journal of Comparative Neurology, 102*, 511–556.

Caspary, D. M., Raza, A., Lawhorn-Armour, B. A., Pippin, J., & Arneric, S. P. (1990). Immunocytochemical and neurochemical evidence for age-related loss of GABA in the inferior colliculus: Implications for neural presbycusis. *Journal of Neuroscience, 10*, 2363–2372.

Centers for Disease Control and Prevention and the Agency for Toxic Substances and Disease Registry. (1999). *Simply put. Tips for creating easy-to-read print materials your audience will want to read and use.* Retrieved October 2, 2008, from http://www.cdc.gov/od/oc/simpput.pdf

Congdon, N., O'Colmain, B., Klaver, C., Klein, R., Munoz, B., Friedman, D., et al. (2004). Causes and prevalence of visual impairment among adults in the United States. *Archives of Ophthalmology, 122*(4), 477–485.

Dillon, H., James, A., & Ginis, J. (1997). The Client Oriented Scale of Improvement (COSI) and its relationship to several other measures of benefit and satisfaction provided by hearing aids. *Journal of the American Academy of Audiology, 8*, 27–43.

Ebert, D. A., & Heckerling, P. S. (1995). Communication with deaf patients: Knowledge, beliefs, and practices of physicians. *Journal of the American Medical Association, 273*(3), 227–229.

Feeney, M. P., & Sanford C. A. (2004). Age effects in the human middle ear: Wideband acoustical measures. *Journal of the Acoustical Society of America, 116*(6), 3546–3558.

Gatehouse, S. (1999). Glasgow Hearing Aid Benefit Profile: Derivation and validation of a client-centered outcome measure for hearing-aid services. *Journal of the American Academy of Audiology, 10*, 80–103.

Gates, G.A., Cobb,J. L., D'Agostino, R. B., & Wolf, P.A. (1993). The relation of hearing in the elderly to the presence of cardiovascular disease and cardiovascular risk factors. *Archives of Otolaryngology-Head and Neck Surgery*, *119*(2), 156-161.

Gates, G. A., Couropmitree, N. N., & Myers R. H. (1999). Genetic associations in age-related hearing thresholds. *Archives of Otolaryngology-Head and Neck Surgery*, *125*, 654-659.

Glorig, A., & Davis, H. (1961). Age, noise, and hearing loss. *Annals of Otology, Rhinology, and Laryngology*, *70*, 556-571.

Gordon-Salant, S., & Fitzgibbons, P. (2001). Source of age-related recognition difficulty for time-compressed speech. *Journal of Speech, Language and Hearing Research*, *44*, 709-719.

Grady, C. L., & Craik, F. I. M. (2000). Changes in memory processing with age. *Current Opinion in Neurobiology*, *10*, 224-231.

Hellstrom, L. I., & Schmiedt, R. A. (1990). Compound action potential input/output functions in young and quiet-aged gerbils. *Hearing Research*, *50*, 163-174.

Hellstrom, L. I., & Schmiedt, R. A. (1996). Measures of tuning and suppression in single-fiber and whole-nerve responses in young and quiet-aged gerbils. *Journal of the Acoustical Society of America*, *100*, 3275-3285.

Helzner, E., Cauley, J., Pratt, S., Wisniewski, S., Zmuda, J., Talbott, E., et al. (2005). Race and sex differences in age-related hearing loss: The Health, Aging and Body Composition Study. *Journal of the American Geriatric Society*, *53*(12), 2119-2127.

Hetu, R., Jones, L., & Getty, L. (1993). The impact of acquired hearing impairment on intimate relationships: Implications for rehabilitation. *Audiology*, *32*, 363-381.

Jerger, J. (1972). Audiological findings in aging. *Advances in Otorhinolaryngology*, *20*, 115-124.

Keithley, E. M., & Feldman, M. L. (1979). Spiral ganglion cell counts in an age-graded series of rat cochleas. *Journal of Comparative Neurology*, *188*, 429-442.

Kirikae, I., Sato, T., & Shitara, T. (1964). Study of hearing in advanced age. *Laryngoscope*, *74*, 205-221.

Kochkin, S. (2005). MarkeTrak VII: Hearing loss population tops 31 million people. *The Hearing Review*, *12*(7), 16-29.

Kochkin, S., & Rogin, C. (2000). Quantifying the obvious: The impact of hearing instruments on the quality of life. *The Hearing Review*, 7, 6-34.

Lee, F. S., Matthews, L. J., Dubno, J. R., & Mills, J. H. (2005). Longitudinal study of pure tone thresholds in older persons. *Ear and Hearing*, 26, 1-11.

McCoy, S., Tun, P., Cox, L., Colangelo, M., Stewart, R., & Wingfield, A. (2005). Hearing loss and perceptual effort: Downstream effects on older adults' memory for speech. *Quarterly Journal of Experimental Psychology. A: Human Experimental Psychology*, *58*(1), 22-33.

Mohr, P., Feldman, J., Dunbar, J.-R. A, Niparko, J., Rittenhouse, R., & Skinner, M. (2000). The societal costs of severe to profound hearing loss in the United States. *International Journal of Technology Assessment in Health Care*, *16*(4), 1120-1135.

Plomp, R., & Mimpen, A. (1979). Speech-reception threshold for sentences as a function of age and noise level. *Journal of the Acoustical Society of America*, *66*(5), 1333-1342.

Reuter-Lorenz, P. A. (2002). New visions of the aging mind and brain. *Trends in Cognitive Sciences*, *6*, 394-400.

Reuter-Lorenz, P. A., Jonides, J., Smith, E., Hartley, A., Miller, A., Marchuetz, C., et al. (2000). Age differences in the frontal lateralization of verbal and spatial working memory revealed by PET. *Journal of Cognitive Neuroscience*, *12*, 174-187.

Schucknecht, H. F. (1974). *Pathology of the ear.* Cambridge, MA: Harvard University Press.

Schucknecht, H. F., & Gacek, M. R. (1993). Cochlear pathology in presbycusis. *Annals of Otology, Rhinology, and Laryngology*, *102* (1 Pt. 2), 1-16.

Schulte, B. A., Gratton, M. A., & Smythe, N. (1996, May). *Morphometric analysis of spiral ganglion neurons in young and old gerbils raised in quiet.* Paper presented at 19th Annual Midwinter Research Meeting of the Association for Research in Otolaryngology, St. Petersburg, FL.

Suryadevara, A. C., Schulte, B. A., Schmiedt, R. A., & Slepecky, N. B. (2001). Auditory nerve fibers in young and aged gerbils: Morphometric correlations with endocochlear potential. *Hearing Research 161*, 45–53.

Tarnowski, B., Schmiedt, R. A., Hellstrom, L. I., Lee, F., & Adams, J. (1991). Age-related changes in cochleas of Mongolian gerbils. *Hearing Research, 54*, 123–134.

U.S. Census Bureau. (2008). *U.S. population projections*. Retrieved September 25, 2008, from http://www.census.gov/population/www/projections/files/nation/summary/np2008-t2.xls

Walden, B., Busacco, D., & Montgomery, A. (1993). Benefit from visual cues in auditory-visual speech recognition by middle-aged and elderly persons. *Journal of Speech and Hearing Research, 36*(2), 431–436.

Willott, J. F. (1991). The aging auditory system. In *Aging and the auditory system: Anatomy, physiology, and psychophysics* (pp. 100–131). San Diego, CA: Singular.

Wingfield, A., McCoy, S., Peelle, J., Tun, A., & Cox, L. (2006). Effects of adult aging and hearing loss on comprehension of rapid speech varying in syntactic complexity. *Journal of the American Academy of Audiology, 17*(7), 487–497.

Working Group on Speech Understanding and Aging. (1988). Speech understanding and aging. *Journal of the Acoustical Society of America, 83*, 859–894.

Zafar, H. (1994). Implications of frequency selectivity and temporal resolution for amplification in the elderly. *Unpublished doctoral dissertation*, Wichita State University, Wichita, KS.

End of Chapter Examination Questions

Chapter 16

1. What is the percentage of people over age 65 years who possess impaired hearing?

2. There are two primary types of auditory involvement that in combination comprise presbycusis. What are they?

3. Schucknecht (1974) referred to four types of inner ear presbycusis. Please list them.

4. How does vision affect a hearing impaired person's ability to communicate?

5. The authors of this chapter suggest five environmental accommodations that can assist the older adult's ability to hear and understand speech. Name *four* that were presented by the authors.

End of Chapter Answer Sheet

Name _____ Date _____

Chapter 16

1. _____%

2. a. _____.

  b. _____.

3. a. _____.

  b. _____.

  c. _____.

  d. _____.

4. _____

  _____

  _____

5. a. _____

  b. _____

  c. _____

  d. _____

17

The Impact of Hearing Loss on Older Adults

RAYMOND H. HULL

Introduction

From the information presented in Chapter 15, it is clear that the effects of aging on individuals are as unique as their response to the process. When the effects of aging begin to impact negatively on sensory processes that previously permitted efficient personal and social functioning, it may become even more difficult to cope with advancing age. The sensory deficit discussed here is presbycusis, or hearing impairment as a result of the process of aging.

The Impact

Whatever the cause or manifestation of the disorder called presbycusis, the effects on the some 24 million older adults who possess it are, in many respects, the same. The disappointment of not having been able to understand what their children and grandchildren were saying at the last family reunion can be frustrating to say the least. It becomes easier to withdraw from situations where communication with others may take place rather than face embarrassment from frequent misunderstandings of statements and inappropriate responses. To respond to the question, "How did you sleep last night?" with "At home of course!" is embarrassing, particularly when other misinterpretations may have occurred within the same conversation and continue with increasing regularity. An older adult who may be an otherwise alert, intelligent individual will understandably be concerned about such misunderstandings. Many older adults who experience such difficulties feel that perhaps they are "losing their mind," particularly when they may not know the cause for the speech understanding problems. Perhaps their greatest concern is that

their family may feel that they are losing the ability to function independently and that the personal aspects of life for which they are responsible will be taken away.

Communication is such an integral part of financial dealings, for example, that older adults may also question their own ability to maintain a responsible position in the family, although in the end they may not wish to withdraw from those responsibilities. The self-questioning that may occur can be further aggravated by well-meaning comments by others. A comment by a concerned son or daughter such as, "Dad, why don't you think about selling the house and moving into an apartment? You know this house is too much for you to care for," can be disquieting. Even though an older family member may be adequately caring for the house, cooking nutritious meals, and looking forward to each spring so that he can work in the garden, a seed of doubt about one's ability to maintain a house and other life requirements adequately because of age has been planted. A statement by his physician such as, "Of course you're having aches and pains, you're not a spring chicken any more," can bring about doubts of survival.

Compounding these self-doubts may be a growing inability to understand what others are saying because of presbycusis. It becomes easier, for lack of other alternatives, to withdraw from communicative situations in which embarrassment or fear of embarrassment may occur. If forced into such a difficult situation, the easiest avenue is to become uncommunicative rather than to attempt responses to questions and fail, thus instilling doubts in younger family members' minds about one's ability to maintain independent living. If forced into responding to questions that are not fully understood because an important word is missed or misunderstood, frustration by both the older adult and the family can result.

How Do Older Adults React to Their Hearing Impairment?

Feelings of embarrassment, frustration, anger, and ultimate withdrawal from situations that require communication are very real among older adults who possess impaired hearing and those who interact with them. When so much else is taken away from many older adults including leadership in their family, a steady income, a spouse or friend who may have recently passed away, convenient transportation, and a regular social life, a gradual decrease in one's ability to hear and understand what others are saying can be debilitating. As one elderly adult told this author, "I would like to participate socially, but I feel isolated when I cannot hear."

Many older adults feel so frustrated by their inability to understand what the minister is saying at church, what their friends are saying at the senior center, or what the speaker at an anticipated meeting is saying, that they withdraw from such situations. They may be described by their family or others with whom they associate as non-communicating, uncooperative, withdrawn, and, most unkind of all, "confused" or "senile." A less than expected benefit from the use of hearing aids may further result in fear by the older adult or his family that, perhaps, the disorder is mental rather than auditory.

It has been observed by this author that, in some instances, a portion of the depression experienced by older persons who have impaired hearing is brought about by feelings that the breakdowns in communication "are all my fault because it is my hearing impairment." It may not occur to them that the disorder of hearing may be magnified by family members who do not speak plainly, or by being placed in communicative environments that are so noisy and otherwise distracting that persons with normal auditory function are also having difficulty hearing and understanding the speech of others. Those, for example, may include attempting to listen to a speaker in an auditorium with poor acoustics when the only seat left when he arrived was toward the rear of the room under the balcony; watching a 20-year-old television set with a distorting speaker system; or attempting to understand what his shy 3-year-old granddaughter is saying.

Some older adults who have hearing impairment become so defeated in their attempts at communication that it does not dawn on them that they might be better able to understand what others are saying if those with whom they are communicating would either improve their manner of speaking or improve the communicative environment. However, many older adults have resigned themselves to "not be a bother" rather than assert themselves by criticizing their family's manner of speaking or the environments in which they are asked to communicate. Rather, older adults may simply visit their families less frequently, even though they desire to be with their daughter or son and grandchildren. Sadly, however, they may withdraw into isolation at home rather than attempt to maintain social or family contacts where they have previously felt frustration and embarrassment.

How Do Others React to Older Adults Who Possess Presbycusis?

One 82-year-old adult quite eloquently stated to this author, "For every poor ear, there's at least one poor speaker and one noisy place where it is difficult to understand what I am supposed to be hearing!" He was probably quite accurate in his appraisal, or perhaps even understated it.

As stated earlier, many older adults have placed themselves in a position of "not being a bother," perhaps not realizing that at least a portion of their difficulties in communication with others may be the result of attempting to talk to persons who do not speak clearly or being asked to communicate in environments that may cause even a person with normal hearing to have difficulty. However, even though an older person's adult child may lack good speech skills, the blame for miscommunication or misunderstanding may be placed on the elderly parent with hearing impairment, and not the speaker, without attempting to analyze the problems of two-way interpersonal communication.

Generally, the initial visible frustration with an older adult's inability to understand what is being said is noticed by a listener. A lesser reaction may have resulted in a simple request for repetition or rephrasing of the statement for clarification. When an elderly listener with hearing impairment fails to understand a statement after several repetitions of a difficult word, it is usually he who first notices the apparent frustration on the face of the speaker, rather than the speaker himself. Increased self-imposed pressure to succeed in understanding a problem word within a speaker's sentence tends to increase anxiety and heighten the probability of failure to understand it. One of two reactions generally follows. (a) The most frequent on the part of an elderly listener is to become frustrated, apologize, and withdraw from the situation. (b) The second probable response is a feeling of anger coupled with frustration and embarrassment and either a covert or overt expression of, "Why don't you speak more clearly!"

Who initiated this trying situation? In all probability it was the *speaker* rather than the listener. The speaker's initial unspoken display of frustration at the older listener's inability to understand the statement or question may have caused heightened anxiety on the listener's part. Anxiety, in that situation, breeds failure, failure breeds frustration, frustration breeds further failure, and on and on, until some resolution to cease the conversation, leave the situation, or continue to display anger and frustration is reached.

Did the initial attempt at the conversation prompt this less-than-tolerable situation? Probably not. The person with impaired hearing who has been frustrated in attempting to hold conversations on previous occasions usually develops a fairly immediate awareness of signs of anxiety, frustration, or concern that are reflected in a speaker when a misunderstood word or phrase leads to a delay or void in the conversation. After failure in various communicative environments on other occasions with other speakers, which perhaps occur with greater regularity, the older adult begins to anticipate a speaker's response, perhaps prematurely in some instances. In any event, a speaker at some time has planted the seed of suspicion that he was frustrated, concerned, and perhaps even angry at the older listener's failure to understand or interpret what he was saying.

The second party's negative response to the older person's obvious difficulty in understanding may be the result of an unanticipated interruption in the flow of a conversation. Otherwise, the reasons may be a lack of desire to really communicate with the older person, a lack of tolerance for a disorder that is not readily visible and therefore disconcerting to the unimpaired person, or a lack of knowledge regarding ways in which the situation could be made more comfortable for both the listener who has hearing impairment and the speaker.

An unimpaired person will typically assist a person who has difficulty walking to safely cross a busy street or guide a person who is visually impaired through a maze of chairs. In that situation, however, the impairment and the manner in which assistance can be offered are both obvious to a person who may, in fact, know little about the handicapping effects of blindness. But verbal communication, which is generally experienced as a rather smooth ongoing set of events, when interrupted by an invisible disorder such as hearing impairment, may be disconcerting to the unimpaired person. This can be particularly true when a hearing aid is not worn or otherwise displayed.

Communication ceases to exist for a brief instant. At that point the person with unimpaired hearing may not know how to resolve the situation. The misunderstood word or phrase is repeated, but perhaps to no avail. The person who has impaired hearing may still misinterpret the verbal message. A natural response is to repeat the word or phrase once again in a louder voice, perhaps with emphasis and facial expression that reveals at least some frustration, as the speaker may have not yet determined why the listener is having difficulty understanding what he is saying. The evident frustration may, in turn, concern the listener who has impaired hearing, and communication is at a standstill.

If the impaired auditory system of a person with impaired hearing was as noticeable as the impaired limbs of a person with a physical injury, perhaps the perplexing frustrations that occur could at least be reduced. Presbycusis is such a complex auditory disorder, however, that simply raising the intensity of one's voice may do little to ease the difficulty. In fact, in some instances, the misinterpretations can actually increase as a result of heightened anxiety. In other words, the frustrations experienced by both persons who possess non-impaired hearing and those with impaired hearing do exist,

and can negatively influence communication when solutions on how to reduce the communication breakdowns are not known.

Hearing Impaired Older Adults versus Others Who Are Hearing Impaired

Why do family members, friends, or spouses of elderly adults with presbycusis appear to be more frustrated than persons who, for example, must communicate with children who have impaired hearing? Adults and children, perhaps, tend to be more compassionate toward children and young adults who have difficulty communicating as the result of hearing impairment. That is not to say that there are not instances in which attempts at getting a message across to a child who has impaired hearing fail in frustration for both the child and the speaker. Accommodations by unimpaired children and adults, however, appear to be made willingly in most instances, because they know a child is likely to have difficulty understanding their verbal message, either because of the hearing impairment per se or as the result of language delay. On the other hand, the unimpaired person who is frustrated at attempts to communicate with an elderly adult who has impaired hearing may rationalize the reason as simply being because the person is "old."

Are the frustrations and resulting tension expressed because a listener is an older person? Perhaps in a few instances this may be true, but probably not as a general rule. Those who may have known an elderly person for some time before the onset of the auditory difficulties may become frustrated because this person "was always quite alert." For reasons unknown to them, however, frustrating and failed attempts at "communicating with Dad" are causing friction within the family. "Dad's mind seems to be failing. I told him yesterday to get the safety inspection sticker for his car renewed and he asked, 'Who was safe?' Maybe we should get him a hearing aid." When a hearing aid is purchased for this elder by a well-meaning son or daughter, he may refuse to wear it because, as he says, "It doesn't help"; he may be then described by his family as stubborn. Or they may feel that, "He refuses to do anything to improve himself," when in reality perhaps the hearing aid did not provide significant improvement because it was not chosen and fit in accordance with the configuration of his hearing and his auditory needs.

So how do others who associate with the elderly person with presbycusis react to him? As one family member said to this writer:

> We are concerned about Dad. We used to have a good time talking about the good old days and about what he wanted to do after he retired. Now that he can't seem to hear us or understand what we say, we all get angry. He can't understand what we are saying no matter how loud we talk, and all he does is get mad because no matter how many times we repeat what we say, he still can't get it. We bought him a hearing aid, but he won't wear it. He says it doesn't help. For $1500, it should do something for him, but we all feel that he just can't get used to something new. Besides, he's just stubborn, we think. Our whole lives have changed since this hearing problem has gotten worse. We don't communicate anymore. We don't even like to have him over anymore and no one goes to visit him. He just sits. We are embarrassed to take him out to restaurants because he can't understand the waiters and then becomes angry when we try to interpret what they are

saying. And, he talks so loud! So we just let him sit at his house. We told him to sell the house and move into an apartment complex where other older persons live. He says that if we try to sell his house he'll lock the doors and windows and never come out until the hearse takes him away. His hearing problem has changed all of our lives for the worse. We really are at our wits' end!

Such statements by concerned and frustrated children, friends, and spouses of older persons who have hearing impairment are heard numerous times in the audiologist's professional life. But the vast majority of these older adults can be helped if those who serve them take the time to listen to their responses to their auditory disorder and their state in life and to carefully evaluate their hearing disorder. From this information viable service programs can be developed, not only for older persons who have hearing impairment, but also for those who most closely associate with them.

Reactions of Older Adults to Their Hearing Loss: A Dialogue

How do older adults with impaired hearing react to the disorder and the difficulties they have in attempting to communicate with others? The following statements from patients reflect their feelings about their hearing loss. They are taken from initial pretreatment interviews with 10 older adults who have hearing impairment and were video recorded by this author. This type of personalized information provides important insights into the feelings and desires of older adults that are not only important in the counseling process, but also in the development of treatment programs on their behalf.

Case Studies

The Interviewees

All of the interviewees are of an average socioeconomic level and are bright, articulate older adults. All, however, possess a frustrating impairment of hearing.

Occupational History. Two women were teachers, one at the elementary and the other at the high school level. One man managed a grain elevator in a rural community. He had no formal education past the sixth grade. One man was a retired agricultural agent for Weld County, CO. One man was a farmer, with no formal education past the third grade. Four women still consider themselves to be housewives and not retired. One man was a retired missionary. Four of these individuals presently reside in health care facilities, and the remainder are living in the community in their own homes.

State of Health and Mobility. The six adults interviewed who reside in the community all described themselves as being well. They described themselves as mobile, although only one of the women drove a car. All of the men who do not reside in a health care facility drive their own car. The women who were not driving a car said that transportation was occasionally a problem, but that city bus service was generally adequate, or friends or relatives would take them where they want to go. All patients interviewed, except one man who was troubled with gout, stated that they sometimes walked where they needed to go, mostly for exercise.

No patients interviewed who resided in health care facilities drove a car. Transportation was stated as being generally adequate through local bus service or by the health care facility's "ambulobus" service. The adults who reside in health care facilities generally described the reason for placement there as health reasons, except for one who felt that she was simply deposited there. Health and physical problems among those confined persons included heart problems, kidney dysfunction, Parkinson disease, visual impairments, and hearing loss. Walking was described by all as somewhat difficult. Two patients were confined to wheelchairs—one because of Parkinson disease and one because of arthritis.

Age. Ages of the patients included here ranged from 74 to 95 years. The mean age was 81 years.

Reason for Referral. All persons interviewed for this discussion had been referred for aural rehabilitation services or had sought out the service. All had consented to participate in aural rehabilitation treatment on an individual or group basis after an initial hearing evaluation and counseling.

The Dialogue. The following are the interviewees' descriptions of themselves and the impact of their hearing impairment on them. The dialogue is taken from video recorded responses by each interviewee to the question, "How do you feel about yourself at this time and your ability to communicate with others?"

Video recorded interviews are routinely held with each patient seen by this author prior to aural rehabilitation services and again at the program's conclusion. The purpose for all pre- and post-video recorded interviews is to allow patients to confront themselves and their feelings about their ability to function in their communicating worlds. Changes in their opinions of themselves and their ability to function communicatively are thus more easily mapped. Patients are further allowed the opportunity to note changes in themselves and their opinions of their ability to communicate with others by watching and listening to their own statements. The following are brief but descriptive excerpts of statements by patients:

Case 1

Age: 76

Sex: Female

Residence: Community (in own house)

Marital status: Never married

Prior occupation: Elementary educator

Health: Good

Mobility: Good

Dialogue. "I try to say, 'What did you say?' but sometimes they begin to appear angry. I become frustrated—so—so frustrated that I then become angry at myself, because I have become angry at those with whom I am talking. Do other people have problems where they cannot understand what people are saying? Am I the only one?

"I didn't realize why I had begun to dislike going to meetings until I realized I was not understanding what they were saying. I had been blaming my friends—and they had been secretly blaming me. I hope I can retain their friendship after I explain to them that the problems weren't all their fault."

Discussion. This woman's comments indicate concern over the difficulties she is experiencing in her attempts at interacting with others. She is, however, not resigned

to continued failure. She is still striving to retain friendships with others. Further, she is still enrolled in aural rehabilitation treatment and making satisfactory progress in learning to make positive change in her communication environments.

Case 2

Age: 77 years

Sex: Female

Residence: Health care facility

Marital status: Widow

Prior occupation: Housewife

Health: Arthritis, renal disease

Mobility: Confined to wheelchair; mobility severely limited

Dialogue. "I feel handicapped. Anymore, I don't know what the demands are, or what capabilities I have. I try so hard to hear that I become very tired. I may pass away any day. Is there hope for me? I want to talk to my children more than anything else, but they are so busy and can't come to see me very often. I want to hear what the minister here is saying at the chapel. Church means a great deal to me now.

"I feel so alone when I can't participate in things I want to do. I can't weed out what I want to hear from the noises around me. The most important thing is communication. I desperately want it. My grandchildren—I pray that I can someday spend a pleasant afternoon with them."

Discussion. This woman feels despondent. She is, however, an alert person and desires that her situation will improve. She is enrolled in an aural rehabilitation treatment program, but her state of depression has not improved significantly. She says that if her family would visit her, it would help. Most importantly, she desires to have someone with whom to communicate. She has currently been referred for counseling.

Case 3

Age: 78 years

Sex: Male

Residence: Community (in own house)

Marital status: Widower

Prior occupation: Grain elevator manager

Health: Generally good; has known cardiovascular problems; some dizziness noted on occasion.

Mobility: Good; drives own car and is physically mobile. He is mentally alert and always seems to have a joke for the occasion. But, in most respects, he is a man of few words.

Dialogue. "It's embarrassing. When people find out that you have trouble hearing, they don't seem to want to talk to you anymore. If you ask them to speak up, sometimes they look angry.

"I feel that time is lost when I go to a meeting I have looked forward to going to and I can't understand a word they are saying. Most people do not seem to have good speech habits. On the other hand, my poor hearing doesn't help a bit either.

"My main goal in coming here is to learn to hear a woman's voice better, maybe a woman's companionship won't be so hard to come by. As they say, a woman's voice may not be as pretty as the song of a bird, but it's awful darn close!"

Discussion. This man possesses a significant speech recognition deficit, and strongly desires that aural rehabilitative services be of help to him. He feels that he has much to live for and is willing to work to improve his auditory problems. Assertiveness training and manipulation of his communicative environments has supported those efforts.

Case 4

Age: 95 years

Sex: Female

Residence: Health care facility

Marital status: Widow

Prior occupation: Housewife

Health: Parkinson disease

Mobility: Severely limited; is confined to a wheelchair.

Dialogue. "I would like to be free, to drive, to go visit children and friends. I would like to get away from confinement. I would like to be able to hear again—to be able to be a part of the conversations that take place in this home. It would be pleasant to hear the minister again or to talk to my children. They live far away, though, and can't come to visit.

"My main concern is death right now. I know that the infirmity I have will end in death. I don't know if I'm ready. If I could hear the minister here at this facility, maybe I would know."

Discussion. These comments are typical of many elderly persons who are confined to a health care facility. They feel many needs, but so few can easily be fulfilled. This woman is alert, however, and can respond to aural rehabilitation services including the use of hearing aids or other assistive listening devices so that she can more efficiently hear what the staff are saying, and importantly, the chaplain of the health care facility. And, if accommodations can be made in the chapel so that she can participate in those services, then one of her other desires would be fulfilled. Further, if learning to manipulate her more difficult communicative environments can be achieved so that she can function better within the confines of the health care facility, then her remaining years will become less isolating.

Case 5

Age: 78 years

Sex: Male

Residence: Health care facility (pos-hospitalization)

Marital status: Married

Prior occupation: County extension agent

Health: Intestinal blockage; arthritis; otherwise in generally good health

Mobility: Generally good; drives own car on occasion; walks to many places

Dialogue. "I feel lost sometimes. If I look at people right straight in the eye, then sometimes I get what they say. I get angry sometimes, but I've finally figured out that for every poor ear, there's at least one poor speaker!

"It's rough to have poor ears. I have trouble hearing women's voices. I wish I could hear them, since I'm around women more now than ever before. Maybe it's me, maybe I don't have good attention.

"I wish I could hear my preacher. I go to church every Sunday, but I don't get much out of it."

"I wish I could understand what people are saying in a crowd, like when our children and our grandchildren come back home to visit. If I'm talking to only one person, sometimes I do okay."

Discussion. This man expresses a great many "wishes," but so far has not extended himself a great deal in aural rehabilitation services. In other words, he desires to improve, but seems to feel that either he does not possess the capability to regain greater communication function, or simply does not want to put forth the effort. He appears to have great communicative needs, but does not yet seem to be convinced of their importance. Counseling is important here, accompanied by the fitting of hearing instruments or other assistive listening devices so that he can communicate more efficiently with others, watch television, and hear the sermons at church.

Case 6

Age: 74

Sex: Male

Residence: Community (in own house)

Marital status: Widower

Prior occupation: Farmer

Health: Excellent, except for gout, which restricts his mobility

Mobility: Not as mobile as desired, because of the gout; drives his own car and is an avid fisherman

Dialogue. "In a crowd—I have my worst trouble. Riding in a car drives me crazy!

"One thing that I have found is that people don't talk with their mouth open.

"My ears hum, and that hurts too, in terms of my ability to understand what people are saying.

"Some people talk with their hands in front of their mouth; that is very disturbing.

"I don't think that my children understand that my problem is my hearing—not my mind.

"It just seems like the voices don't come through. I went to the doctor and he says my hearing is ruined. My hearing is my only handicap. My minister has an English brogue and I can't understand a word of what he is saying! And, groups sound kind of like a beehive. I feel embarrassed. Someone speaks to you and you give them the wrong answer. I like to go to social gatherings, but I still get embarrassed. However, I certainly am not going to give up!"

Discussion. This man represents the almost ideal older patient for aural rehabilitation services. He is alert and active and desires to maintain himself as an active social person. He has also found a female companion who, like him, is an avid fisherman. What an ideal motivational factor for success in aural rehabilitation!

Case 7

Age: 81 years

Sex: Male

Residence: Community (in own house with spouse)

Marital status: Married

Prior occupation: Missionary; still functions as part-time minister for a local church. He receives many requests to serve on community and church committees.

Health: Excellent

Mobility: Excellent; walks a great deal and drives own car

Dialogue. "My greatest concern is my inability to participate in council meetings at church. In some cases, I am in charge of the meeting, but if I cannot understand what the members are saying, then my participation is made almost impossible. It distresses me tremendously that in some instances I cannot perform my duties. Maybe it's me? Maybe my concentration wanders. Maybe my mind is not working as well now, although I feel that it is. I have 20 to 30 members in the Sunday school class that I teach. I find that I have terrible problems determining what their questions are. If I do not know what their questions are, how can I respond to their needs?"

Discussion. These statements are made by an obviously frustrated man. "How can I respond to their needs?" This man has a great deal to offer his community and church, but is beginning to feel defeated. The audiologist must consider this type of older patient as a high priority and intervene as a strategist to assist the person in learning what can be done to function more efficiently in his prioritized communicative environments. This includes counseling, learning to manipulate his communicative environments to his advantage, hearing aids, and others.

Case 8

Age: 83 years

Sex: Female

Residence: Community (in own house with spouse)

Marital status: Married

Prior occupation: Nonretired housewife

Health: Excellent

Mobility: Excellent, but has never learned to drive a car; depends on husband or bus for transportation; walks a great deal

Dialogue. "My hearing loss has been a handicap to me. I ask people to speak up, and they sigh and sometimes I feel terribly embarrassed. Sometimes they shout at me, which hurts in more ways than one.

"I do wish people would speak more distinctly. Even with my family, they sometimes forget to speak up 'for Mom.'

"On the telephone I tell people that I'm wearing a hearing aid whether I am or not. They usually speak up more after that.

"My husband says I am a different person in this later age. I used to be full of fun, but now I don't even want to go to church. I don't like to go because I don't understand what others including the minister are saying.

"It isn't all peaches and cream to be this way. It hurts more than anything when people laugh at you when you give the wrong answer to something they say. I just go home and cry.

"People mumble when they talk.

"I just sometimes want to get out of people's way. I don't want to be a bother to anyone—be a nuisance. I've lost my self-confidence and I don't know if I'll ever get it back."

Discussion. This otherwise vital woman was on the verge of giving up. Further, her husband was talking about placing her in a nursing home. After 15 weeks of individual aural rehabilitation treatment, she learned to manipulate the majority of those communicative environments that were most difficult for her. Further, she has rejoined a women's social group from which she had previously resigned membership. The gradual progression from a depressed woman to one with renewed hope has been rewarding to observe.

Case 9

Age: 76 years

Sex: Female

Residence: Community (in own house)

Marital status: Single

Prior occupation: Elementary educator

Health: Excellent

Mobility: Excellent

Dialogue. "I was feeling concern in as much as when people would ask me a question, I would know they were speaking, but I couldn't make sense out of it. I was afraid that my mind was going. I felt closed in, not comfortable—like I could hear, but little of it made sense—like I was losing my mind!

"I think sometimes that people want me to go away. When I found out that my problem was with my hearing and not my mind, the relief was wonderful. Now I feel that I have something I can try to handle, where before I didn't think I had a chance.

"If people will bear with me, I'll be able to talk with them. I'm going to stay in there just as long as I can."

Discussion. This woman benefited greatly from initial counseling sessions regarding her auditory problem and learning some reasons for the difficulties she was encountering. After she found that the communicative problems she was experiencing were "not the result of her mind," but rather her hearing, she was a ready candidate for a formal aural rehabilitation treatment program including the evaluation for and fitting of hearing aids, environmental design modifications, and others that were important to her treatment plan.

Case 10

Age: 79 years

Sex: Female

Residence: Health care facility; stated that she thought her daughter was looking for an apartment for her, but found herself in the health care facility instead

Marital status: Widow

Prior occupation: Housewife (nonretired)

Health: Generally excellent except for broken hip 2 years ago

Mobility: Somewhat restricted because of fear of falling; otherwise excellent. She takes the bus to those places she desires to go.

Dialogue. "I used to blame others for my inability to hear and understand what was being said, but someone the other day told me it was my fault, me and my inability to hear.

"A speaker at a meeting the other evening spoke for 45 minutes and I did not understand a word she was saying! The disturbing thing was that she refused to use the microphone!

"I was in a car with two friends the other day; I rode in the back seat. They were talking in the front seat. They were talking about a person I had not seen for quite a while. They said something about a ball game, and something about Omaha, and something about someone becoming very ill. I finally felt that I had to say something, so I asked, 'She is well, isn't she?' Well, what they had said was that my friend had died! She became very ill during a ball game in Omaha and died while being taken by ambulance to the hospital. It was terribly embarrassing, but they don't become angry with me. It is frustrating to try to do well, but continually fail. I try not to be irritable. I think I can overcome it."

Discussion. This is an example of an alert, intelligent woman who, because of factors beyond her control, fell as a result of a broken hip and leg, and found herself unable to provide for her personal-physical needs. She was thus placed in a health care facility—hopefully for a relatively short time. She has accepted such placement because of the evident short stay. She is responding well to aural rehabilitation treatment services, particularly in learning to cope within her most difficult environments and those with whom she must communicate. She has analyzed the reasons for many of her communicative difficulties, and is aware of her limitations.

Summary

Auditory deficits as the result of presbycusis are as real as the people who possess the disorder. The disorder, however, affects each person in unique ways. One common denominator is evident, however, and that is that the resulting communication problems can be frustrating and, in many instances, debilitating. The most common strain among the confessions of these older persons, however, involves the isolation and loneliness that they experience.

End of Chapter Examination Questions

Chapter 16

1. The greatest fear described by many hearing impaired older adults is that they are afraid that their family and friends will mistake their hearing loss for _____.

2. What are three emotional reactions an older adult might have to the difficulties experienced as a result of his hearing impairment?

3. As hearing impaired older adults communicate their feelings regarding their hearing loss to the author, the most common thread centers on _____ and _____.

4. The most common goal expressed by older hearing impaired adults to the author involved their desire to better communicate with _____.

5. The inability of some hearing impaired older adults to utilize hearing aids well gives rise to even greater _____.

6. When repeated attempts at communication fail, some hearing impaired older adults simply _____

7. (True/False) Presbycusis affects only older adults. Why?

8. (True/False) One concern of persons with presbycusis is that family members will feel that they are no longer able to function on an independent basis.

9. (True/False) According to the author, presbycusis affects all older persons in essentially the same way. Briefly explain your choice.

End of Chapter Answer Sheet

Name _____ Date _____

Chapter 17

1. _____

2. _____

   _____

   _____

3. _____   _____

4. _____

5. _____

6. _____

7. Circle one: True   False

   _____

   _____

   _____

8. Circle one: True   False

9. Circle one: True   False

   _____

   _____

   _____

18

Special Considerations for the Use of and Orientation to Hearing Aids for Older Adults

RAYMOND H. HULL

Chapter Outline

Introduction

The tests and processes involved in evaluating and prescribing hearing aids, as well as the various styles, component parts, and circuits of hearing aids are covered partially in Chapter 4 of this text and in numerous other texts. Therefore, the focus of this chapter is on how amplification can be considered as part of the aural rehabilitation program for older adults.

The fitting and dispensing of hearing aids and other amplification systems and devices are important aspects of the process of aural rehabilitation. When an older adult's level of auditory acuity is brought to a more efficient level through the appropriate fitting of a hearing aid, then other components of the auditory habilitation or rehabilitation program are facilitated. For many older individuals, a properly fitted and properly used hearing aid will enhance their ability to interact more competently and more enjoyably in their social and personal worlds.

Factors Influencing Successful Hearing Aid Use by Older Adults

As discussed in Chapter 16, hearing loss and accompanying auditory impairment found among many older adults is quite complex. In older individuals who possess both a sensorineural hearing loss and a compounding central auditory impairment, a hearing aid alone may not resolve all of the hearing problems being experienced (Humes, 2008; Rawool, 2007; Stach, 1990). Hull (1992, 1998, 2001) discussed the additive factors that an older person experiences when attempting to understand speech through a peripheral and central auditory system that is no longer programmed for the speed and agility required for comprehending rapid adult speech, and must also cope with less than beneficial environmental/listening influences with which the auditory system must contend. In other words, it is important to consider the possibility that a hearing aid candidate's audiogram may not reveal all that is important when recommending the individual for a hearing aid fitting, because central nervous system (CNS) auditory involvement can negatively influence performance in speech comprehension with and without amplification.

In an early treatise on hearing aid considerations for elderly adults, Kasten (1992) stated that there are nine important factors that go beyond a person's auditory function that must be considered when determining the appropriateness of amplification for older adults. Those are (a) motivation, (b) adaptability, (c) personal appraisal, (d) money, (e) social context, (f) personal influences, (g) mobility, (h) vanity, and (i) dexterity.

Motivation

In their early writings, Rupp, Higgins, and Maurer (1977) consider motivation as being the most important factor in their feasibility scale for predicting successful hearing aid use. They point out that those who show less personal motivation and depend more on the urging of others to procure a hearing aid are less likely to be successful in the use of amplification. Likewise, the individual who has a great desire to continue to lead a mentally, physically, and emotionally active life and to participate in the affairs of society is more likely to be a successful user of hearing aids. On the other hand, those who have lost interest in their surroundings and are willing to withdraw from society may have little motivation or desire to be successful in the use of amplification. Thus, the probability of these persons being successfully rehabilitated through hearing aid use becomes correspondingly less.

Adaptability

One of the more important factors concerning the use of amplification is the expectations of each individual. Until a person becomes hearing impaired and finds that some type of amplification is important, or until the person attempts unsuccessfully to interact communicatively with a spouse or friend who has impaired hearing, it is unlikely that the person will have an understanding of the possible benefits of a hearing aid.

New hearing aid users are sometimes quite surprised when they first experience amplification. It is likely that some people expect a hearing aid to restore their hearing to the efficiency that it had in previous years, and others may expect a hearing aid to be nothing but a nuisance. It is almost certain that neither of these expectations is realistic or correct. If an individual expects essentially complete correction of the hearing deficiency, she will almost certainly be disappointed. Conversely, if an individual has so little optimism as to think that the hearing aid will be of no help, then she is likely to be unwilling to put forth the effort necessary to become oriented to and consequently wear the instruments. In other words, the person may simply be unwilling to give amplification a chance. If a person is unwilling to try something that is new or unusual, then major changes in attitude are necessary before successful hearing aid use will be noted.

Personal Appraisal

An individual's personal assessment and emotional feelings about her communication problems are extremely important factors in the degree of success in the use of amplification. In other words, audiological assessment data are appropriate in determining the degree of hearing loss, but self-assessment is also important. To document the patient's self-appraisal of the impact of the hearing loss, one of the available scales for determining the degree of communication disability may be appropriate. Several scales of communication that are suitable for adults can be found in the Appendices of this text. There is generally good agreement on the degree of disability as determined by audiological data and by a self-inventory using one of the self-assessment scales.

Successful use of amplification is most likely when there is a positive correlation between the two sets of information (audiometric data and self-assessment). One who is able to appraise her personal disability objectively and with accuracy is generally in a position to at least accept the resulting communication problems and assist in developing a realistic approach to the possibilities, as well as to the specific procedures needed to overcome the negative impact of the hearing loss to the degree possible.

Money

The financial status of a person can certainly have a profound effect on her interest in hearing aids. For the majority of potential users, however, the purchase of hearing aids is not impossible. On the other hand, hearing aids still may be in the category of a luxury and would probably be purchased only if the person who has hearing impairment is convinced that they will meet her needs. Many people are aware that their friends and perhaps they themselves have spent hundreds if not thousands of dollars for one or more hearing aids that proved to be unsatisfactory and were relegated to a dresser drawer or closet shelf after the return warranty ran out. Thus, some people are unwilling to spend the money necessary to obtain hearing aids. When an individual is living on a fixed income and is only meeting living expenses, then the matter of hearing aid purchase may become financially difficult.

Those who are eligible for Medicaid assistance can sometimes obtain help from that source in buying a hearing aid (if their state Medicaid laws provide for hearing aids). However, some states (e.g., California, Kansas, and others) only provide one hearing aid every 3 to 5 years unless the patient has special circumstances such as blindness. Hearing aid banks can be an important resource, and there may be other possibilities for financial assistance by civic organizations. However, these sources also may have restrictions that present problems in carrying out a purchase.

Social Context

The older patient who has hearing impairment, as any other person, may fit anywhere along a continuum from one who is socially active to one who is socially withdrawn. Those who are active in various aspects of social life are ones who are likely to desire to maintain contact with other people and to communicate actively. Those who are withdrawn, on the other hand, may have lost interest in such contact. Thus, it becomes the task of the audiologist to determine if a

withdrawal is due to hearing loss and, if so, how to rehabilitate the person.

It seems reasonable to assume that those who are engaged in social activities would be the ones most likely to be successful in rehabilitation utilizing hearing aids. At least they would have the desire and motivation for this type of achievement. Conversely, those who are withdrawn or who lack social awareness might be the ones least likely to be successful in rehabilitation with hearing aids.

The large remaining group includes those who are neither extremely active socially nor completely withdrawn. They are, in fact, the ones who are in the process of losing their interest in social contact, because there is too great an effort needed to maintain communication with their friends. Although their lagging interest in social affairs would make them less than ideal candidates for the use of amplification, it is also highly possible that satisfactory selection of amplification and the use of appropriate rehabilitation procedures can improve the probability of reentry into social activities.

Personal/Functional Influences

The attitudes, interests, and activities of the friends of the older patient who has hearing impairment can have a great deal of influence on her attitudes and desires. If the person is still employed or active in volunteer or avocational activities that involve her with communication, and if the people who are associated with the person who has hearing impairment are sympathetic, understanding, and stimulating in their conversations, then the elderly person's desire to utilize amplification will be enhanced. Conversely, if the living situation and the people involved in the life process of the older person lack stimulating ingredients, then the individual who has hearing impairment is likely to have little reason for wanting to try to obtain or adjust to the use of amplification.

Mobility

Restrictions in physical mobility can have a great impact on older adults and their willingness to use hearing aids and other prosthetic devices. For example, if an individual is able to be involved in various activities including church, theater, musical concerts, and favorite social clubs, then she is likely to be a good candidate for the use of amplification and improved communication. On the other hand, those who are limited in mobility and who rarely leave their immediate vicinity for social or business contacts may have less apparent need for communication and, therefore, less need or desire for amplification. Further, there are those who desire to live alone and may have little motivation for communication with others. They may feel a great deal of loneliness, yet they are unable or unwilling to make the effort to maintain contact with other people. These persons may have a need for the communicative assistance that can be obtained through amplification, yet they often are physically and emotionally limited in their ability or desire to become involved in social activities and, thus, their ability or desire to utilize amplification. They might have other types of debilitating impairments in addition to the hearing impairment, yet they may be able to participate in social activities, for example, if transportation is available. However, the hearing problem presents an additional barrier, and the combination of impairments results in greater isolation. The result is that they may be less successful from the standpoint of improvements in social contact and their ability to communicate then we as rehabilitation specialists expect them to be. However, the lack of improvements may be out of default rather than from their desire to isolate themselves.

Vanity

Vanity is an aspect of human nature that can have a great impact on a person's interest in trying to adjust to hearing aids. Corrective lenses for the eyes are an example of how a prosthetic appliance can be widely accepted. Many people would prefer not to wear eyeglasses, but nevertheless a large majority of our society eventually needs to wear some type of visual correction. In fact, most people accept the use of corrective lenses gracefully at some time in their lives and may even consider it stylish to wear them. Once an individual has accepted the necessity of eyeglasses, she may go to extremes by purchasing large and gaudy eyewear, which definitely calls attention to the prostheses. On the other hand, based on their own opinions of appearance of self or the opinions of others, persons may try to use contact lenses or corrective surgery to conceal a sight problem as completely as possible. Sunglasses are thought of as glamorous and most people, young and old, wear them for both utility to protect their eyes and for style.

Hearing aids have not received the same level of acceptance as eyeglasses. And it is unlikely that anyone would buy overly large or conspicuous hearing aids in the same way that some people buy large or unusual pairs of eyeglasses. On the contrary, people are interested in being fit with hearing aids that are as small and inconspicuous as possible. This seems to be true for most people, regardless of their age or lifestyle. A large behind-the-ear instrument is frequently rejected in favor of smaller all-in-the-ear or miniature open-canal models, simply because the person feels that this would be less conspicuous but still beneficial. Some older persons state strongly that they might accept an in-the-ear instrument, but would not even consider a postauricle aid, even though it might provide them better hearing. On the other hand, some people are unwilling to wear an instrument of any kind, because they do not wish to advertise that they have a hearing problem. They would prefer to try to "get by" and to conceal it. This type of attitude has historically presented a barrier in acceptance of amplification. However, this view appears to be diminishing, as people of our current generation take charge of their own destiny by doing whatever is necessary to reduce barriers to their lives.

Dexterity

Hearing aids and their controls continue to become smaller. This reduction in size has made hearing aids far more acceptable to a larger number of people than ever before. For the vast majority of the population, the smaller size has not presented a great problem. However, with advancing age and physical limitations that can accompany aging, the reduction in the dimensions of instruments and the resulting decrease in the size of the controls and batteries can present difficulties.

With age, the sense of touch may diminish, and people can find it difficult to know precisely if they are correctly seating a hearing aid or earmold into the concha, or if they actually have the battery in place. Elderly adults may be seen with a hearing aid hanging precariously from their ear, or with an earmold that is far from being seated properly. The individual may be unaware about the situation even though she has just inserted the hearing aid. Those individuals may complain that the hearing aid does not work properly or that it hurts the ear; both complaints may be easily resolved by ensuring that the aid is properly seated in the ear. Likewise, an older person may have such a poor sense of touch that she is unable to find the volume control or the off-on switch. When the person tries to move a control to a desired location, the person may not be certain whether the movement was successful. Even though a specific model of hearing aid may have internal controls, and all have been preset at the fitting, one must still insert the hearing aid properly in order for it to work as it is intended.

Thus, good manual dexterity and a good sense of touch can help a great deal in the successful use of amplification. On the other hand, reduced dexterity and sense of touch can be strong deterrents to success, and almost certainly require the assistance of some relative or other person to overcome this difficulty. A mandatory portion of every hearing aid fitting with an older individual should include a dexterity check to determine if the person can use the controls, fit the aids to the ears, and actually handle and change batteries. The fitter should note any problems and consider the need for larger or stacked volume controls, or fitting with internal preset controls.

Modifications According to Different Populations of Older Adults

There are several populations of older adults that must be considered, and the differences among these populations influence the potential use of hearing aids. According to the early treatise by Kasten (1992) referred to earlier, the differences among these populations influence the procedures that can be used for selecting a suitable hearing aid.

The Independent Older Adult

Older individuals in the independent group are frequently the easiest to work with and the most successful in terms of hearing aid use. They continue to be in control of their lifestyles and they enter into the process of hearing aid use with their eyes open, albeit sometimes reluctantly. Among the factors or prognostic areas that predict hearing aid use, individuals in this population are most frequently amenable to change. These individuals often continue to see a great many varied opportunities available themselves of and frequently are willing to modify behavior and attitudes for their own betterment and for the benefit of their spouse or friends.

With the independent living population, motivation is the critical factor. When motivation exists, even to a limited degree, appropriate counseling can bring about positive change in a patient. Sympathetic support on the part of a spouse or friend can clearly help to strengthen the degree of communicative success.

To a large degree, potential success with hearing aids is directly tied to the extent that a potential hearing aid user can see and experience success in significant and meaningful communication situations. Success in communication can cause a heightened social awareness and can lead to a genuine desire to expand social horizons and to modify an individual's personal everyday life.

The Semi-Independent Older Adult

When clinicians work with the semi-independent population they are faced with a different set of circumstances. These individuals frequently have large portions of their lifestyles dictated by those who control the environment in which they live. In some instances this direction is provided by well-meaning but communicatively naïve sons or daughters in whose homes the older person may reside, who are unaware of the special needs of older adults. All too often, this group of older individuals finds themselves living in a relatively comfortable, albeit controlled, environment, and they may think that their only other option is nursing home placement. As a result, their psychological set and their attitude toward the factors relating to successful hearing aid use are consciously or subconsciously dictated to them by the individual or individuals governing their living accommodations.

With this population, it is frequently necessary to spend as much time with the persons who control the living environment as with the older individuals themselves. If the well-meaning son or daughter is not sold on the value of hearing aids, then the older individual may not be convinced that they will help. If the son or daughter feels that hearing aids are too expensive to warrant purchase, the likelihood is high that the older individual will find no way to afford the purchase. If the son or daughter strongly states that the older person does not seem to have enough of a problem to warrant hearing aid use, then chances are that the older person will at least verbalize a similar statement. If the son or daughter feels that the older person does not have a wide enough range of activities or experiences to benefit from a hearing aid, then the likelihood is quite high that the older person will reflect the same belief and, even worse, may demonstrate it.

In spite of the apparent needs of an older individual, decisions about amplification and attitudes toward amplification may be shaped by others who are not directly experiencing the problem. On the other hand, family members can also be a catalyst in the successful use of hearing aids.

The former situation creates an awkward position for the older individual who has impaired hearing. She may readily recognize the need for the kind of assistance that can be obtained from amplification but genuinely fear the consequences of a decision that goes contrary to the power structure in her environment. Although often not intentional, the older individual in the semi-independent population may become the *recipient* of attitudes and decisions rather than the *originator* of her own attitudes and decisions.

The Dependent Older Adult

The dependent living population frequently requires a different approach and demands serious moral judgments on the part of the audiologist or the hearing aid dispenser. Individuals in this population may be almost totally controlled and cared for as the result of their physical, emotional, or mental condition. If this population is viewed objectively in terms of hearing aid use, clinicians are faced with the fact that they may have poor motivation, little adaptability, limited insight in terms of personal appraisement, little available money, poor social awareness, and a restricted social environment, as well as limited mobility and finger dexterity.

In addition to these factors, we must realize that these people often are cared for by well-meaning and hard-working staff members who know almost nothing about hearing aid use and who are primarily concerned with physical factors relating to the maintenance of life. Taken as a group, the prospects for successful hearing aid use are limited. This has been substantiated in early reports of Alpiner (1963), Gaitz and Warshaw

(1964), and Grossman (1955), who discuss three general attitudes that can appear among dependent older individuals who choose not to become involved in hearing aid use: (a) they may deny that a problem is present; (b) they may display a general attitude of hopelessness; and/or (c) they may express a recognition of the hearing loss, but may indicate no desire for any type of rehabilitation.

Successful Hearing Aid Use for Dependent Older Persons

For dependent older persons, a key to successful hearing aid use may, for example, be staff members who care for the individual or the volunteers who help in activities of daily living. These people must be trained in proper hearing aid use and maintenance and must be schooled on the importance of hearing aids for communication. By explaining in detail the methods and procedures they can use to convey information to the older individual who has hearing impairment, they receive extensive knowledge about hearing aid use and care.

Clinicians must realize, however, that there generally is a relatively high turnover of staff in many health care facilities. As a rule, the work is hard, the hours are long, and the pay is often not commensurate with the work involved. As a result, many individuals stay with a particular job only until they are able to find something else that will provide them with more satisfaction or more money. With this in mind, clinicians must realize that in-service training that deals with hearing aid use and care must be performed on a recurring basis and must include a great deal of demonstration and some rather thorough follow-up evaluations.

With the dependent group, clinicians must remember that well-fitted hearing aids are not an end unto themselves. Hearing aid use will be successful only if there is a need for communication, a desire for personal interaction, and support that includes family and staff encouragement and understanding. Hearing aid use will be successful only when older individuals can demonstrate to themselves a real benefit from the process.

A Final Consideration as It Relates to the Extremely Dependent Older Adult

One final factor is essential to consider when dealing with the extremely dependent aged population. By definition, individuals in this group may be incapable of caring for themselves and require the constant attendance of others who provide for their needs. For the hearing aid user within this group, a significant other person must be knowledgeable and proficient in terms of hearing aid use. She must be able to ensure that the hearing aids are working properly, the batteries are appropriate and working, the earmolds or hearing aids are inserted properly, and the hearing aids are set as they should be for the individual. Although these do not seem to be overwhelming tasks, they can be major hurdles for an overworked health care facility staff member who has had limited experience with hearing aid use. The audiologist must maintain close contact with health care facility administrators and nursing staff including nurse aides so that she can be available when staff turnover requires a new staff training program. In this way, continuous care for hearing aid users is assured.

Hearing Aid Orientation

The importance of adequate orientation to one's hearing aid(s) has been stressed throughout this chapter, but a separate dis-

cussion of the essential elements of that important aspect of hearing aid fitting and use is important. Orientation to the use of hearing aids is an essential part of the ongoing aural rehabilitation program. The fitting and dispensing of hearing aids is just the beginning of the process. If a patient is not comfortable with a hearing aid, its uses, benefits, and limitations, it will probably not be successfully employed by the patient.

There are generally seven important components of a hearing orientation program:

1. An understanding of the function of the component parts and adjustments of hearing aids;
2. Practice in fitting, adjusting, and maintaining the hearing aid;
3. An understanding of the limitations of amplification;
4. Knowledge of why the particular hearing aid was selected for a patient;
5. How to begin using a newly selected hearing aid;
6. How to troubleshoot hearing aid problems; and
7. How to exercise a hearing aid user's legal rights.

Depending on the state of health, alertness, and physical ability of the patient, those key elements should guide the hearing aid orientation program. The hearing aid orientation program need not be restricted to a specified time frame. If the patient is part of an ongoing aural rehabilitation program, hearing aid orientation is integral. The patient asks questions, receives answers from the audiologist, requests adjustments regarding the fit of the amplification, and in this regard, receives comprehensive orientation and adjustment service over time.

If the patient is among the dependent population, it becomes critical that her family, significant other, or health care facility staff become integral members of the hearing aid orientation program, as they may be the ones who fit the patient with the hearing aid each day.

Patients and their significant other(s) should be provided practical information about the care and maintenance of the hearing aid(s), and their uses. For example:

1. The patient should receive general information about hearing aids, what they are, what they do, what they do not do, and the component parts. There is so much misinformation presented in advertisements about hearing aids that it behooves the audiologist to provide accurate and informative details.

2. Information on adjusting to one's hearing aid is critical to the orientation process. This involves practicing placing the hearing aid in one's ear and removing it; what to expect from the hearing aid in noisy or otherwise distracting environments; and how to adjust the aid.

3. The care of one's hearing aid, including the potential harm from water, hairspray, excessive heat, perspiration, and other factors are important parts of the orientation process. Receiving information on cleaning and caring for one's hearing aid is as important as learning how to use it.

4. Telephone use with a hearing aid with or without a telecoil should be a part of the orientation process.

5. Information on what causes "whistles and squeals" is also important for patients to receive. This can be a part of the information presented on "When do hearing aids need repair?"

6. Battery sizes, materials, life expectancy, increasing battery life, and other information about batteries is also critical to the orientation process. There is almost as much misinformation available to hearing aid users about batteries as there is about hearing aids themselves.

An effective and efficient hearing aid orientation process is a critically important part of the fitting of hearing aids. The effectiveness of this part of the aural rehabilitation process can enhance or doom the willingness of patients to use their hearing aid(s) in constructive ways.

Summary

The older individual who has hearing impairment may belong to one of several different populations who demonstrate a wide range of skills and abilities. Therefore, it is frequently necessary to modify the procedures for selecting and fitting hearing aids to successfully meet each patient's amplification needs.

It matters little which dependency category an aged person may fit into. Each individual presents a unique set of capabilities and limitations and audiologists must be aware of all as they pertain to each individual to deal effectively with these patients.

The growing population of aged individuals poses a unique challenge to all persons involved in the hearing health care team. The audiologist must be particularly aware that she is not dealing with one large, homogeneous group of individuals, but rather with several subgroups who have advanced age as a common factor and their individual level of ability as a distinctive feature.

References

Alpiner, J. G. (1963). Audiologic problems of the aged. *Geriatrics, 18,* 19–26.

Gaitz, C., & Warshaw, M. S. (1964). Obstacles encountered in correcting hearing loss in the elderly. *Geriatrics, 19,* 83–86.

Grossman, B. (1955). Hard of hearing persons in a home for the aged. *Hearing News, 23,* 11–20.

Hull, R. H. (1992). Introduction to hearing aids. In R. H. Hull (Ed.), *Aural rehabilitation* (pp. 28-41). San Diego, CA: Singular.

Hull, R. H. (1998). *Hearing in aging.* San Diego, CA: Singular.

Hull, R. H. (2001). Consideration for the use and orientation to hearing aids for older adults. In R. H. Hull (Ed.), *Aural rehabilitation* (pp. 373-392). San Diego, CA: Singular.

Humes, L. E. (2008). Aging and speech communication. *ASHA Leader, 13,* 10-13.

Kaplan, H., Bally, S. J., & Brandt, F. D. (1990). *Communication skill scale.* Washington, DC: Gallaudet University.

Kasten, R. N (1992). Considerations for the use and orientation to hearing aids for older adults (pp. 265-277). In R. H. Hull (Ed.), *Aural rehabilitation.* San Diego, CA: Singular.

Pichora-Fuller, M. K. (2006). Effects of age on auditory and cognitive processing: Implications for hearing aid fitting and audiologic rehabilitation. *Trends in Amplification, 10,* 29-59.

Rawool, V. W. (2007). The aging auditory system, Part 3: Slower processing, cognition, and speech recognition. *The Hearing Review, 9,* 38-46.

Ross, M. (1972). Hearing aid evaluation. In J. Katz (Ed.), *Handbook of clinical audiology* (pp. 482-513). Baltimore: Williams and Wilkins.

Rupp, R. R., Higgins, J., & Maurer, J. F. (1977). A feasibility scale for predicting hearing aid use (FSPHAU) with other individuals. *Journal of the Academy of Rehabilitative Audiology, 10,* 81-104.

Stach, B. A. (1990). Central auditory processing disorders and amplification applications. Research Symposium: Communication sciences and disorders of aging. *ASHA Reports, 19,* 150-156.

End of Chapter Examination Questions

Chapter 18

1. The author presents *nine* factors that should be considered when determining the appropriateness of amplification for hearing impaired older adults. Name and describe *six* of those factors.

2. The author presents a number of elements that must be taken into consideration when recommending and fitting hearing aids for older adults who have hearing impairment. Compare and contrast them for the following groups: (a) the independent older adult, (b) the semi-independent older adult, (c) the dependent older adult, and (d) the extremely dependent older adult.

End of Chapter Answer Sheet

Name _____   Date _____

Chapter 18

1. a. _____

b. _____

c. _____

d. _____

e. _____

f. _____

2. a. _____

b. _____

c. _____

d. _____

19

Techniques of Aural Rehabilitation for Older Adults with Impaired Hearing

RAYMOND H. HULL

Chapter Outline

Introduction

The process of aural rehabilitation on behalf of older patients is as exciting as it is rewarding. To be involved in the recovery of communication skills that may have previously caused an adult to withdraw from his communicating world is, indeed, gratifying. Both the patient and the audiologist can rejoice in the recovery of those skills. Some older patients recover skills that allow them to participate on a social basis once again, at least with a greater degree of efficiency. Others may simply regain the ability to communicate with their family with greater ease. In light of those gains and, perhaps, a step toward a reinstatement of communicative independence, a patient and his audiologist have reason to rejoice.

Clinicians cannot, under any circumstances, hope to benefit every older hearing impaired person. But, in attempting to do so, if some are helped who had previously submitted to a self-imposed withdrawal from family and friends because of the embarrassment from responding inappropriately to misunderstood messages, then professionals can be satisfied that our work is worthwhile.

Because most older adults who have hearing impairment have experienced normal to near-normal auditory function during their younger years, and because they are generally fully aware of the communicative difficulties they face, it is important that our services address their specific communicative needs. In light of the fact that it is being confirmed that auditory disorders found in older adults are quite complex (see Chapter 16 and Chapter 17), approaches to aural rehabilitation must accommodate the communication difficulties experienced as a result of compounding problems; many of these are found in a probable combination of both peripheral and central involvement. The audiologist is, indeed, serving complex people who possess complex auditory disorders.

Individual versus Group Treatment

Individual Treatment

Some individuals will require individual aural rehabilitation treatment. In instances in which patients are experiencing communicative difficulties that are not conducive to a group therapy environment because of their individual or personal nature, individual sessions are warranted.

For example, a semiretired physician came to this author with a desire for more efficient communication within his office and examination room. The sessions centered on the specific difficulties he was experiencing in that environment, and he did not desire to open them up to group aural rehabilitation sessions.

Another patient's concern was that her granddaughter's wedding was forthcoming, and she felt that she was not going to be able to hear and understand what people were saying while she stood in the reception line. Her request was to receive some hints on how to "not embarrass herself and her family" by responding inappropriately to what people were saying to her in the reverberant environment of their church fellowship hall. Her aural rehabilitation program was based on two sessions of problem solving and supportive and informational counseling. After successfully working through the potential pitfalls of the communicative demands of her granddaughter's wedding, the woman returned to enter group therapy.

The sessions held for this woman were rather personal in regard to the difficulties she was anticipating and, in that instance and at that time, she felt that they were not conducive to a group therapy environment. So her desire for individual sessions was fulfilled.

Other circumstances in which individual treatment sessions would be appropriate include:

1. The patient's hearing impairment and concomitant communicative difficulties are so severe that the patient requires concentrated effort to resolve them to the greatest degree possible before entering a group environment.
2. The patient's emotional response to the auditory impairment and the resulting communicative difficulties are such that group involvement, at that particular time, is contraindicated.

Group Treatment

Group aural rehabilitative treatment, as discussed later in this chapter, can be extremely motivating for many older adults who are experiencing impaired hearing. Once the problems and difficulties that are specific to individual patients have been resolved to the degree possible through work on an individual basis, patients can move into group treatment, if group services are warranted (Figure 19–1).

Individuals in group treatment find strength in hearing of others' successes and failures in their own communicative environments. They gain insights through group discussions and problem solving into how to best cope in spite of their hearing impairment. The camaraderie that develops can be rewarding to group members as their

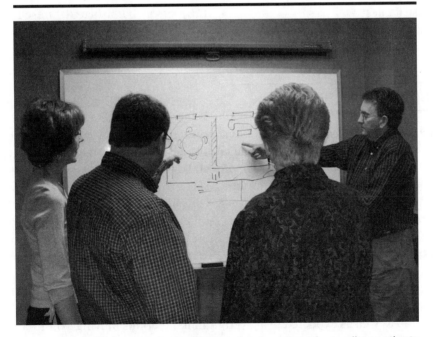

Figure 19–1. Group aural rehabilitation treatment works to allow patients to share frustrations and triumphs.

confidence grows in their ability to take charge of the difficulties that they have been having in their own communicative worlds.

Components of Aural Rehabilitation Services for Older Patients

The following are important elements in aural rehabilitation service programs for older adults that are applicable for either the well adult in the community or those who are confined to a health care facility. They include:

1. Counseling
2. Hearing aid orientation
3. Adjusting the listening environment
4. Development of positive assertiveness
5. Developing compensatory skills in the use of residual hearing and supplemental visual cues
6. Involvement of family and significant others

Counseling

As this author teaches his students about aural rehabilitation services for older adults, it is emphasized that counseling, for lack of a better term, is one of the most important aspects and is intertwined throughout the process of aural rehabilitation. It is not something that occurs alone or out of context. It is an integral part of everything an audiologist does when working with his patients. It is talking. It is instilling confidence in a patient who has become discouraged when he did not do as well as expected in a given communicative environment. It is listening to the feelings a patient reveals about himself, or that person's relationship with an intolerant family member or roommate. And it is trust that must develop between audiologist and patient. Counseling is the discussion that develops when a patient desires to talk about an incident in which he had particular difficulty understanding what another person was saying, and also includes the problem solving that can unravel the possible reasons for the difficulty.

This aspect of the process of aural rehabilitation is, again for lack of a better term, called counseling. But, whatever it is called, it involves listening, talking, problem solving, facilitating adjustment to a frustrating disability, and the development of trust between patient and audiologist.

When an audiologist encounters an older adult who has impaired hearing who says, "I do not desire to be helped. I am old and I do not know how much longer I will live," the attitude of the person certainly will influence how much potential progress that he will make. This is particularly true if the person has isolated himself from the outside world and is resigned to not seek help because of advanced age.

The Audiologist as Counselor

If there are no other significant contraindicating factors that would hinder responsiveness to aural rehabilitation services, the audiologist is in a position to serve in a counseling role. It is possible that this patient has said what was said because he has been told by others that "you are too old." A well-meaning physician may have said, "You know you're no spring chicken any more." Or a child may have said unthinkingly, "Mom, you know you can't care for yourself as well as you used to, so we should start thinking about moving you to a care facility," not realizing that the older adult is convinced that placement in a "care facility" will be terminal. Such statements, even said in a well-meaning way, are understandably unsettling to an older adult.

One of this author's patients, a woman of 89 years, told me that her 50-year-old daughter told her they should sell her house and she should then move into an efficiency apartment. She was so hurt and angry that she could not think of anything to say. She felt convinced that if her mature daughter felt that she could not care for her house, then she must be doing a worse job than she thought. I asked her what she would have said if her daughter had suggested that to her when she was 45 years old and her daughter was 15. She said she would have asked her why she would say such a thing, but she said, "But when you are 89 years old, perhaps it is not worth it."

If the medical records of an individual indicate satisfactory health, and there appears to be nothing that would contraindicate the provision of aural rehabilitative services, then the self-defeating attitude of the potential patient may be the only thing that stands between the provision of services and reasonable progress in aural rehabilitation treatment. Although the person's realistic view of becoming older may be a healthy one, long-term mourning because of age and the possibility of death is not. The audiologist can be a positive catalyst in moving beyond aging, particularly for those who are barred from social interaction as a result of their auditory deficit.

Feelings to Which the Audiologist Must Respond

Phrases exemplifying attitudes typical of many older adults who have hearing impairment have been recorded by this author during initial aural rehabilitation interviews with hundreds of older patients. The feelings that prompted these revealing statements are those that can and do stifle the desire for aural rehabilitative services or the progress they may be capable of. They are, further, those to which the audiologist must respond. The following are a few of those statements, out of context, recorded by this author:

- "I feel that I'm on trial, becoming incompetent."
- "My son is right behind me. He comes down to see me as often as he can, but he has a lot of business to handle there. I don't see him very often anymore."
- "I can't hear and my eyes bother me. Surgery won't help my ears or my eyes. I'm told that I'm too old."
- "My arthritis bothers me all over, especially with the weather. I used to walk a lot. I can't hear now. I'm too old."
- "I fear being alone—being melancholy —with no future to look forward to. I need to find some way to be useful. But I can stand a lot. I'm still sturdy."
- "I would like, more than anything, to be able to get out, to socialize, but I can't hear very well. I would like to go to church, but the children don't come on Sundays and there is no one to take me."

One statement stands out from all of the rest. It is a statement by a physically strong and mentally alert 82-year-old man who possesses impaired hearing and who is torn between giving up and submitting to the opportunity to improve his ability to function communicatively through an audiologist's services. The statement is, "I'd like to put a younger person on my shoulders to function intellectually on my behalf and hear for me, and to go on from there. I suppose I need to learn to rely on myself . . . relationships with people are important, but do I have the potential?"

The above statements are representative of those heard by audiologists who accept the opportunity to provide a significant rehabilitative service on behalf of adults who have impaired hearing. These people, in many ways, wish to be recognized not simply as older persons, but as adults who have grown older, who have something to offer, and who do not want to be left alone. Their resolution to "not be a bother" and their resignation to "being old" is, in some cases, the most logical choice in their minds for lack of alternatives. The audiologist can be a catalyst in developing a desire for self-enhancement.

The audiologist must not be afraid to work with these patients in a close professional manner. He must not be hesitant to intervene in a counseling role, but must be cognizant of those instances when a patient's emotional problems are beyond the scope of the audiologist's service. For those persons, it is the responsibility of the audiologist to refer the individual to other appropriate counseling professionals. Above all, the patient must be confident in the audiologist who is providing the aural rehabilitation service. The patient must be aware that the audiologist understands the communicative impact of presbycusis through his experience in working with other patients. The patient must know that the audiologist feels that he can, indeed, be helped to communicate more efficiently through aural rehabilitative services, and that feeling has justification on the basis of evaluation, not sympathy. A feeling of justified trust is the true key to motivational counseling. The patient pictured in Figure 19–2 trusts that the audiologist understands the frustrations that he has experienced, and that what the audiologist is saying will assist him in learning to cope in his otherwise difficult communicative environments.

Listen-talk-empathize-listen—encourage where appropriate—remember the status and age of the patient—provide support

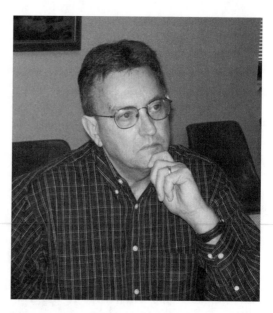

Figure 19–2. Assertiveness training brings out strengths patients may not realize they possess.

—counsel—listen—ask questions—expect answers—listen—provide guidance. Then, add an appropriate amount of inspiration for what may be the key to successful motivational counseling. Counseling as a part of the aural rehabilitation process is presented later in this chapter under The Process of Aural Rehabilitation.

Hearing Aid Orientation

Information in Chapter 18 deals with considerations for hearing aid orientation on behalf of older adults. As stated in that chapter, the process of adjustment to the use of hearing aids and orientation to their efficient use can be facilitated with greater ease for some older patients than others; this depends on prior exposure to and knowledge of the use of hearing aids and factors of memory, manual dexterity, and others. The process of adjustment to hearing aids and orientation to their use can be logically carried into daily or weekly aural rehabilitation treatment sessions, as can the trial use of various assisting listening devices.

Through carryover of hearing aid orientation into the aural rehabilitation treatment program, slight adjustments to the hearing aids can, for example, be made to alleviate communicative problems encountered during the previous week. Questions can be answered regarding their use, and discussions regarding certain difficult listening environments can be entertained that may benefit not only that individual patient, but others in a group session. More experienced hearing aid users can be an important catalyst in a new user's successful adjustment to amplification. Further, experimental adjustments in hearing aid gain and frequency response can be made in accordance with the activities in various treatment sessions.

Carryover of the hearing aid orientation process into aural rehabilitation treatment sessions can be as important as the orientation process itself, and is a logical extension. The consistency of patient contact is a valuable asset in facilitating adjustment to amplification. In group treatment sessions, the catharsis and camaraderie that arise as various patients describe their own difficulties experienced during the initial adjustment period is a healthy environment for efficient adjustment to hearing aid use. Procedures for hearing aid orientation applicable for older adults are outlined in Chapters 13 and 18 in this text.

Adjusting or Manipulating the Listening Environment

As is noted in The Process of Aural Rehabilitation section of this chapter, elderly patients are initially asked to establish priorities for situations in which they desire to function more efficiently. After this is completed, they are asked to choose one or two in which they most desire to learn to communicate more efficiently. They are, of course, requested to be reasonable in their selections. In this way, the aural rehabilitation treatment program can be designed to meet their specific communication needs. In instances in which a patient's auditory difficulties are so severe that group sessions are not practical or cannot be tolerated by the patient, individual treatment is scheduled.

The goal, however, is to integrate the patient into a group situation as soon as possible, if at all possible. Another situation in which it is desirable that individual treatment be instituted is in the case of a patient whose priority communication environment is so different as to warrant individual work. A situation in point is a patient who was provided services individually by this author. His most difficult communication environment as a teacher in a middle school was his classroom. His treatment sessions, therefore, centered on physical/environmental adjustments in that specific room. The author worked with him individually on redesigning his classroom, which was specific to his difficulties and strategies for communication in that environment. He had little difficulty in other more social environments.

Patient Discussions of Problem Environments

Problem solving of difficult listening environments can be extremely productive. Those sessions center on discussions of the patients' chosen prioritized communication environments. Priority environments most frequently center on church (understanding the minister or Sunday school teacher, or participating in church committee meetings), other social environments in which groups of people meet, understanding what women or children are saying, or understanding what people are saying in environmentally distracting environments such as on the street corner, in a restaurant, or at the theater. The inevitable commonality of their choices allows for group sessions that are beneficial for everyone, as the majority of patients can enter into the discussions as they relate to them.

A problem specific to a certain environment, for example, is brought before the group by one of the therapy group members. The patient who presented the communication problem is asked to describe it in detail by giving examples of instances when it has occurred and the physical environment of each. As the physical environment is described, the audiologist or the patient diagrams it on the chalkboard as accurately as possible. The room or other physical environment is drawn on the chalkboard or flip chart (including windows, doors, partitions, furniture, and so on). The remainder of the group is then asked to give suggestions, as they see it, about how the patient may have adjusted to that communication environment by changing it, making physical adjustments, or their opinion of making requests of the speaker to resolve the patient's difficulty understanding what was being said.

As those suggestions are made, the audiologist lists suggestions and makes the suggested adjustments on the diagram, for example, (a) moving the patient's chair into a better situation for listening, (b) changing position away from a window, (c) moving closer to a public address system speaker, (d) asking the person being conversed with to move closer, (e) walking out into a hallway where it is quieter, (f) asking the speaker to move closer to the microphone, and so on.

Participation in this type of treatment activity can be extremely motivating. As the patient joins the group discussion by expanding on the explanation of the difficult environment and as questions or possible solutions are made, ways in which he may have been able to change the listening environment or those within it to his benefit become clearer. Others in the group also benefit because they may have found themselves in a similar environment or may in the future.

Creating Positive Assertiveness

A trait that appears to become more typical as some people grow older is to become less assertive. This is particularly true of older adults who have been placed in a health care facility, or who have moved from their home to a retirement complex not of their own will, or who are trying to maintain their independence by remaining at home. Some may seem "stubborn," but those responses may be out of self-defense, perhaps because they may not have heard or understood what was expected of them, or they may suspect that they are being imposed upon rather than being allowed to make independent decisions about their life.

Then, in all too many instances, older persons in health care facilities are not told what is going to be done to them, and they find that things are being done *to* them rather than *for* them. Rather than continuing to react against the health care facility personnel and, thus, being listed as "uncooperative," such patients may become more passive.

Whether an older person is residing in a health care facility or in the community, it regrettably becomes more common for dramatic and sometimes unpleasant things to occur in that person's life. In light of the unexpected occurrences that may occur, it becomes easier to remain passive and wait rather than to become assertive and say

"No," as one may feel forced to do something anyway. "Dad is getting stubborn in his old age," may be the label placed on the older person. Many older persons feel powerless because of a lack of independence. It is difficult to respond to a rapidly changing world when one does not possess the finances, transportation, physical mobility, quickness of analytical thought, or strength to manipulate one's environment.

Examples of Passive Behavior

One of this author's patients, a 78-year-old man, was asked to chair a committee in his church because of his knowledge of religion. He was flattered to be asked to accept that position, but then shortly resigned because he could not understand what his committee members were saying. When I asked him why he did not ask the members to speak up, he said that he did once. He further stated that it worked for a short time, but then they returned to their previous manner of speaking. When I asked him why he did not change the room arrangements so he could place himself in a more advantageous position for communication, he said that the room had been in that same arrangement for years, and he did not want to disrupt it. Those attitudes can defeat an otherwise potentially productive person.

Another example that illustrates the feelings of older adults who have hearing impairment is one that involved a 72-year-old female patient who had just returned from a lecture on Southeast Asia that she had been looking forward to attending for some time. She explained that the lecturer, a woman who had a rather soft voice, began talking to the audience, and then walked away from the public address system microphone and sat down in front of the podium with the statement, "I'm sure that you can all hear me without the microphone."

The patient said that she hardly understood a word the speaker said throughout the next hour, but she was too embarrassed to leave the auditorium. When I asked her why she did not say, "Please use the microphone; we are having difficulties hearing you," when the speaker moved away from it, her reply was that she just could not bring herself to do it. She wanted to, but was too embarrassed. "Besides," she said, "maybe I was the only person there who couldn't hear her." When I asked her if she was important enough to warrant that speaker's consideration, this patient's response was simply, "I hope so." I said, "Don't you think that the microphone was placed there for a purpose? A public address system generally helps everyone to hear more comfortably. If you would have said something, I am sure that others in the audience would have been pleased that the presenter had returned to the podium and used the microphone." Her reply was that she had not thought of that. "But still," she said, "I didn't want to make a nuisance of myself. I'm just an old woman who can't hear very well." One of the audiologist's challenges is to change that attitude of self-depreciation.

Learning to Help Themselves

The attitude just described is one that must be altered, if possible, if persons who possess impaired hearing are to learn to cope and function more efficiently in their communicative worlds. In light of the fact that some people are simply not willing to accommodate older adults who have hearing impairment or, perhaps, are not aware of what accommodations can be made to facilitate communication, older persons must be taught ways to become assertive enough to manipulate their communication environments and those with whom they desire to communicate.

Altering Passive Behaviors

As stated earlier, one way to alter passivity is by asking individual patients to describe difficult communication situations in which they have found themselves during the past week or month. The situation in which the 72-year-old woman found herself, as described above, is a prime example of the problems that are brought to the treatment sessions. Suggestions by group members are brought forth after individual questions by the group members and the audiologist have been satisfied. When other group members courageously state what they would have done in that situation (e.g., told the woman speaker, "I would appreciate it if you would use the microphone.") in front of the audience, they are asked if they really would have done it. If they hold fast to their commitment, they are challenged to do it at the next lecture they attend when the speaker hesitates to use the microphone. Occasionally, a group member returns after such an experience and triumphantly proclaims, "I did it!" On occasion, another member of the aural rehabilitation treatment group who may have been in attendance at that meeting will confirm that the individual did a very nice job in changing a poor listening situation to a more pleasant one. Also, others at the meeting may have thanked our patient for asking the speaker to use the microphone by saying, "We just did not have the courage to speak up like that!" The triumph is great and does much toward encouraging the other group members to also become more assertive.

Other difficult situations brought before the groups may include family dinners, going to a noisy restaurant, talking to timid grandchildren, talking to one's attorney with other members of the family in attendance, following more than one request in a sequence, and many others. The bywords in these treatment sessions are, "If those with whom we desire to or must communicate do not seem to be accommodating, then we must assert ourselves by showing them *how* they can best communicate with us!" Suggestions or adjustments must be made without hesitation. To do otherwise is to "place ourselves back where we started." These are powerful treatment sessions that instill confidence in patients who may not have had confidence for some time.

Involvement of Family and Significant Others

The patient's family and significant others in the patient's life are critical elements for a successful aural rehabilitation treatment program. This is particularly true if a patient's significant other is willing to become involved in the aural rehabilitation process. This includes attending individual or group treatment sessions and participating in follow-up assignments.

A significant other's involvement in the aural rehabilitation treatment process provides that person with a better understanding of the difficulties and frustrations with which the friend, spouse, or family member undergoing treatment is faced, particularly if he can attend the first sessions when discussions of hearing loss and difficult communication situations are emphasized. It further aids the patient's significant other to understand the commonality of communication difficulties when other patients discuss similar problems. The involvement prompts a realization that the communication difficulties that have arisen because of the auditory deficit are not limited only to his spouse, family member, or friend, but are found in others as well. That enhanced understanding hopefully can be passed on to others who are close to the patient.

This author frequently requests that those who attend the treatment sessions with individual patients be fit with earplugs to at least experience to some degree what depressed hearing "sounds like." Some of the communicative frustrations revealed by the patients are often felt by the significant others at least during that brief period of time. It is explained to them, however, that earplugs do not replicate the speech recognition problems being encountered by the person with whom they are attending the sessions, but simply demonstrate a moderate loss of hearing acuity. Still, their use may enhance a feeling of empathy for the frustrations the hearing impaired person must feel. One important byproduct of encouraging the involvement of a significant other in the aural rehabilitation treatment program is that carryover of the treatment process into the everyday life of a patient can be greatly enhanced. If, for example, an older patient asserts himself before the remainder of the family by suggesting certain adjustments regarding seating arrangements for Thanksgiving dinner so that he can become involved in the conversation with greater efficiency, the significant other can reinforce and strengthen that positive step.

It is, further, not as much fun to go to a restaurant or the movie by oneself. The significant other will not only strengthen and encourage carryover, but also make some potentially apprehensive situations more enjoyable. It helps to have someone there to back you up when the going gets rough!

One of the most discouraging aspects of the provision of any rehabilitative service to elderly patients is the lack of family involvement. In many instances, if a spouse has passed away, the remainder of the family may live quite a distance from the patient. Children may visit only once a year if the distance is great, and that may be for only a few days around a principal holiday, which

can be stressful even with normal hearing. Even if grown children live in the same community, their desire for involvement with their parent on a social basis may be lacking, let alone a desire to become an important part of their mother's or father's rehabilitation program. The excuse is generally, "We just don't have time." In this remarkably advanced society, it is sad that we lose sight of the needs of our family. But it seems to be the case, and alternative means for carryover support for older patients must, in many cases, be sought.

As stated earlier, a patient's spouse can be the most effective significant other, if the spouse is emotionally supportive of his or her husband or wife. If the spouse is not willing or capable of aiding in the support or carryover process, then a friend is appropriate and can be a most effective partner in the aural rehabilitation process. In fact, at times it is common for people to discuss feelings with supportive friends prior to bringing them before a spouse or other family members. In any event, a close friend can be a very significant other.

A case to illustrate this point is that of a 70-year-old male patient who was provided aural rehabilitation services by this author. He had been a widower for 4 years. On the first day of his group aural rehabilitation program, he brought a female companion. Both loved to fish and were almost inseparable. They both enjoyed attending social gatherings together, but the patient was experiencing great difficulty hearing and, in particular, understanding what was being said in those environments. His female companion was willing to explain what was being said, but was becoming frustrated at the consistency with which she had to function in the capacity of interpreter. In this instance, she attended all treatment sessions with the patient, she wearing her earplugs and he his hearing aids. A great deal of warmth and understanding developed between them. And his ability to function communicatively increased, as did her willingness to aid in the treatment process through carryover. The assignments, which included experimentation at social gatherings, were carried out in an excellent manner. Problem situations that were to be discussed during treatment sessions lessened and, likewise, his dependence on his female companion for communicative support became less frequent.

The support and carryover by this significant other was instrumental in the patient's achievements in learning to use his residual hearing with greater efficiency, to use supplemental visual clues, and to change his most difficult listening environments in constructive ways. Without such support and assistance, an audiologist will have great difficulty facilitating such improvements. In the end, he may never be able to assist the patient in making such significant and positive strides as will the significant other.

The Process of Aural Rehabilitation

The aural rehabilitation program for an older adult patient can include:

1. Knowledge of the patient's desires and needs for communication through setting priorities that are those of the patient, not the audiologist;
2. Ongoing motivational counseling as an integral part of the process;
3. Carryover of hearing aid orientation, at least for those who seem to benefit from amplification;
4. Learning how to manipulate one's environment and the speakers in those environments to enhance communication;

5. Learning to become positively assertive;
6. Throughout everything listed, learning to use one's residual hearing and supplemental visual cues to enhance comprehension of verbal messages.

To put all of this together into a meaningful aural rehabilitation treatment program for an older adult is not really difficult. As a matter of fact, the process becomes quite logical once a number of older patients have critiqued your approach in relation to its meaningfulness and benefit to them.

The following is an example of an approach to aural rehabilitation treatment for elderly adult patients, employing and intermingling the six listed areas. This process has been found effective for use with both confined and community-based older adults.

The Ongoing Aural Rehabilitation Program: Reasons for Successful and Unsuccessful Treatment Programs

Some structure in the treatment process is desired by the majority of older patients. But, on the other hand, overly structured sessions can be counterproductive. For example, it is sadly not uncommon for audiologists who utilize traditional speechreading (lipreading) approaches that emphasize a progression from phoneme analysis to syllables, words, phrases, sentences, and stories (which, for example, stress several like phonemes) to begin to realize in a fairly short time that the patients who seemed motivated initially are attending speechreading sessions with less regularity. Soon they may cease attending altogether. Excuses generally range from "My family is coming to visit and I will be spending time with them," to "We have several church suppers coming up, and I have to help with them." It is embarrassing to see such persons downtown later with apparently nothing to do. They may further call to tell your secretary that they really do not feel the need to come to "class" anymore, even though the audiologist knows that they have made little or no progress in treatment.

Those patients are telling us something that we should receive loudly and clearly. That is, if they felt that aural rehabilitation services were benefitting them, they probably would still be attending, as they evidently were motivated when they began.

If the aural rehabilitation treatment program had been geared to the specific needs of those patients, they would probably be taking advantage of the audiologist's services. But, for those reasons, and because the audiologist may have begun the first session from a predetermined approach to speechreading, the patients were not interested in receiving those services any more. A few faithful patients might continue to attend, but they probably will leave the final session as able or unable to communicate with others they were in the beginning. The audiologist may wonder why these otherwise apparently alert older adults have not improved, even though they may say, "I enjoyed your class," and pat the audiologist on the shoulder. Further, why does this audiologist have to coerce patients in health care facilities to attend aural rehabilitation treatment sessions or have to depend on a gracious activity director to bring them from their rooms to attend sessions that should be helping them cope in the everyday world more efficiently? Again, it may be because the audiologist has lost sight of the fact that the treatment must be designed with the needs of the patients in mind. Other treatment procedures used by speech-language pathologists, occupational therapists, physical therapists, physicians, and others are

based on a treatment plan designed around the assessed needs of each patient. Why, then, are some audiologists still opening their lipreading lesson book and beginning at page 1 to provide services to patients who have varied and individual communication deficits and needs? Those speechreading books too often are used as "hymnals," and the session begins with the audiologist saying, "And for the next session we will turn to page 15." That is not treatment.

Individualizing the Approach

How does one develop a meaningful approach to aural rehabilitation treatment for the older patient? More than 30 years ago Hardick (1977) described the basic characteristics of a successful aural rehabilitation program for older adults. They are well defined and provide comprehensive guidance for those who intend to provide services for older patients and in many ways are still current. Those characteristics are:

1. The program must be patient centered.
2. The program must revolve around amplification and/or modifying a patient's communication environment.
3. All programs consist of individual therapy, with some group sessions when necessary.
4. The session must contain normally hearing friends or relatives of the person who has hearing impairment.
5. Aural rehabilitation programs are short-term.
6. The program is consumer oriented.
7. Aural rehabilitation programs and their potential benefits need to be promoted to colleagues and other professionals.
8. "Successful graduates" should be used as resource people in therapy activities whenever possible (Hardick, 1977, pp. 60–62).

These characteristics are extremely important for consideration prior to the initiation of aural rehabilitation programs for older adults. They go far beyond the more traditional lipreading procedures that continue to be employed by some. Even though Hardick (1977) and others recommended group treatment for older patients, some will require individual services. However, as has been noted by this author, there is a tendency among some to hesitate or refuse to participate in individual treatment unless they themselves have requested it.

Other early patient-centered approaches to aural rehabilitation are discussed by Alpiner (1963), Alpiner and McCarthy (1987), Colton (1977), Colton and O'Neill (1976), Giolas (1994), Hull (1982, 1992, 1997, 2001, 2007), McCarthy and Alpiner (1978), M. Miller and Ort (1965), O'Neill and Oyer (1981), Sanders (1982, 1993), and others. The aspect stressed by these authors is that older adult patients possess needs that are specific to them and each patient's aural rehabilitation program must be centered on his needs and priorities.

If the ingredients presented on the previous pages are combined properly, a possible sequence of services emerges. An example of such a sequence is provided below.

Awareness of Reasons for Auditory Dysfunction

Understanding Hearing Loss. Facilitating an awareness of the reason for auditory communication difficulties through an understanding of the process of aging and its effect on the auditory mechanism is an important part of the aural rehabilitation process. Included is a discussion of the central processing of auditory-linguistic information and the effect of aging on the speed and precision of that important component in communication, particularly in noisy or

otherwise distracting environments. The level of terminology is determined by the individual or group in question. The audiologist is cautioned never to speak down to patients. It is important to use the correct technical terminology, but immediately explain it at the level of the persons involved. Clinicians must always remember that the audience is adult, no matter what their educational level or age. They deserve to be treated as such.

Charts need to be used in such discussions, perhaps along with a 35-mm slide or PowerPoint presentation on the ear. If individuals in the group are severely hard of hearing, projected slides should be used only if enough light can remain in the room to facilitate the use of visual clues. Charts, diagrams, slides, and chalkboard drawings are used for these discussions, including presentations on (a) the aging ear, (b) uses, benefits, and limitations of hearing aids, (c) environmental factors that affect communication, (d) poor speakers versus good speakers and their makeup, and (e) a general discussion of the aging process.

The basis for the first session (or sessions) is to facilitate a basis of understanding for the remainder of the treatment program, to develop a better understanding among the patients of what has occurred to them, and to assure them that in all probability they can improve, at least to some degree. Most persons leave such session or sessions with a better understanding and greater acceptance of what is occurring to them and a desire to participate in the aural rehabilitation treatment program.

It cannot be emphasized enough that a significant other in each patient's life should be encouraged to attend these sessions (Figure 19–3). Whether it is a spouse or a family member such as a child or a friend, he will gain much greater insight into the auditory or communication prob-

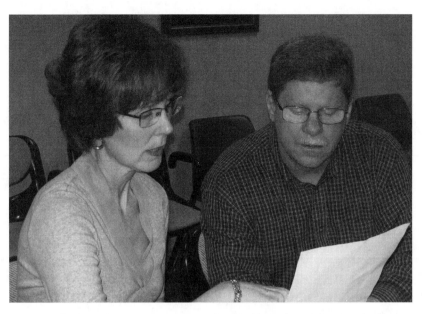

Figure 19–3. A spouse, family member, or significant other can reinforce the aural rehabilitation process.

lems with which the person is attempting to cope.

Prioritized Communicative Needs. The second step in the aural rehabilitation treatment programs is, as stated earlier, to ask each patient to list those difficulties in communication that most affect him. The Wichita State University Communication Appraisal and Priorities Profile (CAPP), as presented in Figure 19-4, can be used in this process. They may include specific communication environments, such as a meeting room, church, certain restaurant, table arrangement at their child's home, and so on. They also may list certain individuals who they have difficulty understanding.

The next step is for patients to set priorities for these situations or persons, from most important to least important and, if they had their choice, in which of those would they most like to improve. They are

asked, of course, to be realistic in their final choices. For some, the choice is a simple one. For others, it is more difficult. It is important to note, however, that if gains are made in one category, there is the probability that patients will observe improvement in others.

They are asked to discuss their choices, present a situation in which they had difficulty, and explain what prompted them to make those choices. Particularly in a group situation, it is interesting to note the general consistency of priority areas that emerge. The patients generally appreciate the camaraderie that develops out of this discussion. For the first time, many of them realize that they are not the only ones who have difficulty in certain environments.

In many instances, patients put part of the blame for their auditory/communicative difficulties on others who display poor speech habits. That is acknowledged and

The WSU Communication Appraisal and Priorities Profile

Date_____

Name_____ Age_____ Sex____

Address_____ Phone_____

Please indicate below those situations in which you are able to communicate best, those that are difficult for you in some instances, and those that are a definite problem. Under "explain," please tell us more if you desire, such as certain instances when you experience more difficulty than others, certain types of speakers, certain places, and so on.

	No problems	Only in specific instances	Definite problem	Priority
1. At parties or other social events	____	____	____	____
Explain_____				
_____				
2. At the dinner table	____	____	____	____
Explain_____				
_____				
3. On the telephone	____	____	____	____
Explain_____				
_____				
4. At home	____	____	____	____
Explain_____				
_____				
5. With males	____	____	____	____
Explain_____				
_____				
6. With females	____	____	____	____
Explain_____				
_____				

Figure 19–4. The WSU Communication Appraisal and Priorities Profile (CAPP).

discussed. The discussion centers on the fact that there are, indeed, many poor speakers in this world. A demonstration of some of the habits that interfere with efficient communication is appropriate. Patients generally immediately recognize poor speaking habits.

Even though there are many poor speakers, persons with impaired hearing must develop ways to cope in those communication environments. The encouraging acknowledgment that they can, in many instances, manipulate such difficult situations to function more efficiently in them, and that they will be working on those situations, ends the discussion on a positive note.

These items generally do not consume more than 1 or 2 full-hour sessions. The discussions of priority difficulties and circumstances that interfere with efficient communication should not be curtailed, however, because the airing of frustrations and concerns will greatly facilitate future progress. For many, this may be the first time those concerns have been discussed. To prematurely conclude such a discussion simply on the basis of a rigid schedule can stifle the airing of emotions and adjustment that may otherwise not be made.

On Becoming Assertive. Weekly assignments for each patient are made and include noting a communication situation in which they had particular difficulty that, in the end, interfered with communication. As discussed earlier, they write about situations and diagram the physical environment if necessary (or simply recall it as accurately as possible). In any event, patients are to bring the specifics of the situation to the next treatment session for presentation and discussion. Each patient (or in the case of individual treatment, the patient) presents his difficult situation, if one has been noted. It is imperative that the patient who was involved in the situation be the one who presents it and not the significant other who may accompany the patient.

After a thorough presentation, with diagrams if desired, the situation is discussed by the group (or in the event of individual treatment, by the patient, the audiologist,

and the accompanying significant other, if he was involved). Suggestions regarding possible ways the patient might have manipulated the communication environment to his best advantage, including the physical environment or the speaker, are made by the group under the guidance of the audiologist and are accepted as viable or discarded.

As stated by this author previously (Hull, 2007), insights into ways of manipulating the communication environment to the best advantage, along with methods of coping with and adjusting to frustrating situations, are in turn developed among patients under the guidance of the audiologist. This form of self- and group analysis is an extremely important part of the aural rehabilitation program. Patients, then, are helped to develop their own insights into methods of adjusting to situations where communication is difficult. If, for some reason, they find that it is impossible for them to make the necessary adjustments, perhaps they can, in a positive, supportive, and assertive manner, ease their difficulty by requesting that others make certain adjustments. Perhaps they could request that the physical environment be adjusted so that they can function more efficiently in it or they can make adjustments on their own.

It becomes difficult for some older patients to develop even mildly assertive behaviors. They do not want to be noticed as a demanding older person. Many do feel rather vulnerable, perhaps feeling that the people who invited them to a party did so more out of obligation than desire. They may feel that if they request those seeking conversation change positions by moving to a quieter place to talk, or request that someone change the position of his chair to be in a better position to talk then, perhaps, the hosts will feel that it is more trouble than it is worth to invite them again. In light of such fears, it becomes quite logical to avoid that possibility by simply remaining quiet and being fearful that if asked a question, he might be embarrassed by answering inappropriately. Those fears are occasionally brought forth by patients and should be discussed as they arise.

Examples of those discussions include one that was initiated by one of this author's patients who was being seen on a group basis. The woman in question was discussing a situation involving another woman with whom she had morning coffee on almost a daily basis for a number of years. The patient's complaint was that her friend was an incessant gum chewer, and as she chewed as she talked, it interfered with precise articulation and two-way conversation. Her friend interpreted the patient's inability to understand what she was saying to be the result of the hearing impairment, not her imprecise manner of speaking from her enthusiastic gum chewing, compounded by the patient's hearing loss. This apparent interpretation of the situation infuriated my patient. But she continued the morning coffee time, because there were few other women her age in that geographic area and, besides, they had been friends since childhood.

This woman's major concern was how to tell her friend that her manner of speaking and gum chewing had, for several years, interfered with her ability to understand what she was saying and, in the end, made what might have been a pleasant conversation a difficult one. She was particularly afraid to say anything because of the embarrassment her friend might feel because the situation had been going on for so long and nothing had previously been said. "Almost like," as the patient said, "being associated with a person for a long time and never knowing her name. As time passes, you become increasingly embarrassed about asking her name, particularly when she knows yours." The suggestions that came from the group varied from an enthusiastic, "Tell her

that if she wants to talk to you, to take her gum out of her mouth!" to a timid, "If you value your friendship, maybe it is best to say nothing and simply tolerate the situation." The latter suggestion was discarded. The ultimate conclusion was to simply tell the truth.

It was the consensus of the group that they would respect their own friend more if he would say something like, "You know, we've been friends for a long time. You realize, as I do, that I have some difficulty hearing what people say to me. I have particular difficulty with men who wear mustaches or beards, people who do not move their lips enough, or people who talk with their hand near their mouth, as I depend upon seeing the face of persons with whom I am talking. You know, I have difficulty understanding what you say sometimes and I think that I may have discovered why. I know that you like to chew gum a great deal and, like me, it helps my mouth not to become so dry. I do think, however, that because you—probably not realizing it—chew your gum while we are talking, it doesn't allow me to see your lips move properly and, besides, you aren't able to talk as plainly when you chew it so hard. I just bet that if you don't chew gum while we are having our coffee, I will be able to understand you better and we'll have a nicer time talking. Do you want to give it a try?" Positive assertiveness are the two key words in this instance. For that patient, the strategy she and the remainder of the group determined as most effective did prove to be successful. She maintained the friendship.

Other Topics to Facilitate Communication. Other topics for discussion and for the development of communicative strategies may include (a) weekly socials at private homes where the furniture arrangements interfere with efficient communication. Some, as experienced through this author's work with older patients, involve (b) the table arrangement at one patient's son's home where they usually had Thanksgiving dinner, (c) the television set at a male patient's friend's home, (d) the seating arrangement and acoustics at a church meeting room, and others. Even though the discussions and thought-provoking suggestions generally aid the individual whose situation is being discussed, they also provide insights for the remainder of the group on how they, too, may be able to manipulate similar communicative environments.

These assertiveness sessions can be extremely stimulating for the patients involved and for their significant others in attendance. Patients have told this author that those sessions are probably the most valuable for them, particularly because we are working and sharing about their problems in communication. As patients identify with other patients' difficult communication situations and relate to solutions as they see them, insights into solutions for their own difficult situations emerge and are strengthened.

Self-confidence reawakens when patients return to state that the solution contrived during the last session did not work as planned, but with a few adjustments developed by him, it did. Most older patients, no matter the level of hearing impairment or how distraught they may be as a result of their inability to communicate, can benefit from these assertiveness sessions. The topics of self-worth and "I'm important too" that become a part of the discussions are an extremely important part of the total aural rehabilitation program.

Use of Residual Hearing with Supplemental Visual Clues

Even though the use of visual clues and every possible bit of residual hearing individual patients can muster is discussed and practiced throughout all aspects of the aural rehabilitation program, sessions should also emphasize those aspects of communication. Again, it is suggested that strict approaches to speechreading and auditory training not be emphasized. Rather, the fact that the majority of older patients possess normal to near-normal language function should be capitalized on to encourage the use of innovative and useful approaches toward increased efficiency in the use of a very natural complement to communication, that is, the complement of vision to audition.

The premise on which these sessions are based is that speech (including the phonemic patterns of words in the English language, the use of gestures, inflectional clues, and the English language itself) is generally quite predictable, although, understandably, there are differences among individual's speech patterns, use of gestures, words, and so on. A further premise is that the average listener has been taking advantage of the redundancies inherent in American English speech and language patterns to aid in verbal comprehension for the majority of his life. When hearing declines with age, along with the precision and speed of the processing of phonemic verbal and linguistic elements of speech, it becomes more difficult to comprehend what others are saying. This is particularly true in environmentally distracting or otherwise difficult listening situations.

The purpose of these sessions, therefore, is to remind patients of what they have been doing for years at an almost subliminal level—that is, using important parts of auditory/verbal messages, when heard, and supplementing what was not heard with visual clues. By visual clues, this author means the face of the speaker, including lip, tongue, and mandibular movements, gestures, facial expression, shoulder movements, and so on used to "fill in the gaps" between what was heard, what was not heard, and what was observed visually.

A further purpose of these sessions is to discuss the redundancies of the phonemic and linguistic aspects of spoken American English and to encourage patients to take advantage of them when they are communicating with others. This aspect of the aural rehabilitation treatment program is called, for lack of a better descriptive title, "A Linguistic Approach to the Teaching of Speechreading" described by this author over 30 years ago (Hull, 1976). It essentially depends on patients possessing normal language function. Further, a great deal of time is spent using the chalkboard. If, however, a patient has visual impairment, these sessions help to enhance auditory closure. The term *closure* is the byword during these sessions, as the reader soon will realize.

Linguistic Closure

As the reader will observe in this section, patients are asked to determine the correct information within sentences from the least number of words provided. Patients are asked to imagine that the word or words written on the chalkboard are those that were heard. Blanks are placed between words, representing those not heard or not heard well. Patients are, first of all, asked to tell the audiologist what the sentence is about (out of context), when perhaps only one word is provided out of a total of seven, with six blanks indicating those words that were not heard.

Patients are encouraged to venture guesses as to what the sentence might be. Let us say, for example, that the word presented is *street*, located as the last word in the sentence. The patients are asked to let their minds wander: "Take a guess." As patients accept that encouragement and begin to guess, the fear of being wrong appears to decrease. Many are genuinely surprised, in fact, to find that their "educated" guesses are often extremely close, if not correct. Guesses in this instance may, for example, range from "The man was walking down the street," to "The stoplight fell into the street." They are, however, encouraged to be rational in their decisions. The question may appropriately be asked, "How many times have you heard someone say, 'The stoplight fell into the street?' Probably not frequently. The word 'street' as the last word in a sentence tells you what? It tells you, generally, that something is happening. If the word came as the second word in a sentence, maybe after the word 'the,' I may have been describing the street, such as, 'The street was very bumpy.' But, because it is located at the end of the sentence, we know that something is probably happening either on or to the street.

"Now, let's set the stage for an example of this activity. Let us say that your neighbor's child, Billy, has run away. You and other people from around the neighborhood are searching for him. Suddenly, someone runs to you and says something about, "_____ _____ _____ _____ _____ _____ street!" You observed that the speaker had obviously been running, and was pointing up the street as he was talking. Now, what do you imagine the speaker was telling you?" Because the audiologist has now set the stage for the patients, their guesses will probably be quite close to what he had intended.

The audiologist's next step is to say, "Now I am going to allow you to fill in the gaps by observing my face and gestures as I take the place of the excited neighbor who is talking to you. I will be using the chalkboard (or flip chart) as you fill in the gaps." The audiologist then presents the sentence in a slightly audible manner and with full visible face and gestures. If patients are not able to "make closure," then another word is added to the blanks on the chalkboard, and the patients are allowed to try again. An example of the sequence of presentation, if additional words are required, is presented below.

1. ____ ____ ____ ____ ____ ____
   street!
2. I ____ ____ ____ ____ ____ street!
3. I ____ ____ ____ ____ our street!
4. I saw ____ ____ ____ our street!
5. I saw ____ ____ down our street!
6. I saw ____ running down our street!
7. I saw Billy running down our street!

As patients become aware of what the message contains, the audiologist continues by discussing (a) the importance of the position of each word within the sentence that was required before they were able to determine its content, (b) their linguistic value in terms of the probability of situations in the meaning of the sentence, (c) the importance of the environmental clues that were available to them, and (d) the supplemental use of visual clues.

An important element involved in any of these sessions is the audiologist's enthusiasm for the fact that, perhaps, the patients needed only to "hear" one or two words out of the sentence to make closure and grasp the meaning of the sentence. It is encouraging for older patients to understand that, with their knowledge of the English language and their successful use of visual and auditory clues, they were able to determine what a message was.

On more difficult sentences and more complex contrived situations, patients may require more heard words to be provided via the chalkboard. Nevertheless, they are being reminded that with a relatively small amount of visual, auditory, and environmental information, they are generally able to determine at least the thought of what is being said.

Linguistic, Content, and Environmental Redundancies

Formal usage of American English is redundant in the position of various parts of speech. In other words, the positions of principal words, such as nouns, pronouns, and direct objects, are generally constant, as are function words, descriptors such as adjectives and adverbs, and action words such as verbs. Some dialects within the United States do, however, deviate from those standard rules. During these sessions, although the technical names of the parts of speech are not stressed, the importance of those words that fall within various positions in verbal messages are discussed as they relate to deriving the meaning of those messages.

This aspect of treatment capitalizes on the fact that most older patients who have hearing impairment will possess at least near-normal language function. It stresses that as people listen to others, they zero in on words within conversations that permit them to at least derive the thought of what is being said, so that the conversation can be followed. In some distracting environments, less of the message may actually be heard, but most persons can still maintain the content or intent of what is being said. It is normal in those circumstances to ask a speaker to repeat a word, if one was missed, because it appeared to be an important one regarding the content of the statement.

The point that is stressed to the patients is that the reason a listener was able to determine that the word was an important one in following the conversation is that most listeners have an almost innate knowledge of the structure of the American English language that has progressively expanded since early childhood. This provides the listener with a distinct advantage even in light of a loss of hearing.

The treatment sessions that stress this important aspect of efficient listening revolve around bringing that functional language capability to a more conscious level. Occasionally, patients have become so despondent over an inability to communicate with others that such otherwise natural compensatory skills have become repressed.

Content and Environmental Redundancies

These discussions stress that, as we observe human behavior, it is discovered that not only do the same people generally say similar things on similar occasions, but they also say them in similar places. In other words, in a given environment, depending on who the person is with whom one will be speaking, what the listener knows about him, and if the listener is aware of those influences, the general content of some conversations can be predicted with reasonable accuracy.

Patients are asked to describe the environments they frequent. In all probability they will be those that were set as priorities earlier. They are also asked to describe those persons who are generally there, including their speaking habits, their facial characteristics, and their known interests. During these treatment sessions, the patients also are asked to write down the most frequent topics of conversations that are observed among those whom they have described. These not only include frequent topics, but also words and phrases that those people may use habitually. They are asked to keep those lists and add to them as they remember additional items or as they find out more about the person after speaking with him. Patients also are asked to begin new lists as they meet new people. The more one knows and remembers about a person, the more communication is enhanced.

An awareness of the predictability, or redundancy, of people and what they will say within known environments is sometimes surprising to older adults who have hearing impairment. If it is surprising, it is generally because they had not really thought about it prior to that time. If nurtured, however, this awareness can facilitate increased efficiency in communication.

Reducing Auditory or Visual Confusions

Other activities that, by necessity, are important for adults may include sharing information on why certain confusions of words occur in conversations. This particularly concerns older adults, because word confusions may occur with some frequency. These discussions not only mention the fact that the nature of the majority of auditory disorders that older adults face enhances the probability of auditory confusions, but also that the nature of certain sound and visual elements within many words enhances the probability of confusions because they either sound like or look like other words. When words are confused with others, the meaning of a sentence or conversation may appear to be different than what was intended. Words used as examples of homophenous (visually similar) and potentially confusing words include, for example:

1. found-vowed
2. purred-bird
3. head-hen
4. vine-fried
5. geese-keys
6. neck-deck

An example of an activity that can bring about an awareness of how these confusions can occur is based on typed lists of sentences or sentences written on the chalkboard. It is generally best to use those sentences that contain visually or auditorily confusing words within mock conversations to exemplify most accurately the patients' real-world difficulties. In this instance, the first sentence on the patients' list may be presented by the audiologist within a short "conversation." The conversation is presented with voice, but as close to the patients' auditory thresholds as possible. Full-face observations and gestures are used.

When the sentence within the conversation is presented, the patients are asked to determine if the sentence the audiologist said was the same as or different from the one on their list. If they determine that there was, indeed, a word that was different than observed in the sentence on their list, then they are asked to explain why they felt that there were differences. On the other hand, if they felt that the sentence presented by the audiologist was the same as the one on their sheet or on the chalkboard, they also are asked to explain why.

If in the context of the short conversation the patients determine what word or words in that sentence "threw them off course," they are asked not only to analyze those confusing words, but attempt to determine why they were confusing. They also are asked, in light of what they derived from the remainder of the conversation, to determine the words (or the thought) that the sentence should have contained so that it makes sense. When that analysis is completed, the patients again are asked to listen to and observe the conversation and the possibly confusing sentence to determine if it then appears to be what they thought it should have been within the context of the intended message. If the word or words within the sentence still do not appear to be what they should have

been to complete the thought of the conversation, then they again are asked to attempt to determine what the confusion was.

An example of the type of brief conversation and stimulus sentence used in this exercise is:

1. Stimulus sentence: "She bought a new coat."
2. Stimulus conversation: "Alice came over yesterday to see me, and had some news to share. She said that she now has a new friend who is soft, black and white, and weighs about 1 pound. Well, she bought a new coat. She named him Mike."

In this stimulus conversation, the possible visual confusion occurs with the word *coat*, which was given to the patients within the stimulus sentence they were expecting from their list of sentences. Again, if patients in this instance determine that the word in the sentence they were expecting did not make sense within the context of the conversation, they are asked to explain why that word seemed to be misplaced, and what the word should have been. Further, the visual and auditory similarities and differences between the word they were expecting and the one they saw and heard are discussed.

These exercises should progress toward truly homophenous (visually similar) and homophonous (acoustically similar) words within sentences. The "mental gymnastics" required during these sessions allows for practice in making on-the-spot decisions regarding misunderstood messages by determining why a sentence within a conversation was visually or auditorily confusing, or otherwise did not make sense. The process generally involves:

1. Analyzing the information derived from the previous portions of a conversation;

2. Determining that a confusing word has been received that may change the content of what is being said;

3. Sifting mentally through other words that look or sound like one that would make more sense in light of the previous portions of the conversations;

4. Simultaneously projecting what that word should have been from the ongoing conversation.

Communicating under Adverse Conditions

One of the most frequent communication problems that older adult patients view as their most difficult is communication in noisy environments, including social events and meetings. Many patients' primary complaint, after finding themselves in an adverse listening environment, is that the noise and the resulting difficulties they experience in attempting to sort out the primary message from the chatter of other voices makes them tense and nervous. They describe the nervousness as perhaps the greatest detriment to their ability to manage a conversation successfully in those environments. They tell this author that as they begin to experience difficulty within a noisy communicative environment, they begin to feel nervous. The nervousness, as they describe it, results in a further deterioration of their ability to cope in that environment and, thus, their ability to sort the primary message from the noise.

For many, the only alternative that appears to be available is to excuse themselves from the situation by ceasing the conversation. By submitting to that less-than-satisfactory option, however, they generally feel some embarrassment. Unless they are quite resilient, many will simply avoid those situations in which they consistently fail.

Because situations include social events, meetings, the theater, church, and other desirable environments, the decision to avoid them can be self-defeating. The torment of those with hearing impairment may continue, as they still want to function communicatively in those environments and are torn between making another attempt at coping and giving up altogether.

In an attempt to ease such communication problems, treatment sessions need not only be designed to aid patients in the development of skills for communicating in those distracting environments, but also to develop coping strategies. The terms *desensitization*, *reciprocal inhibition*, and others may be appropriate to use here, but *coping behaviors* stands as the most meaningful for this discussion.

Within this framework, patients again choose as priorities those environments in which they have most difficulty or those within which they most desire to function with greater efficiently. Those situations are recreated within the treatment room as accurately as possible, based on individual patients' description of their chosen difficult environments. It is stressed that in the treatment environment, no one can fail but can feel free to discuss his concerns or frustrations as they arise. Use of the language-based speechreading instruction previously discussed is further emphasized during these sessions. The areas stressed in the discussions during these noise exercises are outlined in Table 19–1, but not in order of importance.

These sessions are used as the culminating treatment experience. Patients are asked to take everything that they have gained from the previous sessions and put it to use here. Some may never learn to cope in environmentally distracting situations. Others develop such self-confidence that they feel more comfortable in the most adverse environments.

TABLE 19–1. Topics for Discussion Stressed during Treatment Sessions

- Relaxation under stressful conditions.

- Confidence that clients can piece together the thought of the verbal message, even though not all of it was heard.

- Remembering that, because of their normal language function and their knowledge of the predictability of American English, they can determine what is being said if supplemental visual cues are used along with as much auditory information as is possible under the environmental circumstance.

- Knowledge that other people in the same environment may also be having difficulty understanding what others are saying and that they also may or may not be coping successfully with the stress.

- Freedom to manipulate the communication environment as much as possible by, for example, asking the person with whom they are speaking to move with them to a slightly quieter corner where they can talk with greater ease or move his chair to a more advantageous position so the speaker can be seen and heard more clearly, or other positive steps to enhance communication.

- Remembering that if difficulty in a communication environment seems to be increasing, and feelings of concern or nervousness begin to become evident, they should feel free to interrupt the conversation and talk about the noise or the activity around them that seems to be causing the difficulties. The other person will probably agree with that observation and, in talking about it, feelings of stress may be reduced and communication may be enhanced.

- Remembering that the amount of recorded noise used in treatment sessions is probably greater than will be found in other environmentally stressful situations. If success was noted in their treatment sessions, then similar success may be carried over into other stressful listening environments.

One aspect of coping is stressed. That is that few persons, whether they possess normally functioning auditory mechanisms or have hearing impairment, can tolerate every noise environment. They must learn to recognize their limits in attempting to develop coping behaviors.

Introducing Noise into the Treatment Environment

As each patient's difficult communication environment is recreated by the audiologist and other members of the treatment group, taped noise that is the same as or similar to the environment the patient(s) described is introduced into the room. It is best to use a tape or CD with multiple speakers system to recreate the noise environment most accurately. The noise is introduced gradually at the beginning of these sessions and increased as tolerance and coping behavior likewise increase, until the noise is presented at such a level as to become difficult to tolerate. If patients wear hearing aids, they also are asked to experiment with them as they participate in the mock noisy communication environments.

The patients are told that the situation during treatment is going to be made more difficult in regard to noise levels and/or visual distractions than they will probably experience in the real world. Patients inevitably desire such an approach, as they would rather practice in such difficult situations in the friendly environment of the treatment room than among less tolerant people.

Discussions of Adverse Listening Environments

Discussions of noise itself and its natural effect on speech perception are introduced before the actual recreations begin. An awareness of different types of noise, the general acoustical characteristics, emotional impact, and other factors give patients a better understanding of the situation as they see it. When one begins to gain an understanding of feared elements, the fear generally subsides.

Almost without fail, some persons begin to become nervous and frustrated during the noise sessions. The susceptibility of certain patients to intolerance for noise can be observed by an alert audiologist, even when low levels of noise are introduced.

If the group (or individuals) begins to become obviously frustrated, the audiologist, rather than ceasing the activity immediately, terminates it momentarily at a logical point and begins to discuss general feelings about the noise rather than attempting to pinpoint individual personal feelings about it. The audiologist might appropriately say, "Noise makes me feel nervous. How about you? Sometimes during these sessions I want to turn it off. When I'm in a situation where I can't turn it off, it even makes me upset sometimes. Is that a little like the feelings you have when you find yourself in a situation like that?" Generally, the response will be affirmative and patients will agree that those feelings are real for them, also.

The time-out periods are used to talk about feelings about noise. When feelings

of frustration and even anger are expressed freely among patients, the reality that those feelings are not uncommon among others occasionally brings relief to those who perhaps thought that they were among only a few who had such difficult time. These persons are thus learning to cope with their feelings and realize that they are normal reactions to adverse and frustrating communication environments.

Discussing those feelings freely, without fear of negative responses from others, is an important part of the aural rehabilitation process. As frustrations and anger are expressed regarding their difficulties tolerating and communicating in a noisy world —and occasionally at the whole process of growing older—the way opens for the aural rehabilitation program to move forward toward the development of coping behaviors and techniques for manipulating their own communication environments as positive, assertive attributes. As one of this author's patients so aptly stated, "In a noisy world of generally poor speakers, we usually have to fend for ourselves. But we are looking to you to teach us how, and to give inspiration to use what we learn."

Other Approaches to Aural Rehabilitation Treatment

Other components of effective aural rehabilitation sessions as utilized by this author (Hull, 2001) involve the following elements.

The Use of Time-Compressed Speech

In light of the probability of a slowing of the speed of central nervous system processing of auditory-linguistic information with advancing age (Humes, 2008; Madden, 1985; Marshall, 1981; Schmitt & McCroskey, 1981;

Stach, 1990; Welsh, Welsh, & Healy, 1985; and others), the use of time compression of speech has been found by this author to be a method through which patients can learn to compensate to some degree for that decline. Some older patients can increase their ability to comprehend speech with speed and precision that is greater than they had before the training.

Patients practice by listening to progressively time-compressed sentences and paragraphs, attempting over an 8- to 10-week sequence of sessions to increase the speed with which they are able to synthesize and make auditory-linguistic closure. Some patients have increased their accuracy of speech comprehension for sentences and paragraphs up to 40% at time-compression levels of 35% (65% of the message received over time). These same older patients have been found to correspondingly increase their accuracy of auditory-only speech recognition by as much as 24% (Hull, 1988).

This is a very exciting and tangible method for enhancing the speed and accuracy of speech comprehension among individual patients who can tolerate the demands of the process. Usable aided or unaided hearing is a prerequisite, however, because this is an auditory-only task.

Interactive Laser Video Training in Speed and Accuracy of Visual Synthesis and Closure

Interactive laser video technology recently has evolved for use in training Olympic athletes, Air Force fighter pilots, and air traffic controllers to increase their speed and accuracy in making visual closure, visual tracking, and visual synthesis. This technology also has been found by this author to be an effective and motivational way of training adults who have hearing impairment to increase their visual compensatory skills, particularly as it relates to speed, accuracy, and visual vigilance (Hull, 1989).

Environmental Design

Hull (1989, 2001) has described avenues for educating older patients who have hearing impairment regarding techniques and strategies of environmental design. This involves modifying the acoustical or environmental design of their homes, offices, and other communicative environments to their listening and communicative advantage. Training also involves how to make modifications in those and other situations in which they find themselves, including social environments, meetings, and business environments that otherwise may have placed them at a communicative disadvantage. These can be very powerful aural rehabilitation sessions that provide patients with tangible methods for modifying their most difficult communication situations.

Summary

It is important for older patients to be given the opportunity to make decisions regarding areas of communication in which they desire to improve. Even though many may feel discouraged because of the embarrassing difficulties they experience in their attempts at understanding what others are saying, they have communicative priorities that must be addressed through their aural rehabilitation programs.

As adults who probably possessed normal hearing during the majority of their life and whose case histories may reveal nothing more than that they have become older, they deserve to participate in the decisions regarding their treatment program. However, guidance must be provided by the audiologist.

References

Alpiner, J. G. (1963). Audiological problems of the aged. *Geriatrics, 18*, 19–26.

Alpiner, J., & McCarthy, P. (Eds.). (1987). *Rehabilitative audiology: Children and adults* (Vol. 3.). Baltimore: Williams & Wilkins.

Bergman, M. (1980). *Aging and the perception of speech*. Baltimore: University Park Press.

Colton, J. (1977). Student participation in aural rehabilitation programs. *Journal of the Academy of Rehabilitative Audiology, 10*, 31–35.

Colton, J., & O'Neill, J. (1976). A cooperative outreach program for the elderly. *Journal of the Academy of Rehabilitative Audiology, 9*, 38–41.

Downs, M. (1970). *You and your hearing aid.* [Unpublished manual.] University of Colorado Medical Center, Department of Otolaryngology, Division of Audiology, Denver.

Giolas, T. G. (1994). Aural rehabilitation of adults with hearing impairment. In J. Katz (Ed.), *Handbook of clinical audiology* (pp. 776–792). Baltimore: Williams and Wilkins.

Hardick, E. J. (1977). Aural rehabilitation programs for the aged can be successful. *Journal of the Academy of Rehabilitative Audiology, 10*, 51–66.

Hull, R. H. (1976). A linguistic approach to the teaching of speechreading: Theoretical and practical concepts. *Journal of the Academy of Rehabilitative Audiology, 9*, 14–19.

Hull, R. H. (1980). Aural rehabilitation for the elderly. In R. L. Schow & M. A. Nerbonne (Eds.), *Introduction to aural rehabilitation* (pp. 311–348). Baltimore: University Park Press.

Hull, R. H. (1982). *Rehabilitative audiology.* New York: Grune & Stratton.

Hull, R. H. (March, 1988). *Hearing in aging.* Paper presented at the National Invitational Conference on Geriatric Rehabilitation. Department of Health and Human Services, PHS, Washington, DC.

Hull, R. H. (1989, November). *The use of interactive laser/video technology for training in visual synthesis and closure with hearing impaired elderly clients.* Paper presented at the Annual Convention of the American Speech-Language-Hearing Association, St. Louis, MO.

Hull, R. H. (1992). Techniques for aural rehabilitation with elderly clients. In R. H. Hull (Ed.), *Aural rehabilitation* (pp. 278–292). San Diego, CA: Singular.

Hull, R. H. (1997). Techniques for aural rehabilitation treatment for older adults who are hearing impaired. In R. Hull (Ed.), *Aural rehabilitation: Serving children and adults* (pp. 367–393). San Diego, CA: Singular.

Hull, R. H. (2001). Aural rehabilitation for older adults with impaired hearing. In R. Hull (Ed.), *Aural rehabilitation* (pp. 393–424). San Diego, CA: Singular/Thomson Learning.

Hull, R. H. (November, 2006). *Addressing central auditory processing in aural rehabilitation for older adults.* Paper presented at the Annual Convention of the American Speech-Language-Hearing Association, Miami, FL.

Hull, R. H. (2007). Fifteen principles of consumer-oriented audiologic/aural rehabilitation. *ASHA Leader, 12*, 6–7.

Humes, L. E. (2008). Aging and speech communication. *ASHA Leader, 4*, 10–13.

Jerger, J., & Chmiel, R. (1997). Factor analytic structure of auditory impairment in elderly persons. *Journal of the American Academy of Audiology, 7*, 269–276.

Kasten, R. N. (1981). The impact of aging on auditory perception. In R. H. Hull (Ed.), *The communicatively disordered elderly* (pp. 33–51). New York: Thieme-Stratton.

Madden, D. (1985). Age-related slowing in the retrieval of information from long-term memory. *Journal of Gerontology, 40*, 208–210.

Marshall, L. (1981). Auditory processing in aging listeners. *Journal of Speech and Hearing Disorders, 46*, 226–240.

McCarthy, P. A., & Alpiner, J. G. (1978). The remediation process. In J. G. Alpiner (Ed.), *Handbook of adult rehabilitative audiology* (pp. 88–111). Baltimore: Williams and Wilkins.

McCroskey, R. L., & Kasten, R. N. (1981). Assessment of central auditory processing. In R. Rupp & K. Stockdell (Eds.), *Speech protocols in audiology* (pp. 121-132). New York: Grune & Stratton.

McLauchlin, R. (1992). Hearing aid orientation for hearing impaired adults. In R. H. Hull (Ed.), *Aural rehabilitation* (pp. 178-201). San Diego, CA: Singular.

Miller, M., & Ort, R. (1965). Hearing problems in a home for the aged. *Acta Oto-Laryngologica, 59,* 33-44.

Miller, W. E. (1976, November). *An investigation of the effectiveness of aural rehabilitation for nursing home residents.* Paper presented at the Annual Convention of the American Speech and Hearing Association, Houston, TX.

O'Neill, J. J., & Oyer, H. J. (1981). *Visual communication for the hard of hearing.* Englewood Cliffs, NJ: Prentice-Hall.

Sanders, D. A. (1982). *Aural rehabilitation.* Englewood Cliffs, NJ: Prentice-Hall.

Sanders, D. A. (1993). *Management of hearing handicap.* Englewood Cliffs, NJ: Prentice-Hall.

Schmitt, J. F., & McCroskey, R. L. (1981). Sentence comprehension in elderly listeners: The factor rate. *Journal of Gerontology, 36,* 441-445.

Smith, C. R., & Fay, T. H. (1977). A program of auditory rehabilitation for aged persons in a chronic disease hospital. *Journal of the American Speech and Hearing Association, 19,* 417-420.

Stach, B. A. (1990). Central auditory processing disorders and amplification applications. Research symposium: Communication sciences and disorders and aging. *ASHA Reports, 19,* 150-156.

Traynor, R., & Peterson, K. (1972). *Adjusting to your new hearing aid.* [Unpublished manual]. Greeley, CO: University of Northern Colorado.

Welsh, J., Welsh, L., & Healy, M. (1985). Central presbycusis. *Laryngoscope, 95,* 128-136.

End of Chapter Examination Questions

Chapter 19

1. The author describes two circumstances in which individual treatment sessions would be appropriate for adult patients. What are they?
   a.
   b.

2. Some older adults begin to exhibit passive behaviors in communication situations in which one would expect them to "take charge" of the environment or person causing the problem. Why may passivity begin to take the place of positive assertiveness among older persons who are hearing impaired?

3. Describe the role of a significant other in the aural rehabilitation process.

4. List and describe the six components of aural rehabilitation services for adult patients as described in this chapter.
   a.
   b.
   c.
   d.
   e.
   f.

5. Briefly explain the process that seeks to help a patient be less passive and more assertive in making positive change in difficult listening environments.

6. The author describes reasons why some approaches to aural rehabilitation work and why others do not. Briefly describe those reasons.

7. To improve a patient's communicative environment, the audiologist might suggest:
   a. that the patient move closer to the speaker.
   b. that the patient move away from a window that may be casting shadows on the speaker's face.
   c. that the patient move to a quieter place, where communication can take place.
   d. all of the above.

8. **Individualizing an aural rehabilitation treatment program for a patient involves:**
   a. focusing on the family's concerns.
   b. group therapy.
   c. a long-term aural rehabilitation program.
   d. focusing first on the patient's communication concerns and priorities.

9. **"Counseling" involves:**
   a. listening.
   b. building the patient's confidence in himself.
   c. all members of the family.
   d. giving the patient current information about hearing loss and hearing aids.
   e. all of the above.

10. **What is the complement of vision to audition?**

End of Chapter Answer Sheet

Name _____ Date _____

Chapter 19

1. a. _____

    b. _____

2. _____

_____

_____

3. _____

_____

_____

4. a. _____

    b. _____

    c. _____

    d. _____

    e. _____

    f. _____

5. _____

_____

_____

6. _____

_____

_____

7. Which one(s)?   a   b   c   d

8. Which one(s)?   a   b   c   d

9. Which one(s)?   a   b   c   d   e

10. _____

20

Special Considerations in Aural Rehabilitation for Older Adults in Health Care Facilities

RAYMOND H. HULL

Chapter Outline

Introduction

Approximately 6% of all persons beyond age 65 years reside in various levels of health care facilities (Ignatavicius & Bayne, 1995). Of the some 40 million persons over age 65 years, that percentage represents more than 2.4 million persons (Health Care Financing Administration, personal communication, May 24, 2004). Placement rates for the young-old persons aged 65 to 74 seem to have fallen recently, especially for older men, many of whom are remarrying. But among persons aged 75 to 84, rates have increased, particularly for women. Older women who are most likely to be placed in a health care facility are poor, widowed, living alone, and very old. In 1972, Atchley reported that over 14% of persons age 85 or over were institutionalized. Of those, most were placed in nursing homes or other personal care facilities. On the other hand, in 1987, Stone, Cafferata, and Sangl reported that 21% of persons age 85 years and beyond were recipients of specialized care either in nursing homes, by home health care agencies, or by family. In 1996, the Administration on Aging placed the number of persons over age 70 years who were residing in nursing homes at more than 2 million. Currently, as persons continue to live to greater ages, these numbers have reached over 2.5 million.

In 1996, more than 20% of older persons were limited in their activity because of chronic health conditions, that is, 14% for persons age 65 to 74 years, 26% for persons 75 to 84 years, and 48% for those beyond age 85 years (Administration on Aging, 2002). Further, about 92% of older persons wear glasses and approximately 50 to 60% have hearing impairment to a sufficient degree to interfere with their activities of daily living (Administration on Aging, 2002; Hull, 2001). According to Hull (2001), approximately 92% of persons residing in health care facilities possess hearing impairment of sufficient degree to interfere with their activities of daily living. In an earlier survey (Schow & Nerbonne, 1980), an incidence of hearing loss among health care facility residents was found to be 80%.

Although many of these persons will, for all practical purposes, remain confined for the remainder of their lives because of chronic illness and other physical or mental problems, many can benefit from aural rehabilitation services from an audiologist. They deserve the opportunity for enhanced communicative skills in spite of impaired hearing and to experience the heightened social and personal communication that may result.

Further, with effective in-service education for health care facility personnel on the topics of hearing impairment, the use of hearing aids, and communication with older adults who have hearing impairment, the daily lives of elderly persons (and the staff) within a health care facility can be enhanced. However, these services must be coordinated with educational programming for elderly persons and their families.

Types of Health Care Facilities

Before this discussion of services for confined older persons proceeds, a description of what is meant by *health care facility* is appropriate.

Health care facility is a currently accepted term denoting any facility that provides long- or short-term residential care for older adults who require medical or other health services other than that provided by hospitals. The facilities may provide intensive care services, including 24-hour-a-day nursing care for posthospitalized stroke patients or simply a place to live near nursing or other health care.

Outpatient Residential Facilities

These facilities may include apartment or condominium living for ambulatory older persons. The apartments, or condominiums in this instance, are a part of a health care facility, perhaps in a separate wing or simply on the same grounds. Health care is usually a button push away. Older persons who reside in an outpatient or residential facility may have been ill enough at some recent time to desire the proximity of those services. These facilities most nearly resemble what are generally called *retirement communities*. The only difference is they may be a part of a health care facility complex.

Short-Term Care Facilities

Many health care facilities have an intensive care or a skilled nursing wing or may be an intensive care or skilled nursing facility. These are generally considered short-term care facilities. A stroke patient, for example, when known to be recovering but still too ill to return to her own home because of the need for rather constant monitoring and nursing care, may be released from the hospital and taken to the short-term care facility. The stay may be only a few days or may last for several weeks. These facilities play an important role, not only for recuperative purposes, but also as an alterative to higher-cost extended hospital stays. For stroke patients and others who may require other services, rehabilitation personnel such as

occupational therapists, audiologists, speech-language pathologists, and others are generally available, at least on a contractual basis.

When placed in a short-term facility, it is expected that the patient will be released within a fairly short time. The most desirable destination is the patient's home. Unfortunately, however, for some older adults, the destination is to an intermediate or long-term care facility, for lack of other alternatives.

Intermediate and Long-Term Care Facilities

The most frequently observed facilities for older adults are most often called *nursing homes*. They are facilities where older adults reside who may require nursing or other health care. The primary reason for placement is generally a health or other debilitating problem. However, intermediate care facilities all too frequently become long-term in nature. For example, placement in these health care facilities may be because (a) there is no place else to live, (b) a spouse has passed away and the elderly survivor fears living alone, or (c) the most frustrating to older persons: the elderly person's family "feels that it is best." As one older woman told this author, "I thought my daughter was out looking for an apartment for me and I ended up here!"

These facilities offer a room (often with a roommate), balanced meals, some social and recreational activities, and a nursing staff. Larger health care facilities may have a social services director, an activity director, and rehabilitative services such as occupational therapy, speech-language therapy, and physical therapy. Some facilities are Medicare- and/or Medicaid-approved, but for those programs to provide payment for services and residence, a medically related problem must be the reason for placement in the facility. Further, some health care facilities do not want to be approved by either program because of the relatively low rate of reimbursement for care of the residents, particularly from Medicaid.

The Residents of Health Care Facilities

The older adults who are placed in skilled or intensive care wings of health care facilities or in skilled nursing care facilities are there because of specific health or mental reasons. They may have been transferred from a hospital to the skilled nursing facility because they are still too weak or unable to care for themselves at home, but well enough to be released from the hospital. It is anticipated that the facility and the 24-hour-per-day nursing care that is available will, in that respect, be the "halfway house" for the patient between hospitalization and home. In some instances, however, because of lack of sufficient recovery, older patients must be transferred to an extended care facility because they are not able to care for themselves sufficiently to live at home and, further, there may not be others at home to help the person. Therefore, the adult is placed in a longer term health care facility so that the necessary services for daily needs are available. In all too many instances, an elderly person views such placement as terminal. It is a fear that can interfere with the person's desire for rehabilitative services if those are needed. The audiologist and other health care professionals must be aware of this, as well as other responses and feelings that can interfere with patient desire for supportive services.

Reasons for Placement

What are the reasons for placement in extended care facilities? Because placement for any reason can result in a lessening of desire for self-maintenance or improvement, the audiologist should be aware of them. According to early discussions by Atchley (1972) and Gatz, Bengston, and Blum (1990), the major factor in placement of persons in health care facilities (nursing homes or other residences) appears to be their state of mental or physical health, their previous residential setting, or the family system. Older people in nursing and other health care facilities tend not to have a spouse or children who live nearby, although many have living children. Indications are that many older people would be able to avoid institutionalization if they had relatives to help care for them (Gatz et al., 1990) and if they had adequate finances. A breakdown in the support system appears to be the primary cause for placement in nursing homes or other forms of residential facilities. Others include loss of residence because of urban renewal projects, or perhaps a child who has urged them to sell a house (that according to the child is just too much for the elderly family member to care for).

The placement of an older adult in a health care facility does not generally occur suddenly. A series of events usually takes place prior to placement. Those events may include serious illness. They may include attempts at residence with relatives who, in the end, find the older person to be too much of an emotional or financial burden. For whatever reason, placement in a health care facility (nursing home) was felt to be a necessity and the factors leading to that decision frequently may affect the morale of the older person and her family.

The Impact of Placement

As the majority of older adults view residence in a nursing home as a last resort—in all probability terminal placement—its impact on an older person can have a number of negative implications, which the audiologist or other health professionals who may attempt to provide diagnostic and rehabilitative services must recognize. The negative effects include:

1. Depression
2. Loneliness
3. A growing lack of desire to receive rehabilitative services when they may be indicated
4. The shock and stress associated with the move from a residence where the person may have lived for many years
5. A lessening of self-image due to the routine of the nursing home
6. Gradual dependency on persons who, no matter how caring and helpful, are strangers
7. A lessening of awareness of occurrences in the outside world due to the isolating effect of the nursing home
8. Personality changes resulting from isolation and/or certain medications
9. A loss of independence
10. A loss of personal control, including who her roommate will be, time for sleeping and eating, and other aspects of life
11. The depressing influence of illness
12. The dehumanization of people that can occur in more institutionalized nursing homes
13. A lack of personal stimulation, which occurs from a loss of close interpersonal communication
14. A reduction of sensory capabilities that comes with age, including sense of smell, touch, sight, and hearing

These effects and many others not mentioned are difficult to overcome. Therefore, the elderly resident of a nursing home may not readily accept an audiologist's or any service provider's services.

Establishing Aural Rehabilitation Programs in Health Care Facilities

The large population of persons who have hearing impairment who reside in various levels of health care facilities was, for many years, either ignored or avoided because it was felt they possessed little rehabilitative potential. Others believed they were experiencing so many other problems that it was probably best to leave them alone. Further, many audiology services on behalf of elderly nursing home patients have been provided as parts of practicum experiences by graduate students in audiology training programs. In the greatest majority of instances, however, those students did not possess the insights into aging and aging persons to provide effective aural rehabilitation services. Rather, they may have begun with "lesson number one" in a book of speechreading lessons and proceeded to provide "speechreading instruction" that may have had little or no meaning for the patients involved. The majority of patients, then, had to be rounded up before each weekly session, and the gradually disillusioned graduate student clinician wondered why so many would not leave their room to come to "class." The student clinician may have felt that the book of speechreading lessons must contain something that would benefit the older patients or else it would not have been written. More importantly, the patients were told that the aural rehabilitation program may help them learn to communicate more efficiently with others in spite of their impaired hearing, only to realize later that it did not. It is no wonder, then, that audiologists graduating from training programs may have little desire to initiate audiology service programs in health care facilities. The fact is that many of those graduate students may not have had a positive practicum experience in that setting and found it to be less than stimulating.

Addressing the Needs of Health Care Facility Residents

It is important to remember that residents of health care facilities are individuals who have specific goals and needs. Among the 92% of health care facility residents who possess some degree of hearing impairment, the sense of need and urgency for interpersonal communication is as great as for other persons. After all, verbal communication is one of the traits that identify us as humans. The isolation that occurs as the result of impaired hearing can be even more devastating to persons who are already isolated because of their confinement in a nursing home. Their sense of urgency to break through the barriers to communication caused by an inability to hear and understand what others are saying or, at least, to watch television and understand what is being said may be much greater than evidenced by their statements or emotions. They also may have suppressed a desire to accept those services, as they may feel that perhaps nothing will help at their late stage of life.

In Chapter 19, suggested procedures for aural rehabilitation services for older adult patients were presented. If geared toward the specific priorities of the patient, those procedures will also benefit residents of health care facilities who have impaired

hearing. Before beginning rehabilitation, however, the patients must be encouraged to develop a desire to at least "give it a try." Within reason, depending upon their state of health and mental competence, improvements can be made if they also accept responsibility as adults to participate.

Above and beyond the service aspect is the important fact that the audiologist is working with adults, no matter what their age or temperament. They are adults who, without their desire or control, have become older. And with age, an increasing inability to efficiently hear and understand what others are saying has added to the isolation and depression they may be experiencing. If the audiologist offers the time, energy, and commitment to learn about the process of aging and listen to what her patients are saying about their needs, desires, and concerns, then viable aural rehabilitation treatment programs can be developed.

Developing Realistic Expectations

Another important aspect of this fascinating work must be acknowledged. That is, the audiologist must be realistic in her efforts and expectations when serving this population. No matter how much we would like to effectively serve all persons, there are some who, because of physical or mental problems, do not have the potential to benefit from aural rehabilitation services and others may benefit only marginally. On the other hand, the audiologist must refrain from providing services only on behalf of those who will benefit most to the exclusion of those who may benefit slightly. Even a terminally ill, bedridden person's last weeks or months may be brightened by a health care facility nursing staff who have learned from the audiologists' in-services how to communicate more efficiently with persons who have impaired hearing. This, in itself, can be a significant service. These are quality (not quantity) of life issues.

Determining the Need for Services

Establishing the Benefits

In most health care facilities, it can be assumed there are at least a number of persons who reside there who are hearing impaired and can benefit from some aspect of an assessment and aural rehabilitation program. The benefits of initiating an aural rehabilitation program should be presented to the director and her staff. The benefits stressed in that meeting include:

1. The fact that effective in-service education can enhance communication between health care facility personnel and residents who have hearing impairment and thus ease one reason for frayed nerves on both parts.
2. Recommendations for alterations in the furniture arrangement in a lounge area or other central gathering place that can enhance communication will be of great service to a health care facility. Otherwise, residents may avoid an important area where the greatest amount of activity and communication could take place.
3. Effective hearing aid orientation programs can provide the impetus for previously inefficient users of hearing aids to benefit from them in their daily activities.
4. An effective assessment program can identify persons who have hearing impairment who may have been thought to be uncommunicating or confused for other reasons.
5. A well-designed aural rehabilitation treatment program can provide enhanced

communicative skill for those who can benefit from that service, which can reduce stress both for caregivers and the patient. For others, the aural rehabilitation program may consist of discussions of their most difficult communication environments and suggestions for manipulation of the physical environment or those persons with whom they have difficulty communicating.

These programs, if geared toward patients' specific communication needs, can be extremely beneficial for confined elderly residents. It is also generally found that most persons in the health care facility environment can benefit from at least some aspect of these services either directly or indirectly.

Surveying for Hearing Impairment

The determination of the need for any of the services discussed previously must begin with a survey of the residents of the health care facility and, in specific terms, a presentation of the results of the survey to the health care facility administration. Those include the director, the head of nursing, the activity director, and the social services director. It is suggested that all residents who can respond to a hearing evaluation should be included in the survey.

A typical hearing screening at a fixed intensity level has generally not been found to be a satisfactory method for use in a health care facility, because such large numbers fail. An efficient procedure includes establishment of pure-tone thresholds and the use of immittance audiometry to confirm the type of loss. Even if a quiet environment for assessment can be found, the use of immittance audiometry is important because even low noise levels can interfere with bone-conduction testing.

For those who are found to have impaired hearing, assessment of speech recognition ability with and without visual clues provides relevant information for initial discussions with the health care facility staff about each individual patient's disability and the need for aural rehabilitation services. Speech recognition, in the absence of a sound-treated room and audiometer with speech capabilities, can be assessed with relative accuracy by live voice, with the audiologist seated approximately 4 to 6 feet from the patient. Monosyllabic words, CID Everyday Sentences, and a brief conversation with and without visual clues administered at a comfortable listening level for the patient can provide some important information about the person's speech recognition abilities. However, this should only be conducted by a skilled audiologist who can interpret the results of those rather informal testing procedures.

Presentation of Survey Results

Results of the survey are presented to the administration of the health care facility and, if that facility is a part of a corporate body, a representative of the corporation. If the administration is convinced that an aural rehabilitation program is desired, the program format is outlined.

The survey alone will provide important information for the health care facility staff. Residents who may have previously been described as confused or disoriented may be found to possess a severe enough hearing impairment to account for at least a portion of that behavior. Modifications in patterns of communication by health care facility staff alone may result in positive behavior change on the part of both the staff and those residents. Those modifications in communication strategies by the staff, for example, can result from an effective staff in-service program. An elderly man,

previously described as stubborn, inattentive, withdrawn, and antisocial, may begin to interact more with his environment when communication with staff is likewise improved. Others may demonstrate positive personality change as the result of properly fitted hearing aids, combined with modifications of speaking habits by health care facility staff as the result of an effective in-service program. Being able to hear one's TV by way of an assistive listening device so that the resident can once again enjoy her favorite shows can be a life-changing event.

With information on the incidence, severity, and communicative impact of hearing loss within a health care facility that will be available for discussion with the administration, a full assessment and aural rehabilitation program can be outlined and initiated. This includes a discussion of the possible positive impact of a viable aural rehabilitation program on the residents, on the health care facility staff, and on the other programs within the facility.

Patient Records

Records of progress for each patient must be maintained on an ongoing basis, along with records of physician, staff, family contact, and referrals. Records of social progress, continuing service, medical records, staff notification of audiometric test results, physician and family notification, and progress in the aural rehabilitation program are integral parts of the audiologist's record-keeping procedures. Such reports should be kept both in the patient's master file in the health care facility and as a part of the audiologist's file on each patient.

Patient Care Plan

A patient care plan is developed in cooperation with the audiologist, the speech-language pathologist, social services personnel, and other staff who have daily contact with the person, including the activities director. The plan contains the goals and objectives for each aural rehabilitation patient, along with methods and approaches and the problem or concern. An example of a patient care plan is found in Figure 20-1.

KENTON MANOR

AUDIOLOGY CARE PLAN

RESIDENT: ROOM LOCATION:

A. PROBLEM OR CONCERN:

B. GOALS OF CARE TEAM:

C. METHODS AND APPROACHES:

D. COMMENTS:

NAME:

TITLE:

DATE:

Figure 20–1. Example of patient care plan for aural rehabilitation programs in a health care facility.

Continuing Service Records

Continuing service records must be maintained on an ongoing basis. Each note, dated and signed, relates, for example, to progress in specific aural rehabilitation efforts, a contact made by the audiologist with that patient for hearing aid maintenance, statements regarding communicative progress, or a contact by a family member or the patient's physician.

Communication Progress Forms

Communication progress forms are also integral to the record-keeping efforts on behalf of the health care facility program. The patient's baseline of communicative behavior is noted on each form. Each form for each member of the evaluation team is placed in a patient's file. As each person notes specific changes in communicative behavior, they are noted on her own form for each patient. At weekly or monthly staff meetings, the ratings for each patient are compared, and a consensus as to progress or lack of it is noted in the patient's continuing service record.

Reimbursement for Services

In discussing the auditory assessment program, the aural rehabilitation program, and reimbursement issues with the health care facility administration, it should be emphasized that Medicare and, in some states, Medicaid cover auditory diagnostic evaluations, including special assessment procedures, in accordance with billing procedures and charges that are reasonable and typical in that geographic area. The testing must be justified on an individual basis. Routine testing may not be reimbursed. Audiologists who are certified, or are eligible for certification as audiologists by the American Speech-Language-Hearing Association, or licensed by states having licensure laws, are eligible to become Medicare approved providers of audiology services by award of a Medicare provider number. If the health care facility is Medicare approved, its own accounting office can bill for the service. In whatever manner, an agreement for the avenue of reimbursement for services should, in all instances, be arranged before the initial survey.

The Ongoing Aural Rehabilitation Program

In-Service Training for Health Care Facility Personnel and Families of the Residents

In-service training for health care facility administration, staff, and the residents' families not only supports an assessment and aural rehabilitation treatment program, but also provides carryover of the treatment aspects into the daily life of the residents. In-service provides administration, staff, and families with insights into (a) the cause and effects of presbycusis on residents' ability for communication, (b) the resulting psychosocial impact, (c) the structure of the aural rehabilitation program, (d) what hearing aids can and cannot do, (e) troubleshooting procedures for hearing aid malfunction, and (f) methods for more efficient communication with residents who have hearing impairment.

Included during staff and administration in-services are discussions of individual residents who are involved as patients in the program. Discussions include the hearing impairment those patients possess, the impact of the hearing impairment on their communicative function, their progress (or lack of it) as a result of the aural rehabilitation treatment program, and the development of plans for follow-through and carryover of those patients' programs into their daily lives in the health care facility. The health care facility staff, including the director of nurses, activity director, physical therapist, occupational therapist, and other personnel, including the cooks and custodians, can all be vital forces in the carryover process. This, importantly, includes the families of the residents.

Techniques offered through in-service for more efficient communication with older persons who have hearing impairment can enhance the lives of the staff, the residents' families, and the residents. It is generally found, to everyone's relief, that the emotional encounters resulting from futile attempts at communication between residents who have hearing impairment and staff members are sometimes soothed after utilization of the techniques for communication that the staff learned during in-service and that the elderly patients are learning during their treatment sessions.

Topics for in-service training should include:

1. The basic structure of the auditory mechanism and possible reasons as to the causes of presbycusis.
2. The manifestations of presbycusis and its potential impact on an elderly person's ability to function communicatively. This discussion includes presentations of audiometric configurations and examples of what the patient who possesses presbycusis might hear, compared with a normally hearing person.
3. Hearing aids and their uses and misuses, are discussed relative to what hearing aids are, what they sound like, what they can do, and what they cannot do. The reasons why some persons cannot benefit from hearing aids are also dis-

cussed, along with the necessity for a thorough hearing aid evaluation by a hearing professional.

4. Instruction on the use of hearing aids, placing the earmold properly in the ear, the switches (including the use of the gain control), the battery, the care of earmolds, and others are presented in turn to alleviate some of the difficulties some elderly residents have because of manual dexterity or memory problems. The staff of health care facilities can further aid the carryover of hearing aid orientation for recently fitted residents, if they are familiar with the component parts and their use.
5. Hearing aid troubleshooting procedures also are stressed and include:

   a. Knowledge of the causes of acoustic feedback
   b. Battery longevity and placement
   c. Checking for cerumen in earmolds or receiver tubing
   d. Procedures for cleaning earmolds
   e. Correct use of the telephone switch and other controls

Instructions to the staff of the health care facility on the care of hearing aids can be invaluable. The staff should be instructed to check to see that hearing aids do not go into the shower, the laundry, or denture cups, and that the hearing aids do not accidently get tossed out with soiled tissue paper.

The nurse aide, for example, can reduce a patient's stresses involved in adjusting to hearing aids by having the knowledge required to conduct a quick check on hearing aids that a frustrated elderly resident feels are not working. A simple adjustment of battery placement or reminding the resident that the earmolds need cleaning can eliminate disuse of otherwise beneficial hearing aids. Because these adjustments and reminders may be necessary when the audiologist is not in the health care facility, this aspect of in-service is extremely important. Loss of a hearing aid and malfunction are two of the most frequently observed problems for health care facility residents who have hearing impairment.

6. The components of an aural rehabilitation program are discussed so that administration and staff are aware of the intricacies involved not only in the assessment of auditory function, but also in treatment sessions. These insights and a staff that is knowledgeable of the role of the audiologist permit an enhanced working relationship between audiologist and staff.

   The role of the staff in carryover is also discussed. This includes the fact that the staff can be the vital catalyst in providing an enhanced climate for communication in the health care facility.

7. Discussing methods for effective communication with hearing-impaired older adults is a critical part of in-service training. The stresses that grow out of frustrated attempts at communication, both on the part of residents and staff, can stifle an otherwise pleasant living environment. The suggestions provided the staff include the Thirteen Commandments for Communicating with Hearing Impaired Older Adults presented in Table 20–1.

Provision of Aural Rehabilitation Treatment Services in the Health Care Facility

The specific strategies for providing aural rehabilitation treatment services on behalf of older adult patients in the health care facility remain essentially the same as those outlined in Chapter 19. They are procedures that lend themselves to any level of patient impairment. There are, however, some considerations that will benefit both a patient and the audiologist when providing aural rehabilitation services for confined elderly patients, including:

1. Motivation of residents,
2. The communicative and listening environment of the health care facility,
3. The health state of individual residents,
4. Family involvement, and
5. Compounding visual problems.

Motivation

Some audiologists prefer not to attempt to provide aural rehabilitation services on behalf of older persons who reside in health care facilities. They reason that many potential patients lack the motivation necessary to benefit from their services. As clinicians observe these persons, many of them have good reason for their lack of motivation. Clinicians can, however, blame themselves in some instances for not being able to provide motivation. Cohen (1990) has described a number of reasons for lack of motivation among many elderly persons. Those may include, among others, a lack of available finances, the death of a spouse or friends, lack of efficient modes of transportation, children living a great distance away, and physical problems that may restrict mobility.

Reasons for Lack of Motivation. As clinicians view elderly residents of health care facilities, they observe other more dramatic effects that impact on this population's motivation to receive rehabilitation services. According to early writings in Atchley (1972) and Smyer, Zarit, and Qualls (1990), the most depressing aspect of placement in a health care facility (nursing home) is the move

TABLE 20–1. The Thirteen Commandments for Communicating with Hearing Impaired Older Adults

- Speak at a slightly greater than normal intensity.

- Speak at your normal rate, but not too rapidly.

- Do not speak to the elderly person at a greater distance than 6 feet but no less than 3 feet.

- Concentrate light on the speaker's face for greater visibility of lip movements, facial expression, and gestures.

- Do not speak to the elderly person unless you are visible to her (e.g., not from another room while she is reading the newspaper or watching TV).

- Do not force the elderly person to listen to you when there is a great deal of environmental noise. That type of environment can be difficult for a younger, normally hearing person. It can, on the other hand, be defeating for the hearing impaired elderly.

- Never, under any circumstances, speak directly into the person's ear. Not only can the person not make use of visual clues, but the speaker may be causing an already distorting auditory system to distort the speech signal further. In other words, clarity may be depressed as loudness is increased.

- If the elderly person does not appear to understand what is being said, rephrase the statement rather than simply repeating the misunderstood words. An otherwise frustrating situation can be avoided in that way.

- Do not overarticulate. Overarticulation not only distorts the sounds of speech, but also the speaker's face, thus making the use of visual clues more difficult.

- Arrange the room (living room or meeting room) where communication will take place so that no listener is more than 6 feet from a speaker, and all are completely visible. Using this direct approach, communication for all parties involved will be enhanced.

- Include the elderly person in all discussions about her. Hearing impaired persons sometimes feel quite vulnerable. This approach will help alleviate some of those feelings.

- In meetings or any group activity where there is a speaker presenting information (church meetings, civic organizations, etc.) make it mandatory that the speaker(s) use the public address system. One of the most frequent complaints among elderly persons is that they may enjoy attending meetings of various kinds, but all too often the speaker, for whatever reason, tries to avoid using a microphone. Many elderly persons do not desire to assert themselves by asking a speaker to please use the microphone who has just said, "I am sure that you can all hear me if I do not use the microphone." Most persons begin to avoid public or organizational meetings if they cannot hear what the speaker is saying. This point cannot be stressed enough.

- Above all, treat elderly persons as adults. They, of all people, deserve that respect.

Note. From "The Thirteen Commandments for Talking to the Hearing Impaired Older Person," by R. H. Hull, 1980, *Journal of the American Speech and Hearing Association, 22,* p. 427. Reproduced with permission.

from a home where the person may have lived for many years to a strange and, to that person, a probable final residence. The events leading to placement in the health care facility were, in all probability, equally stressful, including perhaps the loss of a spouse, the loss of a home due to rezoning laws or lack of finances, severe enough illness to require constant nursing care, or slowly declining health simply because of advancing age. If the elderly resident has read the statistics on the longevity of residents of nursing homes, she will know that the probability of survival after the first month of placement is only about 73%. Further, only about 20% ever leave health care facilities except for burial (Moss & Halamandaris, 1997).

The well elderly in the community may not experience the reasons for depression, nor are they experiencing that particular dramatic change in their lives. The fear of the necessity for a move to a health care facility can, however, result in motivation to work toward preventing it.

For those who can benefit from aural rehabilitation services, efforts toward motivation should be made. If for no other reason than to enhance communication abilities with family and friends in the confined environment of the health care facility, to be able to enjoy watching television once again, or to participate more efficiently in social activities within the health care facility, motivation for receiving aural rehabilitation services should be given a high priority. It must be kept in mind, however, as was discussed in Chapter 19, that the aural rehabilitation treatment program must be developed around the patients' prioritized needs for communication, and no others.

Treatment Environment

Discovering an area within the health care facility where aural rehabilitation services can be provided in a pleasant and least restrictive environment can be challenging. Most health care facilities do have an area that is, at least, a pleasant place to be. That area may be an activity room, a lounge that is not the main lounge or lobby area, a staff dining room, or other sections of the health care facility that are not considered by the residents as ones where, for example, people go when they are "not well." Places to avoid include the infirmary and the chapel.

The only available space where frequent disturbances may not occur may be an esthetically undesirable space, such as the laundry room or the rear portion of the cafeteria. In that instance, modifications will be necessary. This is not always greeted with enthusiasm by health care facility administrators, particularly with the tight budgets faced by many. Such modifications for improvement of the therapy environment, however, may be necessary for the aural rehabilitation program to be effective to any degree.

Some remodeling of an otherwise drab room can be done inexpensively. Some wallpaper, a moveable partition, some paint, and carpeting can do wonders for the environment. There are few health care facilities that do not have at least a small amount of money for such improvements. If an audiologist has some talent for painting and minor carpentry, then labor costs may be reduced. Even some of the health care facility residents may enjoy chipping in on the labor. A retired carpenter or painter may find it a joy to lend an experienced hand. Women who can make curtains may enjoy reawakening that skill for the good of the "Audiology Room." If the health care facility agrees to hire professionals to do the remodeling work, then such innovations may not be necessary.

At the University of Northern Colorado Aural Rehabilitation Program for the Aging that began in the middle of 1970s (Hull &

Traynor, 1976), installation of sound-treated rooms and audiometers, including carpentry, electrical work, painting, and other work were funded by the health care facilities involved. When one health care facility was being constructed, the corporate owner's plans included a sound-treated room as part of the initial construction in support of their aural rehabilitation program. Further, the room was to double as a staff lounge. That aspect, for obvious reasons, was not a satisfactory arrangement and the staff later found other quarters for coffee and conversation.

Another health care facility remodeled a large linen closet, one remodeled a large vacant resident room, and yet another built walls for a new room for the audiology services that was previously unused except for storage. Interest level in the program varies from facility to facility, but the general commitment remains the same. Figure 20–2 illustrates a desirable room arrangement for the

provision of aural rehabilitation services, including counseling, hearing aid orientation, and discussions of difficult communication situations that patients face and their resolution.

The Health Status of Patients

As stated earlier, an audiologist must be realistic regarding an elderly patient's potential to respond to aural rehabilitation services. A terminally ill resident of a skilled nursing wing of a health care facility may possess impaired hearing, but not be able to respond to a complex system of diagnostic evaluation. It is not reasonable to ask that person to participate in a complex aural rehabilitation program that involves problem solving and assertiveness training. A knowledgeable staff, however, as the result of effective inservice, may ease some of the frustrations the resident may be having because of an

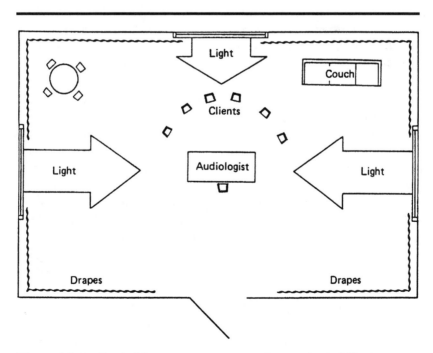

Figure 20–2. Desirable room arrangement for aural rehabilitation services in a health care facility.

inability to understand what they are saying. If the state of health of some individuals was the catalyst for placement in the health care facility, but those persons can indeed benefit from audiology services, additional considerations will be necessary. For example, accommodations for persons who are confined to a wheelchair are mandatory. Ramps into sound-treated testing booths, tables used in therapy that conform to the height of wheelchairs, and doors that permit maneuvering in and out of the rooms are necessary.

Attention Span. Many elderly persons cannot tolerate long periods of concentrated effort on any task. Audiometric evaluations in which attention to an almost inaudible pure tone is required, or aural rehabilitation sessions that instruct on more efficient means for communication, can become intolerable for some very elderly persons, even when the program is specifically designed around their needs. This is equally frustrating to some audiologists who have difficulty understanding the reason for the low attention or tolerance span. The problem does exist, however, and it must be accounted for.

It may be necessary to break audiological evaluations into two or even three short periods, particularly if discussions regarding hearing aids are included. Aural rehab sessions should not last for more than 45 minutes. If patients appear to be less tolerant on a specific day, short breaks during which time something else is talked about may be necessary. An alert audiologist will realize when the "stretch breaks" are required.

Number of Patients for Group Auditory Rehabilitation Sessions. The number of patients for optimal group interaction ranges from six to eight. Aural rehabilitation groups should not exceed this number. If at all possible, it is important to control admittance to specific groups to assure that hearing levels and levels of mental functioning among participants are as equal as possible. It can become frustrating for the group members, the audiologist, and the patient if one patient has extreme difficulty communicating and participating in the group and demands the majority of attention. The audiologist, out of necessity, will tend to spend most of the group time attempting to facilitate that person's participation. The latter does not enhance positive and facilitatory group interaction. As the patients make progress in their communicative skill, the development of advanced classes may be warranted, depending on the needs of the patients.

Individual versus Group Treatment. The more severely hearing impaired residents will require individual aural rehabilitation treatment. If a person progresses to the point that group involvement is possible, then she should be referred to that treatment setting. Some audiologists prefer to begin all patients' treatment on an individual basis so as to attend to any immediate needs they may have. And some may never enter group treatment when their needs are met on an individual basis.

Acoustics and Lighting. Consideration of the acoustic and visual environment of an aural rehabilitation treatment facility is critical. At least initially, the environment should be a quiet one, free of undue reverberation, and with adequate lighting. Because older eyes will generally require as much as twice as much light as younger eyes, lighting is an important consideration.

Visual Aspects. Fluorescent lighting is not suggested for use with older patients. Both the hue of the light and the flicker can cause visual difficulties, inattentiveness, and even seizures. Indirect and incandescent lighting is suggested, but glare from hard tables, floors, walls, and ceilings is to be avoided at all costs. Aging results in a thickening of the lens of the eye and a narrowing of the pupil aperture. Further, the muscles of the eye do not function as well, so accommodations for light changes are not as efficient.

Fozard (1990) and Woodruff (1975) have wisely advised that it takes almost twice the light energy to have the same effect on the older eye as the younger eye. In other words, the older eye is less responsive to light and cannot compensate for changes in light as quickly as it could when it was younger. It behooves the audiologist, therefore, to avoid moving from light to shadows as she is involved in aural rehabilitation treatment sessions.

Acoustic Needs. The suggested acoustic environment is one that consists of non-plush carpeted floors, textured walls or walls whose bottom third is carpeted, spackled acoustic tile ceilings or spackled drywall, and chairs that at least have a padded seat and back. The audiologist can modify this initial design to suit her own acoustic desires relative to aural rehabilitative tasks.

The room should not become so padded that it becomes anechoic, nor should it become too reverberant. A little reverberation gives sound "life." But too much causes distortion of the acoustic aspects of speech. Unfavorable acoustics (reverberated speech) contributes greatly to difficulties in speech discrimination among older persons who have impaired hearing.

Time. The process involved in aural rehabilitation treatment can be fatiguing for both the patient and the audiologist. In providing services, particularly on behalf of older adult patients, the factors of fatigue and alertness must be kept in mind. That includes

remembering that most people function better at certain times of the day and that attention span and periods of maximum alertness are different as one becomes older.

When working with older adults, the period immediately following lunch and anytime in the evening provides the least benefit. The inefficiency of those times is seen most dramatically among the confined or less active older person.

The time periods most advantageous for older adults are those toward the middle of the morning and perhaps 2 hours after lunch. The audiologist should be alert to the behaviors of her patients and change times as needed. It is generally best to ask the patient to suggest the time of day when she feels best.

The length of aural rehabilitation sessions must also be considered. This author has found that most alert, active older adults can work for at least 1 hour, as long as periodic breaks are taken that include brief chats about things other than the treatment session. Many older patients will not be able to tolerate strenuous sessions for longer than 30 minutes. The alert audiologist will be able to judge the tolerance levels of her patients.

Family

Although the role of the family or significant others in the aural rehabilitation process is discussed throughout this text, it is a critically important aspect to be presented concerning the elderly adult who is confined to the health care facility. The discouraging component of this discussion, however, is that many family members of these persons either do not wish to become involved or live such a great distance away that they cannot be involved in any consistent manner. It is disheartening, not only on the part of the audiologist, but more so on the part of the elderly patient, to observe a family member who agreed to come to the health care facility to become involved in the aural rehabilitation process who eventually dissolves the commitment. If such a possibility exists, it is generally better to not ask the family member to participate at all. A *genuine* commitment is necessary before such participation is initiated, mostly for the mental health of the elderly resident. The anguish felt by elderly persons, who eventually realize that their child or other family member apparently did not genuinely desire to become involved, is heartbreaking.

If family involvement is possible, however, the enhanced awareness about the potential for communication by and with the family member can enhance family bonds. The importance of this involvement cannot be stressed enough.

Compounding Problems of Vision

The multiple handicaps of vision and hearing impairment are very real among elderly persons. Many of those with significant visual problems can be found within health care facilities, particularly if they have not been able to remain mobile and self-sufficient in their own homes.

For persons who have rehabilitative potential, the aural rehabilitation process revolves around working toward enhancement of auditory function, as visual clues may be of little advantage. The audiologist's efforts must be combined with those of a vision specialist who can work to assist a person in becoming more mobile, including correcting furniture arrangements in her room, safe use of cosmetics, and self-help skills. That team effort, along with the help of the activity director of the health care facility, can supplant the isolation that may otherwise face the elderly resident. The audiologist can play a vital role in providing input to the person's rehabilitation programs.

Summary

This chapter has presented considerations for the provision of services on behalf of persons who reside in health care facilities. It is stressed that, as with other patients, these persons' communication needs must be addressed as priorities. Even though they are residing within the confines of a health care facility, they are still individuals and, most importantly, they are individual adults with unique goals and concerns. The audiologist and other professionals who serve these people must be constantly aware of that fact. On the other hand, patients must be fully aware that they are involved in treatment, not simply another activity within the health care facility. They must be aware of the reasons for the communication problems they are experiencing, the steps that will be taken to help them, and the strategies involved. Only then will the services and the audiologist be accepted.

References

Administration on Aging and the American Association of Retired Persons. (1996). *Profile of older Americans: 1996* (Pub. No. PF3049, 1090). Washington, DC: Author.

Administration on Aging. (2002). *Profile of older Americans* (Pub. No. PF3049.1090). Washington, DC: Author.

Atchley, R. C. (1972). *The social forces in later life.* Belmont, CA: Wadsworth.

Bayles, K. A., & Kaszniak, A. W. (1987*). Communication and cognition in normal aging and dementia.* Boston: Little, Brown.

Cohen, G. D. (1990). Psychopathology and mental health in the mature and elderly adult. In J. E. Birren & K. W. Schaie (Eds.), *Handbook of the psychology of aging* (pp. 642–667). New York: Academic Press.

Fozard, J. (1990). Vision and hearing in aging. In J. E. Birren & K. W. Schaie (Eds.), *Handbook of the psychology of aging* (pp. 329-342). New York: Academic Press.

Gatz, M., Bengtson, V. L., & Blum, M. J. (1990). Caregiving families. In J. Birren & K. W. Schaie (Eds.), *Handbook of the psychology of aging* (pp. 886-914). New York: Academic Press.

Hull, R. H. (1977). *Hearing impairment among aging persons.* Lincoln, NE: Cliff Notes.

Hull, R. H. (1980). The thirteen commandments for talking to the hearing impaired older person. *Journal of the American Speech and Hearing Association, 22,* 427.

Hull, R. H. (1988). *Hearing in aging.* Paper presented at the National Invitational Conference on Geriatric Rehabilitation. Washington, DC: PHS, Department of Health and Human Services.

Hull, R. H. (1993). *Incidence of hearing loss in a nursing home population.* Unpublished study, Wichita State University, Wichita, KS.

Hull, R. H. (1997). *Hearing in aging.* San Diego, CA: Singular.

Hull, R. H. (2001). Aural rehabilitation for older adults with impaired hearing. In R. Hull (Ed.), *Aural rehabilitation* (pp. 393-424). San Diego, CA: Singular/Thomson Learning.

Hull, R. H., & Traynor, R. (1976). A community-wide program in geriatric aural rehabilitation. *Journal of the American Speech-Language-Hearing Association, 14,* 33-34.

Ignatavicius, D. D., & Bayne, M. V. (1995). *Medical-surgical nursing.* Philadelphia: W. B. Saunders.

Moss, F. E., & Halamandaris, F. E. (1997). *Too old, too sick, too bad: Nursing homes in America.* Germantown, MD: Aspen Systems.

Schow, R. L., & Nerbonne, M. A. (1980). Hearing levels in elderly nursing home residents. *Journal of Speech and Hearing Disorders, 45,* 124-132.

Smyer, M. A., Zarit, S. H., & Qualls, S. H. (1990). Psychological intervention with the aging individual. In J. E. Birren & K. W. Schaie (Eds.), *Handbook of the psychology of aging* (pp. 375-394). New York: Academic Press.

Stone, R., Cafferata, G. L., & Sangl, J. (1987). Caregivers of the frail elderly: A national profile. *The Gerontologist, 36,* 616-626.

Traynor, R. L. (1975). *A method of audiological assessment for the non-ambulatory geriatric patient.* Unpublished doctoral dissertation, University of Northern Colorado, Greeley.

Woodruff, D. S. (1975). A physiological perspective of the psychology of aging. In D. S. Woodruff & J. E. Birren (Eds.), *Aging: Scientific perspectives and social issues* (pp. 179-198). New York: Van Nostrand.

End of Chapter Examination Questions

Chapter 20

1. Among persons residing in health care facilities, approximately _____ possess hearing impairment of sufficient degree to interfere with communication.
   a. 15%
   b. 38%
   c. 56%
   d. 92%

2. Describe the possible benefits a resident of a health care facility may realize from aural rehabilitation treatment.

3. Define the term *health care facility* and briefly compare and contrast the three levels of care that these facilities may provide.

4. Briefly discuss how the attitude of a person toward residing in a health care facility may affect her desire for rehabilitative services.

5. Which of the following is not felt to be a major factor in placement of persons in health care facilities?
   a. Their previous residential setting
   b. Their children regarding them as "inconvenient"
   c. Their state of mental or physical health
   d. Their family setting

6. The scope of the audiologist's services in health care facilities should include:
   a. he resident's family.
   b. the medical/support staff.
   c. the resident.
   d. all of the above.

7. The most efficient screening process recommended for the identification of residents with hearing impairment includes:
   a. fixed intensity level screening.
   b. a conversational voice test.
   c. pure-tone thresholds and impedance audiometry.
   d. interviewing family members and caregivers.

8. **List five possible in-service training topics that the audiologist could share with facility staff members and administrators.**

   a.

   b.

   c.

   d.

   e.

9. **The author suggests two optimal time periods for scheduling aural rehabilitation. What are those times and why might they prove advantageous?**

   a.

   b.

10. **The author describes five considerations that should guide the establishment of aural rehabilitation services on behalf of the residents. What are they? Briefly describe each.**

    a.

    b.

    c.

    d.

    e.

End of Chapter Answer Sheet

Name _____ Date _____

Chapter 20

1. Which one(s)?   a   b   c   d

2. _____

_____

_____

3. _____

_____

_____

4. _____

_____

_____

5. Which one(s)?   a   b   c   d

6. Which one(s)?   a   b   c   d

7. Which one(s)?   a   b   c   d

8. a. _____

b. _____

c. _____

d. _____

e. _____

9. a. _____

b. _____

10. a. _____

b. _____

c. _____

d. _____

e. _____

APPENDICES

Materials and Scales for Assessment of Communication for the Hearing Impaired

The following appendices present an array of assessment tools and scales of handicap that are appropriate for use with adults and elderly clients who are hearing impaired. All are designed for use with either adult or elderly clients, except for The Communication Scale by Kaplan, Bally, and Brandt (1990), which is designed also for younger adults, including high school and college-age students. However, it is also designed to be utilized with adults beyond college age.

The tools and scales in the Appendices include the following:

A. CID Everyday Sentences

B. The Denver Scale Quick Test

C. The WSU Sentence Test of Speechreading Ability

D. Hearing-Handicap Scale

E. The Denver Scale of Communication Function

F. Test of Actual Performance

G. The Hearing Measurement Scale

H. Profile Questionnaire for Rating Communicative Performance in a Home and Social Environment

I. The Denver Scale of Communication Function for Senior Citizens Living in Retirement Centers

J. Wichita State University (WSU) Communication Appraisal and Priorities Profile (CAPP)

K. The Hearing Handicap Inventory for the Elderly

L. The Communication Profile for the Hearing Impaired

M. Communication Skill Scale

N. The Shortened Hearing Aid Performance Inventory

O. Communication Scale for Older Adults (3-Point Response Format)

APPENDIX A

CID Everyday Sentences

List A

1. Walking's my favorite exercise.

2. Here's a nice quiet place to rest.

3. Our janitor sweeps the floors every night.

4. It would be much easier if everyone would help.

5. Good morning.

6. Open your window before you go to bed!

7. Do you think that she should stay out so late?

8. How do you feel about changing the time when we begin work?

9. Here we go.

10. Move out of the way!

List B

1. The water's too cold for swimming.

2. Why should I get up so early in the morning?

3. Here are your shoes.

4. It's raining.

5. Where are you going?

6. Come here when I call you!

7. Don't try to get out of it this time!

8. Should we let little children go to the movies by themselves?

9. There isn't enough paint to finish the room.

10. Do you want an egg for breakfast?

List C

1. Everybody should brush his teeth after meals.

2. Everything's all right.

3. Don't use up all the paper when you write your letter.

4. That's right.

5. People ought to see a doctor once a year.

6. Those windows are so dirty I can't see anything outside.

7. Pass the bread and butter please.

8. Don't forget to pay your bill before the first of the month.

9. Don't let the dog out of the house.

10. There's a good ball game this afternoon.

List D

1. It's time to go.

2. If you don't want these old magazines, throw them out.

3. Do you want to wash up?

4. It's a real dark night so watch your driving.

5. I'll carry the package for you.

6. Did you forget to shut off the water?

7. Fishing in a mountain stream is my idea of a good time.

8. Fathers spend more time with their children than they used to.

9. Be careful not to break your glasses.

10. I'm sorry.

List E

1. You can catch the bus across the street.

2. Call her on the phone and tell her the news.

3. I'll catch up with you later.

4. I'll think it over.

5. I don't want to go to the movies tonight.

6. If your tooth hurts that much you ought to see a dentist.

7. Put the cookie back in the box!

8. Stop fooling around!

9. Time's up.

10. How do you spell your name?

List F

1. Music always cheers me up.

2. My brother's in town for a short while on business.

3. We live a few miles from the main road.

4. This suit needs to go to the cleaners.

5. They ate enough green apples to make them sick for a week.

6. Where have you been all this time?

7. Have you been working hard lately?

8. There's not enough room in the kitchen for a new table.

9. Where is he?

10. Look out!

List G

1. I'll see you right after lunch.

2. See you later.

3. White shoes are awful to keep clean.

4. Stand there and don't move until I tell you.

5. There's a big piece of cake left over from dinner.

6. Wait for me at the corner in front of the drugstore.

7. It's no trouble at all.

8. Hurry up!

9. The morning paper didn't say anything about rain this afternoon or tonight.

10. The phone call's for you.

List H

1. Believe me!
2. Let's get a cup of coffee.
3. Let's get out of here before it's too late.
4. I hate driving at night.
5. There was water in the cellar after that heavy rain yesterday.
6. She'll only be a few minutes.
7. How do you know?
8. Children like candy.
9. If we don't get rain soon, we'll have no grass.
10. They're not listed in the new phone book.

List I

1. Where can I find a place to work?
2. I like those big red apples we always get in the fall.
3. You'll get fat eating candy.
4. The show's over.
5. Why don't they paint their walls some other color?
6. What's new?
7. What are you hiding under your coat?
8. How come I should always be the one to go first?
9. I'll take sugar and cream in my coffee.
10. Wait just a minute!

List J

1. Breakfast is ready.
2. I don't know what's wrong with the car, but it won't start.
3. It sure takes a sharp knife to cut this meat.
4. I haven't read a newspaper since we bought a television set.
5. Weeds are spoiling the yard.
6. Call me a little later!
7. Do you have change for a $5 bill?
8. How are you?
9. I'd like some ice cream with my pie.
10. I don't think I'll have any dessert.

Note. From "The Testing of Hearing in the Armed Services," Technical Report to the Office of Naval Research CHABA (National Research Council Committee on Hearing and Bio-Acoustics), 1951, CHABA No. 5, Bethesda, MD, from the Central Institute for the Deaf under Contract No. 1151 (10) NR 140-069. Reproduced with permission.

APPENDIX B

The Denver Scale Quick Test

1. Good morning.

2. How old are you?

3. I live in (state of residence).

4. I only have one dollar.

5. There is somebody at the door.

6. Is that all?

7. Where are you going?

8. Let's have a coffee break.

9. Park your car in the lot.

10. What is your address?

11. May I help you?

12. I feel fine.

13. It is time for dinner.

14. Turn right at the corner.

15. Are you ready to order?

16. Is this charge or cash?

17. What time is it?

18. I have a headache.

19. How about going out tonight?

20. Please lend me 50 cents.

Note. From "Evaluation of Communication Function," by J. G. Alpiner, in J. G. Alpiner (Ed.), *Handbook of Adult Rehabilitative Audiology*, 1978, p. 36, Baltimore, MD, Williams and Wilkins. Reproduced with permission.

APPENDIX C

The WSU Sentence Test of Speechreading Ability

List 1

1. It was such a great day for hiking.
2. Have you read the sports page this morning?
3. The cost of living will make you poor.
4. He serves excellent food in all his restaurants.
5. What kind of a car do you drive?
6. The weather for the game was almost perfect.
7. Why was the picnic called off this time?
8. I like white houses with large covered porches.
9. Did the white-and-black cat have kittens?
10. Slow music always makes me feel like sleeping.
11. Why did you go there for your vacation?
12. How much snow did we have last night?

List 2

1. Will you come with me to see him?
2. Snow always looks pretty on the mountainside.
3. Is your whole family getting together for Thanksgiving?
4. Do you have an umbrella with you today?
5. Fathers should spend more time with their children.
6. Are you going grocery shopping while in town?
7. The wind is blowing from the northeast again.
8. It is time to go back home now.
9. Did you forget to shut off the water?
10. Hockey has been considered this state's favorite sport.
11. Where do you usually work during the winter?
12. It is a good day for playing golf.

List 3

1. What time was it when you arrived?

2. Have you any brothers or sisters at home?

3. It has rained for the past 3 days.

4. Do you have a dog or a cat?

5. What does the judge say about him now?

6. A soft rain makes grass grow in spring.

7. Did you buy a new car this year?

8. You should brush your teeth three times daily.

9. Children go to school at around age 6.

10. He let the dog out of the house.

11. Soccer is often a rough and tumble sport.

12. Would you like to go to the show?

Note. From "WSU Sentence Test of Speechreading Ability," by R. H. Hull, 2001, in R. H. Hull (Ed.), *Aural Rehabilitation: Children and Adults*, p. 477–478. San Diego, CA: Singular/Thomson Learning. Reproduced with permission.

APPENDIX D

Hearing-Handicap Scale

Form A

1. If you are 6 to 12 feet from the loudspeaker of a radio do you understand speech well?

2. Can you carry on a telephone conversation without difficulty?

3. If you are 6 to 12 feet from a television set, do you understand most of what is said?

4. Can you carry on a conversation with one other person when you are on a noisy street corner?

5. Do you hear all right when you are in a streetcar, airplane, bus, or train?

6. If there are noises from other voices, typewriters, traffic, music, etc., can you understand when someone speaks to you?

7. Can you understand a person when you are seated beside him and cannot see his face?

8. Can you understand if someone speaks to you while you are chewing crisp foods, such as potato chips or celery?

9. Can you carry on a conversation with one other person when you are in a noisy place, such as a restaurant or at a party?

10. Can you understand if someone speaks to you in a whisper and you can't see his or her face?

11. When you talk with a bus driver, waiter, ticket salesman, etc., can you understand all right?

12. Can you carry on a conversation if you are seated across the room from someone who speaks in a normal tone of voice?

13. Can you understand women when they talk?

14. Can you carry on a conversation with one other person when you are out of doors and it is reasonably quiet?

15. When you are in a meeting or at a large dinner table, would you know the speaker was talking if you could not see his lips moving?

16. Can you follow the conversation when you are at a large dinner table or in a meeting with a small group?

17. If you are seated under the balcony of a theater or auditorium, can you hear well enough to follow what is going on?

18. When you are in a large formal gathering (a church, lodge, lecture hall, etc.) can you hear what is said when the speaker does not use a microphone?

19. Can you hear the telephone ring when you are in the room where it is located?

20. Can you hear warning signals, such as automobile horns, railway crossing bells, or emergency vehicle sirens?

Form B

1. When you are listening to the radio or watching television, can you hear adequately when the volume is comfortable for most other people?

2. Can you carry on a conversation with one other person when you are riding in an automobile with the windows closed?

3. Can you carry on a conversation with one other person when you are riding in an automobile with the window open?

4. Can you carry on a conversation with one other person if there is a radio or television in the same room playing at normal loudness?

5. Can you hear when someone calls to you from another room?

6. Can you understand when someone speaks to you from another room?

7. When you buy something in a store, do you easily understand the clerk?

8. Can you carry on a conversation with someone who does not speak as loudly as most people?

9. Can you tell if a person is talking when you are seated beside him and cannot see his face?

10. When you ask someone for directions, do you understand what he or she says?

11. If you are within 3 or 4 feet of a person who speaks in a normal tone of voice (assume you are facing one another), can you hear everything he or she says?

12. Do you recognize the voices of speakers when you don't see them?

13. When you are introduced to someone, can you understand the name the first time it is spoken?

14. Can you hear adequately when you are conversing with more than one person?

15. If you are in an audience, such as in a church or theater and you are seated near the front, can you understand most of what is said?

16. Can you carry on everyday conversations with members of your family without difficulty?

17. If you are in an audience such as in a church or theater and you are seated near the rear, can you understand most of what is said?

18. When you are in a large formal gathering (a church, lodge, lecture hall, etc.) can you hear what is said when the speaker does use a microphone?

19. Can you hear the telephone ring when you are in the next room?

20. Can you hear night sounds, such as distant trains, bells, dogs barking, trucks passing, and so forth?

Note. From "Scale for Self-Assessment of Hearing Handicap," by E. S. High, G. Fairbanks, & A. Glorig, 1964, *Journal of Speech and Hearing Disorders, 29*, pp. 215–230. Reproduced with permission.

APPENDIX E

The Denver Scale of Communication Function

(Circle One)   Preservice   Postservice

Date _____   Case No. _____

Name _____   Age _____ Sex _____

Address _____
                    (City)   (State)   (Zip)

Lives Alone _____   In Apartment _____   Retired _____
         (if no, specify)

Occupation _____

Audiogram (Examination Date _____   Agency _____

Pure Tone:

	250	500	1000	2000	4000	8000 Hz	
RE							dB (re: ANSI)
LE							

Speech Reception

   SRT =   Discrimination Score (%) =

                              Quiet Noise (S/N = _____)

   RE   dB   RE

   LE   dB   LE

Hearing Aid Information:

   Aided _____ For How Long _____ Aid Type _____

   Satisfaction _____

   Name of Examiner _____

Denver Scale of Communication Function

The following questionnaire was designed to evaluate your communication ability as you view it. You are asked to judge or scale each statement in the following manner.

If you judge the statement to be very closely related to either extreme, please place your check mark as follows:

Agree __✓__ _____ _____ _____ _____ _____ _____ Disagree

or

Agree _____ _____ _____ _____ _____ _____ __✓__ Disagree

If you judge the statement to be closely related to either end of the scale, please mark as follows:

Agree _____ __✓__ _____ _____ _____ _____ _____ Disagree

or

Agree _____ _____ _____ _____ _____ __✓__ _____ Disagree

If you judge the statement to be only slightly related to either end of the scale, please mark as follows:

Agree _____ _____ __✓__ _____ _____ _____ _____ Disagree

or

Agree _____ _____ _____ _____ __✓__ _____ _____ Disagree

If you consider the statement to be irrelevant or unassociated to your communication situation, please mark as follows:

Agree _____ _____ _____ __✓__ _____ _____ _____ Disagree

Please Note: Check an answer for every statement. Put only one checkmark on each statement. Make a *separate* judgment for each statement.

Also: You may comment on each statement in the space provided.

1. The members of my family are annoyed with my loss of hearing.

   Agree _____ _____ _____ _____ _____ _____ _____ Disagree

   Comments:

2. The members of my family sometimes leave me out of conversations or discussions.

Agree _____ _____ _____ _____ _____ _____ _____ Disagree

Comments:

3. Sometimes my family makes decisions for me because I have a hard time following discussions.

Agree _____ _____ _____ _____ _____ _____ _____ Disagree

Comments:

4. My family becomes annoyed when I ask them to repeat what was said because I did not hear them.

Agree _____ _____ _____ _____ _____ _____ _____ Disagree

Comments:

5. I am not an "outgoing" person because I have a hearing loss.

Agree _____ _____ _____ _____ _____ _____ _____ Disagree

Comments:

6. I now take less of an interest in many things as compared to when I did not have a hearing problem.

Agree _____ _____ _____ _____ _____ _____ _____ Disagree

Comments:

7. Other people do not realize how frustrated I get when I cannot hear or understand.

Agree _____ _____ _____ _____ _____ _____ _____ Disagree

Comments:

8. People sometimes avoid me because of my hearing loss.

Agree _____ _____ _____ _____ _____ _____ _____ Disagree

Comments:

9. I am not a calm person because of my hearing loss

Agree _____ _____ _____ _____ _____ _____ _____ Disagree

Comments:

10. I tend to be negative about life in general because of my hearing loss.

Agree _____ _____ _____ _____ _____ _____ _____ Disagree

Comments:

11. I do not socialize as much as I did before I began to lose my hearing.

Agree _____ _____ _____ _____ _____ _____ _____ Disagree

Comments:

12. Since I have trouble hearing, I do not like to go places with friends.

Agree _____ _____ _____ _____ _____ _____ _____ Disagree

Comments:

13. Since I have trouble hearing, I hesitate to meet new people.

Agree _____ _____ _____ _____ _____ _____ _____ Disagree

Comments:

14. I do not enjoy my job as much as I did before I began to lose my hearing.

    Agree _____ _____ _____ _____ _____ _____ _____ Disagree

    Comments:

15. Other people do not understand what it is like to have a hearing loss.

    Agree _____ _____ _____ _____ _____ _____ _____ Disagree

    Comments:

16. Because I have difficulty understanding what is said to me, I sometimes answer questions wrong.

    Agree _____ _____ _____ _____ _____ _____ _____ Disagree

    Comments:

17. I do not feel relaxed in a communicative situation.

    Agree _____ _____ _____ _____ _____ _____ _____ Disagree

    Comments:

18. I do not feel comfortable in most communication situations.

    Agree _____ _____ _____ _____ _____ _____ _____ Disagree

    Comments:

19. Conversations in a noisy room prevent me from attempting to communicate with others.

    Agree _____ _____ _____ _____ _____ _____ _____ Disagree

    Comments:

20. I am not comfortable having to speak in a group situation.

Agree _____ _____ _____ _____ _____ _____ _____ Disagree

Comments:

21. In general I do not find listening relaxing.

Agree _____ _____ _____ _____ _____ _____ _____ Disagree

Comments:

22. I feel threatened by many communication situations due to difficulty hearing.

Agree _____ _____ _____ _____ _____ _____ _____ Disagree

Comments:

23. I seldom watch other people's facial expressions when talking to them.

Agree _____ _____ _____ _____ _____ _____ _____ Disagree

Comments:

24. I hesitate to ask people to repeat if I do not understand them the first time they speak.

Agree _____ _____ _____ _____ _____ _____ _____ Disagree

Comments:

25. Because I have difficulty understanding what is said to me, I sometimes make comments that do not fit into the conversation.

Agree _____ _____ _____ _____ _____ _____ _____ Disagree

Comments:

Note. From unpublished materials by J. G. Alpiner, W. Chevrette, G. Glascoe, M. Metz, & B. Olsen, 1971, Denver, CO, University of Denver. Reproduced with permission.

APPENDIX F

Test of Actual Performance

How well does he or she:

	Poor	Adequate	Good	Excellent
1. Pay attention in the group? (daydreams, restlessness, changes the subject)	_____	_____	_____	_____
2. Communicate ideas verbally?	_____	_____	_____	_____
3. Use speech intelligibly?	_____	_____	_____	_____
4. Respond to others? (shares similar experiences, agrees, disagrees)	_____	_____	_____	_____
5. Hear speech when noise was going on around him/her? (like at parties)	_____	_____	_____	_____
6. Understand speech when not able to see the speaker?	_____	_____	_____	_____
7. Monitor the loudness of his or her own speech?	_____	_____	_____	_____

Note. From "The Use of Hearing Test to Provide Information about the Extent to Which an Individual's Hearing Loss Handicaps Him, by C. Y. Konditsiotis, 1971, *Maico Audiological Library Series, 9,* p. 10. Produced with permission.

APPENDIX G

The Hearing Measurement Scale

SECTION 1: Speech Hearing

1. Do you ever have difficulty hearing in the conversation when you're with one other person at home?

2. Do you ever have difficulty hearing in the conversation when you're with one other person outside?

3. Do you ever have difficulty in group conversation at home?

4. Do you ever have difficulty in group conversation outside?

5. Do you ever have difficulty hearing conversation at work?

   5a. Is this due to your hearing, due to the noise, or a bit of both?

6. Do you ever have difficulty hearing the speaker at a public gathering?

7. Can you always hear what's being said in a TV program?

8. Can you always hear what's being said in TV news?

9. Can you always hear what's being said in a radio program?

10. Can you always hear what's being said in radio news?

11. Do you ever have difficulty hearing what's said in a film at the cinema?

SECTION 2: Acuity for Nonspeech Sounds

1. Do you have any pets at home? (Type _____) Can you hear it when it barks, mews, etc.?

2. Can you hear it when someone rings the doorbell or knocks on the door?

3. Can you hear a motor horn in the street when you're outside?

4. Can you hear the sound of footsteps outside when you're inside?

5. Can you hear the sound of the door opening when you're inside that room?

6. Can you hear the clock ticking in the room?

7. Can you hear the tap running when you turn it on?

8. Can you hear water boiling in a pan when you're in the kitchen?

SECTION 3: Localization

1. When you hear the sound of people talking and they're in another room, would you be able to tell from where this sound was coming?

2. If you're with a group of people and someone you can't see starts to speak, would you be able to tell where that person was sitting?

3. If you hear a motor horn or a bell, can you always tell in which direction it's sounding?

4. Do you ever turn your head the wrong way when someone calls to you?

5. Can you usually tell from the sound how far away a person is when he calls to you?

6. Have you ever noticed outside that a car you thought, by its sound, was far away turned out to be much closer in fact?

7. Outside, do you always move out of the way of something coming up from behind, for instance a car, a trolley, or someone walking faster?

SECTION 4: Reaction to Handicap

1. Do you think that you are more irritable than other people or less so?

2. Do you ever give the wrong answer to someone because you've misheard them?

3. When you do this, do you treat it lightly or do you get upset?

4. How does the other person react? Does he get irritated or make little of it?

5. Do you think people are tolerant in this way or do they make fun of you?

6. Do you ever get bothered or upset if you are unable to follow a conversation?

7. Do you ever get the feeling of being cut off from things because of difficulty in hearing?

    7a. Does this feeling upset you at all?

SECTION 5: Speech Distortion

1. Do you find that people fail to speak clearly?

2. What about speakers on TV or radio? Do they fail to speak clearly?

3. Do you ever have difficulty, in everyday conversation, understanding what someone is saying even though you can hear what's being said?

SECTION 6: Tinnitus

1. Do you ever get a noise in your ears or in your head?

2. 2a. to 2e. [A series of items on the nature and incidence of tinnitus.]

3. Does it ever stop you from sleeping?

4. Does it upset you?

SECTION 7: Personal Opinion of Hearing Loss

1. Do you think your hearing is normal?

2. Do you think any difficulty with your hearing is particularly serious?

3. Does any difficulty with your hearing restrict your social or personal life?

4. 4a. to 4f. [A series of items on temporary threshold shift, specifically for those with chronic acoustic trauma, on the relative importance of eyesight over hearing and on other difficult hearing situations not mentioned in the interview.]

Note. From "The Hearing Measurement Scale: A Questionnaire for Assessment of Auditory Disability," by W.G. Noble & G. R. C. Atherley,1970, *Journal of Audiological Research*, *10*, pp. 229-250. Reproduced with permission.

This scale cannot be used without reference to the manual of instructions. Copies of the Scale and the manual of instruction can be obtained from Dr. William Noble, Department of Psychology, University of New England, Armidale, NSW, 2351, Australia.

APPENDIX H

Profile Questionnaire for Rating Communicative Performance in a Home and Social Environment

Home Environment

1. a. In my living room, when I can see the speaker's face, I have:

+2	+1	−1	−2
little or no difficulty in understanding.	some difficulty (but not a lot) in understanding.	a fair amount of difficulty (quite a lot) in understanding.	great difficulty in understanding.

   b. This happens:

1	2	3
seldom.	often.	very often.

2. a. If I am talking with a person in my living room or family room while the television, radio, or record player is on, I have:

+2	+1	−1	−2
little or no difficulty in understanding.	some difficulty (but not a lot) in understanding.	a fair amount of difficulty (quite a lot) in understanding.	great difficulty in understanding.

   b. This happens:

1	2	3
seldom.	often.	very often.

3. a. In a quiet room in my house, if I cannot see the speaker's face I have:

+2	+1	−1	−2
little or no difficulty in understanding.	some difficulty (but not a lot) in understanding.	a fair amount of difficulty (quite a lot) in understanding.	great difficulty in understanding.

b. This happens:

1	2	3
seldom.	often.	very often.

4. a. If someone in my home speaks to me from another room on the same floor, I experience:

+2	+1	−1	−2
little or no difficulty in understanding.	some difficulty (but not a lot) in understanding.	a fair amount of difficulty (quite a lot) in understanding.	great difficulty in understanding.

b. This happens:

1	2	3
seldom.	often.	very often.

5. a. If someone calls me from upstairs when I am downstairs, or from the window when I am in the garden, I will experience:

+2	+1	−1	−2
little or no difficulty in understanding.	some difficulty (but not a lot) in understanding.	a fair amount of difficulty (quite a lot) in understanding.	great difficulty in understanding.

b. This happens:

1	2	3
seldom.	often.	very often.

6. a. Understanding people at the dinner table gives me:

+2	+1	−1	−2
little or no difficulty in understanding.	some difficulty (but not a lot) in understanding.	a fair amount of difficulty (quite a lot) in understanding.	great difficulty in understanding.

  b. This happens:

1	2	3
seldom.	often.	very often.

7. a. When I sit talking with friends in a quiet room I have:

+2	+1	−1	−2
little or no difficulty in understanding.	some difficulty (but not a lot) in understanding.	a fair amount of difficulty (quite a lot) in understanding.	great difficulty in understanding.

  b. This happens:

1	2	3
seldom.	often.	very often.

8. a. Listening to the radio or record player or watching TV gives me:

+2	+1	−1	−2
little or no difficulty in understanding.	some difficulty (but not a lot) in understanding.	a fair amount of difficulty (quite a lot) in understanding.	great difficulty in understanding.

  b. This happens:

1	2	3
seldom.	often.	very often.

9. a. When I use the phone at home, I have:

+2	+1	−1	−2
little or no difficulty in understanding.	some difficulty (but not a lot) in understanding.	a fair amount of difficulty (quite a lot) in understanding.	great difficulty in understanding.

b. This happens:

1	2	3
seldom.	often.	very often.

Social Environment

1. a. If we are entertaining a group of friends, understanding someone against the background of other talking gives me:

+2	+1	−1	−2
little or no difficulty in understanding.	some difficulty (but not a lot) in understanding.	a fair amount of difficulty (quite a lot) in understanding.	great difficulty in understanding.

b. This happens:

1	2	3
seldom.	often.	very often.

2. a. If we are playing cards, understanding my partner gives me:

+2	+1	−1	−2
little or no difficulty in understanding.	some difficulty (but not a lot) in understanding.	a fair amount of difficulty (quite a lot) in understanding.	great difficulty in understanding.

b. This happens:

1	2	3
seldom.	often.	very often.

3. a. When I am at the theater or the movies, I have:

+2	+1	−1	−2
little or no difficulty in understanding.	some difficulty (but not a lot) in understanding.	a fair amount of difficulty (quite a lot) in understanding.	great difficulty in understanding.

   b. This happens:

1	2	3
seldom.	often.	very often.

4. a. In church, when the minister gives the sermon, I have:

+2	+1	−1	−2
little or no difficulty in understanding.	some difficulty (but not a lot) in understanding.	a fair amount of difficulty (quite a lot) in understanding.	great difficulty in understanding.

   b. This happens:

1	2	3
seldom.	often.	very often.

5. a. When I eat out, following the conversation I have:

+2	+1	−1	−2
little or no difficulty in understanding.	some difficulty (but not a lot) in understanding.	a fair amount of difficulty (quite a lot) in understanding.	great difficulty in understanding.

   b. This happens:

1	2	3
seldom.	often.	very often.

6. a. In the car, I find that understanding what people are saying gives me:

+2	+1	−1	−2
little or no difficulty in understanding.	some difficulty (but not a lot) in understanding.	a fair amount of difficulty (quite a lot) in understanding.	great difficulty in understanding.

b. This happens:

1	2	3
seldom.	often.	very often.

7. a. When I am outside talking with someone I have:

+2	+1	−1	−2
little or no difficulty in understanding.	some difficulty (but not a lot) in understanding.	a fair amount of difficulty (quite a lot) in understanding.	great difficulty in understanding.

b. This happens:

1	2	3
seldom.	often.	very often.

Note. From "Hearing Aid Orientation and Counseling," by D. A. Sanders, in M. C. Pollack (Ed.), *Amplification for the Hearing Impaired*, 1975, pp. 363–372, New York: Grune and Sratton. Reproduced with permission.

APPENDIX I

The Denver Scale of Communication Function for Senior Citizens Living in Retirement Centers

Name _____ Date of Pretest _____

Address _____ Date of Post-Test _____

Age _____ Examiner _____

Sex _____

1. Do you have trouble communicating with your family because of your hearing problem?

   Yes _____ No _____

Probe Effect I

Does your family make decisions for you because of your hearing problem?   Yes _____ No _____

Does your family leave you out of discussions because of your hearing problem?   Yes _____ No _____

Does your family get angry or annoyed with you because of your hearing problem?   Yes _____ No _____

Exploration Effect

Do you have a family?   Yes _____ No _____

How often does your family visit you? _____

How far away does your family live? _____ In a city ____ Other ____

How often do you visit your family? _____

2. Do you get upset when you cannot hear or understand what is being said?

Yes _____ No _____

Probe Effect I (to be used only if person responds Yes)

Do your friends know you get upset?	Yes _____	No _____
Does your family know you get upset?	Yes _____	No _____
Does the staff know you get upset?	Yes _____	No _____

Probe Effect II (to be used only if person responds No)

Do your friends realize you are not upset?	Yes _____	No _____
Does your family realize you are not upset?	Yes _____	No _____
Does the staff realize you are not upset?	Yes _____	No _____

Exploration Effect (to be used only if person responds Yes)

How does your behavior change when you become upset?

3. Do you think your family, your friends, and the staff understand what it is like to have a hearing problem?

Yes _____ No _____

Probe Effect

Do they avoid you because of your hearing problem?	Yes _____	No _____
Do they leave you out of discussions?	Yes _____	No _____
Do they hesitate to ask you to socialize with them?	Yes _____	No _____

Exploration Effect

Family	Yes _____	No _____
Friends	Yes _____	No _____
Staff	Yes _____	No _____

4. Do you avoid communicating with other people because of your hearing problem?

   Yes _____   No _____

   Probe Effect

   Do you communicate with people during meal times?   Yes _____   No _____

   Do you communicate with your roommate(s)?   Yes _____   No _____

   Do you communicate during the social activities in the home?   Yes _____   No _____

   Do you communicate with visiting family or friends?   Yes _____   No _____

   Do you communicate with the staff?   Yes _____   No _____

   Exploration Effect

   Is your roommate capable of communication   Yes _____   No _____

   What are the social activities of the home?

   Which ones do you attend?

5. Do you feel that you are a relaxed person?

   Yes _____   No _____

   Probe Effect

   Do you think you are an irritable person because of your hearing problem?   Yes _____   No _____

   Do you think you are an irritable person because of your age?   Yes _____   No _____

   Do you think you are an irritable person because you live in this home?   Yes _____   No _____

   Exploration Effect

   Do you have to live in this home?   Yes _____   No _____

6. Do you feel relaxed in group communication situations?

   Yes _____ No _____

Probe Effect

Do you get nervous when you have to ask people
to repeat what they have said if you have not
understood them?   Yes _____ No _____

Do you feel nervous if you have to tell a person
that you have a hearing problem?   Yes _____ No _____

Exploration Effect

Do you watch facial expressions?   Yes _____ No _____

Do you watch gestures?   Yes _____ No _____

Do you think you are a good listener?   Yes _____ No _____

Do you have a hearing aid?   Yes _____ No _____

Do you wear your aid?   Yes _____ No _____

7. Do you think you need help in overcoming your hearing problem?

   Yes _____ No _____

Probe Effect

If lipreading training was available, would you
attend?   Yes _____ No _____

Do you think this home provides adequate
activities to make you want to communicate?   Yes _____ No _____

Exploration Effect I

Can a person improve communication ability by
using lipreading (or speechreading), which means
watching the speaker's lips, facial expressions,
and gestures when he or she is speaking?   Yes _____ No _____

Do you agree with the above as a definition of
lipreading?   Yes _____ No _____

Exploration Effect II

Is your vision adequate?   Yes _____ No _____

Are you able to get around unassisted?   Yes _____ No _____

Note. From "The Denver Scale of Communication Function for Senior Citizens Living in Retirement Centers," by J. M. Zarnoch & J. G. Alpiner, in J. G. Alpiner (Ed.), *Handbook of Adult Rehabilitative Audiology*, 1978, pp. 166–168, Baltimore: Williams and Wilkins. Reproduced with permission.

APPENDIX J

Wichita State University (WSU) Communication Appraisal and Priorities Profile (CAPP)

Date _____

Name _____ Age _____ Sex _____

Address _____

Phone _____

Please indicate below those situations in which you are able to communicate best, those that are difficult for you in some instances, and those that are a definite problem. Under Explain, please tell us more if you desire, such as certain instances when you experience more difficulty than others, certain types of speakers, certain places, and so on.

	No problems	Only in specific instances	Definite problem	Priority
1. At parties or other social events	_____	_____	_____	_____
Explain				
2. At the dinner table	_____	_____	_____	_____
Explain				
3. On the telephone	_____	_____	_____	_____
Explain				

	No problems	Only in specific instances	Definite problem	Priority
4. At home	_____	_____	_____	_____
Explain				
5. With males	_____	_____	_____	_____
Explain				
6. With females	_____	_____	_____	_____
Explain				
7. With children	_____	_____	_____	_____
Explain				
8. In groups	_____	_____	_____	_____
Explain				
9. With certain important individuals	_____	_____	_____	_____
Explain				
10. At church	_____	_____	_____	_____
Explain				

	No problems	Only in specific instances	Definite problem	Priority
11. At meetings	_____	_____	_____	_____
Explain				
12. Watching TV	_____	_____	_____	_____
Explain				
13. At the theater	_____	_____	_____	_____
Explain				
14. At work	_____	_____	_____	_____
Explain				
15. Other (please specify)	_____	_____	_____	_____
Explain				

Do you have *specific preferences* in regard to things you would like to improve as they relate to your ability to communicate with others? Please present those here:

Note. From "Techniques for Aural Rehabilitation for Aging Adults Who Are Hearing Impaired," by R. H. Hull, in R. H. Hull (Ed.), *Aural Rehabilitation: Children and Adults*, 2001, pp. 401–402, San Diego, CA: Singular/Thomson Learning. Reproduced with permission.

APPENDIX K

The Hearing Handicap Inventory for the Elderly

The purpose of this scale is to identify the problems your hearing loss may be causing. Answer *yes*, *sometimes*, or *no* for each question. Do not skip a question if you avoid a situation because of your hearing problem. If you use a hearing aid, please answer the way you hear without the aid.

		Yes (4)	Sometimes (2)	No (0)
S-1.	Does a hearing problem cause you to use the phone less often than you would like?	____	____	____
E-2.	Does a hearing problem cause you to feel embarrassed when meeting new people?	____	____	____
S-3.	Does a hearing problem cause you to avoid groups of people?	____	____	____
E-4.	Does a hearing problem make you irritable?	____	____	____
E-5.	Does a hearing problem cause you to feel frustrated when talking to members of your family?	____	____	____
S-6.	Does a hearing problem cause you difficulty when attending a party?	____	____	____
E-7.	Does a hearing problem cause you to feel "stupid" or "dumb?"	____	____	____
S-8.	Do you have difficulty hearing when someone speaks in a whisper?	____	____	____
E-9.	Do you feel handicapped by a hearing problem?	____	____	____
S-10.	Does a hearing problem cause you difficulty when visiting friends, relatives, or neighbors?	____	____	____

	Yes (4)	Sometimes (2)	No (0)
S-11. Does a hearing problem cause you to attend religious services less often than you would like?	_____	_____	_____
E-12. Does a hearing problem cause you to be nervous?	_____	_____	_____
E-13. Does a hearing problem cause you to visit friends, relatives, or neighbors less often than you would like?	_____	_____	_____
E-14. Does a hearing problem cause you to have arguments with your family members?	_____	_____	_____
S-15. Does a hearing problem cause you difficulty when listening to TV or radio?	_____	_____	_____
S-16. Does a hearing problem cause you to go shopping less often than you would like?	_____	_____	_____
S-17. Does any problem or difficulty with your hearing upset you at all?	_____	_____	_____
S-18. Does a hearing problem cause you to want to be by yourself?	_____	_____	_____
S-19. Does a hearing problem cause you to talk to family members less often than you would like?	_____	_____	_____
E-20. Do you feel that any difficulty with your hearing limits or hampers your personal or social life?	_____	_____	_____
S-21. Does a hearing problem cause you difficulty when in a restaurant with relatives or friends?	_____	_____	_____
S-22. Does a hearing problem cause you to feel depressed?	_____	_____	_____
S-23. Does a hearing problem cause you to listen to TV or radio less often than you would like?	_____	_____	_____
E-24. Does a hearing problem cause you to feel uncomfortable when talking to friends?	_____	_____	_____
E-25. Does a hearing problem cause you to feel left out when you are with a group of people?	_____	_____	_____

For Clinicians Use Only: Total Score: _____

Subtotal E: _____

Subtotal S: _____

Note. From "The Hearing Handicap Inventory for the Elderly: A New Tool," by I. J. Ventry and B. Weinstein, 1982, *Ear and Hearing*, *3*, pp. 128–134. Reproduced with permission.

APPENDIX L

The Communication Profile for the Hearing Impaired

The purpose of this questionnaire is to find out how your hearing loss affects your daily life and what problems, if any, you may be having as a result. Most of the items deal in some way with communication and your interactions with other people, but there are also items that describe your feelings and your reactions in a variety of situations.

Part I

This section of the questionnaire asks you to describe how often you feel you are able to communicate effectively with others. Mark 1 if you Rarely or Almost Never communicate effectively in that situation. Use 2 for Occasionally or Sometimes; use 3 for About Half the Time; use " for Frequently or Often; and use 5 if you Usually or Almost Always communicate effectively.

We would also like to know how important these situations are to you. That is, we would like to know which types of situations really matter to you and which ones don't. If a particular situation occurs quite often, or if it's essential for you to communicate effectively in that situation, indicate this by marking 5 for Essential on the response sheet. On the other hand, if the situation occurs rarely, or if it does not really matter if you communicate in that situation, then mark 1 for Not Important on the response sheet. Use 2 for Somewhat Important, use 3 for Important; and use 4 for Very Important.

1. Someone in your family is talking to you while you're driving or riding in a car.

2. You're at a social gathering with music or other noise in the background.

3. You're at the dinner table with your family.

4. You're at work and someone is talking to you from another room.

5. You're at a restaurant ordering food or drink.

6. You're talking on the telephone when you're at work.

7. You're at an outdoor picnic.

8. Someone's talking to you while you're watching TV or listening to the stereo.

9. You're listening for information at a lecture, briefing, or class.

10. You're talking with someone in an office.

11. You're at home talking on the telephone.

12. You're at a dinner party with several other people.

13. You're listening to someone speak at religious services.

14. You're at a meeting with several other people.

15. You're at home and someone is talking to you from another room.

16. You're having a conversation at a social gathering while others are talking nearby.

17. You're talking with a friend or family member in a quiet room.

18. You're giving or following work instructions outdoors.

Part II

In this section of the questionnaire you're asked to describe the kinds of experiences you have when you're communicating with others. What kinds of things happen when you're trying to carry on a conversation? What do you do when you have trouble understanding what someone has said? What kinds of things do other people do that make it harder or easier for you to communicate with them?

Mark 1 if the item describes something that Rarely happens or that is Almost Never true for you. Mark 2 for Occasionally or Sometimes; mark 3 for About Half the Time; mark 4 for Frequently or Often; and mark 5 for Almost Always.

19. One way I get people to repeat what they said is by ignoring them.

20. If someone repeats what they've said and I still don't understand, I ask them to repeat again.

21. I have to talk with others when there's a lot of background noise.

22. If I hear part of what someone has said, I only ask them to repeat what I didn't hear.

23. My family gets annoyed when I don't hear things.

24. I try to give the impression of normal hearing.

25. Others think I'm ignoring them if I don't answer when they speak to me.

26. In difficult listening situations, I try to position myself so that I can hear as well as possible.

27. I have conversations with others when I'm home.

28. People think I'm not paying attention if I don't answer them when they speak to me.

29. I have to communicate with others in a group situation.

30. I interrupt others when listening to them is difficult.

31. I've asked my family to get my attention before speaking to me.

32. I tend to dominate conversations so I don't have to listen to others.

33. Members of my family speak to me when they're not facing me.

34. When I don't understand what someone has said, I ask them to repeat it.

35. People who know I have a hearing loss accuse me of hearing only what I want to hear.

36. When I have trouble understanding someone, I pay close attention to his or her face.

37. If someone seems irritated at having to repeat, I stop asking them to do so and pretend to understand.

38. I tend to avoid situations where I think I'll have problems hearing.

39. I get bothered or upset when I'm unable to follow a conversation.

40. I have to talk to others in noisy areas.

41. I avoid conversing with others because of my hearing loss.

42. If I'm sitting where I can't hear, I'll move to another seat.

43. My job required me to use the telephone.

44. When I don't understand what someone has said, I pretend that I understood it.

45. At parties or other social gatherings I try to stay in a well-lighted area so I can see the speaker's face.

46. People treat me as if I'm stupid because I can't understand what they say.

47. When I'm having trouble understanding friends or family members, I remind them that I have a hearing problem.

48. I avoid talking to strangers because of my hearing loss.

49. People get annoyed when I ask them to repeat what they've said.

50. During the day I have to communicate with others.

51. My job involves talking to people who speak quietly.

52. Members of my family leave me out of conversations or discussions.

53. When I must listen in a group, I try to sit where I'll be able to hear better.

54. Others become impatient because I don't always understand.

55. Members of my family refuse to repeat what they've said more than once or twice.

56. Members of my family talk to me from another room.

57. I feel stupid when I have to ask someone to repeat what they've said.

58. When I don't understand what someone has said, I ignore them.

59. People act frustrated when I don't understand what they say.

60. People who know I have a hearing loss don't speak clearly enough when they're speaking to me.

61. People don't remember to get my attention before speaking.

62. My job involves communicating with others.

63. I try to hide my hearing problem.

64. When there's background noise I position myself so that it's less distracting.

65. I've asked friends and people I work with to get my attention before speaking to me.

66. People who know I have a hearing loss don't speak up when they're talking to me.

67. When I don't understand what someone has said, I explain that I have a hearing loss.

68. People say, "Never mind" or "Forget it" if I ask them to repeat more than once.

69. When I'm having trouble following a conversation, I listen carefully and try to catch the main points.

70. I feel foolish when I misunderstand what someone has said.

71. When I think a person is speaking too softly, I ask them to speak up.

72. If possible, I try to watch a person's face when he or she is speaking.

73. People mumble when they're talking to me.

74. I get mad at myself when I can't understand what people are saying.

75. Others think I'm not interested in what they're saying.

76. I feel embarrassed when I have to ask someone to repeat what they've said.

Part III

The items in this section describe a variety of feelings, attitudes, and beliefs about hearing loss and communication. If the statement accurately describes your beliefs, feelings, attitudes, or experiences, mark 4 on the response sheet for Agree or 5 for Strongly Agree. If the statement doesn't accurately describe your feelings or reactions, mark 2 for Disagree or 1 for Strongly Disagree. Mark 3 if you're Uncertain or if you partly agree and partly disagree.

77. Sometimes I have trouble understanding what's being said when someone speaks to me from another room.

78. I feel threatened by many communication situations due to difficulty hearing.

79. My hearing loss is my problem and I hate to bother others with it.

80. I feel left out of conversations because I have trouble understanding.

81. People should be more patient when they're talking to me.

82. My hearing loss makes me mad.

83. Sometimes I'm ashamed of my hearing problems.

84. I withdraw from social talk because of my hearing loss.

85. I'm not very relaxed when conversing with others.

86. Others feel I use my hearing loss as an excuse for not paying attention.

87. Communicating with others is an important part of my daily activity.

88. I sometimes have trouble understanding others when there's background noise.

89. I feel guilty about asking people to repeat for me.

90. Sometimes I feel left out when I can't follow the conversation of those I'm with.

91. I sometimes get annoyed when I have trouble hearing.

92. I hate to ask others for special consideration just because I have a hearing problem.

93. There's a lot of background noise where I work.

94. When I have trouble hearing, I feel frustrated.

95. Because of my hearing loss, I sometimes have trouble communicating with others.

96. I'm not very comfortable in most communication situations.

97. Sometimes it's hard for me to understand what's being said in meetings, conferences, or other large groups.

98. At social gatherings I sometimes find it hard to follow conversations.

99. At times my hearing loss makes me feel incompetent.

100. It's frustrating when people refuse to repeat what they've said.

101. I get very tense because of my hearing loss.

102. Sometimes when I misunderstand what someone has said I feel foolish.

103. I get aggravated when others don't speak up.

104. Because of my hearing loss I keep to myself.

105. I'm sensitive about my hearing loss.

106. When I have trouble hearing, I become nervous.

107. I feel depressed as a result of my hearing loss.

108. I find it difficult to admit to others that I have a hearing problem.

109. Since I have trouble hearing, I don't enjoy going places with friends as much.

110. If people speak where I can't see them, they shouldn't expect me to answer them.

111. My family doesn't understand the strain and stress I feel from trying to understand what they say.

112. I get discouraged because of my hearing loss.

113. I worry about looking stupid when I can't understand what someone has said.

114. Straining to hear upsets me.

115. Communicating with others is an important part of my job.

116. I feel bad about the inconvenience I cause others because of my hearing loss.

117. I get impatient with people who aren't willing to repeat for me.

118. Because of my hearing loss I have feelings of inadequacy.

119. Questions about my hearing loss really irritate me.

120. It bothers me to admit that I have a hearing loss.

121. The problems I have communicating with others really get me down.

122. I sometimes get angry with myself when I can't hear what people are saying.

123. When I can't understand people, sometimes I just don't care anymore.

124. Sometimes it's difficult for me to follow a conversation when others are talking nearby.

125. I can't talk to people about my hearing loss.

126. If people want me to understand them, it's up to them to speak more clearly.

127. Sometimes I feel tense when I can't understand what someone is saying.

128. If someone talks to me while I'm watching TV, I sometimes have trouble understanding them.

129. Others should be more understanding about my hearing problems.

130. I sometimes feel embarrassed when I misunderstand what someone has said.

131. Sometimes I miss so much of what's being said that I feel left out.

132. I let my hearing problems get me down.

133. I have a hard time accepting the fact that I have a hearing loss.

134. I really get annoyed when people shout at me as if I'm deaf.

135. I try not to bother anyone else when I'm having trouble hearing.

136. I feel self-conscious because of my hearing loss.

137. When people mumble, they shouldn't expect me to understand them.

138. Feeling isolated is part of having a hearing impairment.

139. When I can't understand what's being said, I feel tense and anxious.

140. I'd rather miss part of a conversation than admit that I have a hearing loss.

141. I sometimes have trouble understanding what's being said when I can't see the speaker's face.

142. Not being able to understand is very discouraging.

143. I get angry when I can't understand what someone is saying.

144. I don't like to ask other people to help me with my hearing problems.

145. The difficulties I have with my hearing restrict my social and personal life.

Note. From "Development of the Communication Profile for the Hearing Impaired," by M. E. Demorest and S. A. Erdman, 1987, *Journal of Speech and Hearing Disorders, 52*, pp. 129–143. Reproduced with permission.

The CPHI is not reproduced in its entirety here, but rather as an example of the profile. Those who intend to use the CPHI clinically should become thoroughly familiar with the items, scales, and interpretation of the instrument. This information is available in: S. A. Erdman and M. E. Demorest (1990). *CPHI manual: A guide to clinical use.* Simpsonville, MD: CPHI Services.

APPENDIX M

Communication Skill Scale

Identifying Information

Name _____
              Last   First   Middle Initial

Social Security # _____
              (Gallaudet Student use ID Number)

Age _____   Sex   ( ) Male   ( ) Female

When did you become deaf:

    ( )   1)   Birth–2 years of age

    ( )   2)   Age 3–6 years of age

    ( )   3)   Age 6–12 years of age

    ( )   4)   Age 12–18 years of age

    ( )   5)   After age 18

Education:

    ( )   1)   Less than High School

    ( )   2)   High School Graduate

    ( )   3)   Some College

    ( )   4)   College Undergraduate Degree

    ( )   5)   Postgraduate

    ( )   6)   Ph.D.

How long did you attend each of the following:

(Enter 0 if you did not attend and .5 if you attended less than a full year.)

Residential School for the Deaf	_____ year(s)	_____ months
Private School for the Deaf	_____ year(s)	_____ months
Public School—Mainstreamed	_____ year(s)	_____ months
Public School—Special Class	_____ year(s)	_____ months
Private School—Mainstreamed	_____ year(s)	_____ months
Private School—Special Class	_____ year(s)	_____ months

How long did you attend each of the following:

(Enter 0 if you did not attend and .5 if you attended less than a full year.)

Gallaudet University	_____ year(s)	_____ months
National Technical Institute for the Deaf	_____ year(s)	_____ months
Other program for hearing impaired	_____ year(s)	_____ months
Hearing Jr. College, College, or University	_____ year(s)	_____ months
Program not specifically for hearing impaired	_____ year(s)	_____ months

How do you communicate most of the time:

At Home:	( ) ASL	( ) PSE	( ) Speech
At School:	( ) ASL	( ) PSE	( ) Speech
At Work:	( ) ASL	( ) PSE	( ) Speech
In the Community:	( ) ASL	( ) PSE	( ) Speech

How often do you use a hearing aid now:

( )   1)   Do Not Own a Hearing Aid

( )   2)   Not At All

( )   3)   Occasionally

( )   4)   All the Time

Do you wear an aid in:

( )   One ear

( )   Both ears

Type of aid currently in use:

( ) 1) Behind-the-ear aid

( ) 2) In-the-ear aid

( ) 3) Body-worn or eyeglass aid

( ) 4) Vibrotactile aid

( ) 5) Cochlear implant

Indicate the degree of your hearing loss:

( ) 1) Mild

( ) 2) Moderate

( ) 3) Severe

( ) 4) Profound

Instructions

We want to find out how your hearing loss affects your daily life. The following questions are about different communication situations, ways of managing situations, and attitudes about different situations. If you have never experienced the situation do not answer the question. Go on to the next question.

Some of the items ask you whether you understand conversation. The word *understand* means knowing enough of what is said or signed to be able to answer appropriately. Always assume you are interested in what is being said.

We know that some people are easier to understand than others. Please answer the questions according to the way most people talk to you or understand you. We know that sounds and speakers vary. Please answer the questions as best you can.

If you wear a hearing aid, answer the questions as though you were wearing your aid.

SECTION I: Difficult Communication Situations

Please read each situation. Decide if the situation is true:

1. Almost always,
2. Sometimes, or
3. Almost never.

Then indicate if the situation is:

1. Very important to you,
2. Important to you,
3. Not important to you.

If you have not experienced this situation *do not* answer the question. Go on to the next question.

Question #1.

You are in class. The teacher is easy to lipread but is not signing. You understand

_____ (frequency)   _____ (importance)

Question #2.

You meet a stranger on the street and ask for directions. He does not sign. You understand him

_____ (frequency)   _____ (importance)

Question #3.

You are at work. It is quiet. Your supervisor gives you an order. She is not signing but her face is clearly visible. You understand her

_____ (frequency)   _____ (importance)

Question #4.

You are at work. It is noisy. A hearing coworker asks you to eat lunch with her. She does not sign but you can see her face. You understand her

_____ (frequency)   _____ (importance)

Question #5.

You are visiting a friend. His hard-of-hearing child speaks to you about his school. The child does not sign. You understand

_____ (frequency)   _____ (importance)

Question #6.

You are at a meeting. A hearing person speaks but does not sign. You know the subject. You understand

_____ (frequency)   _____ (importance)

Question #7.

You are in class. A hearing person speaks but does not sign. You know the subject. You understand

_____ (frequency)   _____ (importance)

Question #8.

You are at the dinner table at home. All your relatives are hearing. Your grandmother is talking. She does not sign. You do not know the topic. You understand her

_____ (frequency)   _____ (importance)

Question #9.

You are introduced to a hearing person. You sign and speak at the same time. He understands you

_____ (frequency)   _____ (importance)

Question #10.

You are at a meeting with five hearing people. No one signs but everyone's face can be seen. One person talks at a time. You understand the conversation

_____ (frequency)   _____ (importance)

Question #11.

You are watching a movie on television. There is no captioning. It is quiet in the room. You understand

_____ (frequency)   _____ (importance)

Question #12.

You are talking to the doctor. It is quiet. She does not sign. You can see her face clearly. You understand her

_____ (frequency)   _____ (importance)

Question #13.

You are ordering lunch at McDonald's. You speak to the person behind the counter. She understands you

_____ (frequency)   _____ (importance)

Question #14.

You are talking to one person at a noisy party. The person does not sign. You understand

_____ (frequency)   _____ (importance)

Question #15.

You are talking to a family member on the telephone. It is quiet in the room. You understand

_____ (frequency)   _____ (importance)

Question #16.

You are reading in a quiet room. Someone calls you from the next room. You hear the person's voice

_____ (frequency)   _____ (importance)

Question #17.

You are sitting in a car next to the driver. The driver is talking. He is not signing. You understand him

_____ (frequency) _____ (importance)

Question #18.

You must give directions to hearing people at work. They understand your speech

_____ (frequency) _____ (importance)

Question #19.

I have trouble hearing fire alarms in buildings when other people can hear them

_____ (frequency) _____ (importance)

Question #20.

I have trouble hearing fire engines and ambulances when other people can hear them.

_____ (frequency) _____ (importance)

Question #21.

I have trouble hearing cars or buses when other people can hear them

_____ (frequency) _____ (importance)

Question #22.

I have trouble hearing the telephone when I am in the same room

_____ (frequency) _____ (importance)

Question #23.

I have trouble hearing the telephone when I am in the next room

_____ (frequency) _____ (importance)

Question #24.

I have trouble hearing the doorbell when other people can hear it

_____ (frequency) _____ (importance)

Question #25.

I have trouble hearing a knock on the door when other people can hear it

_____ (frequency) _____ (importance)

Question #26.

I have trouble hearing music when it is loud enough for other people

_____ (frequency) _____ (importance)

Question #27.

I have trouble hearing a person's voice when he is talking in the same room

_____ (frequency)   _____ (importance)

SECTION II: Communication Strategies

Please read each situation. Decide if the situation is true:

1. Almost always,
2. Sometimes, or
3. Almost never.

If you have not experienced this situation *do not* answer the question. Go on to the next question.

Question #28.

You are talking with someone you do not know well. You do not understand. You ask her to repeat.

_____ (frequency)

Question #29.

You are talking with two people. You are not understanding. You change the topic so that you can control the conversation.

_____ (frequency)

Question #30.

You ask a stranger for directions. You understand part of what he says. You tell him the part you understand and ask him to repeat the rest.

_____ (frequency)

Question #31.

You answer a question but the other person doesn't understand. You repeat the answer.

_____ (frequency)

Question #32.

You are at work. Your boss gives you instructions. You do not understand. You ask him to say the instructions in a different way.

_____ (frequency)

Question #33.

A friend introduces you to a new person. You do not understand the person's name. You ask the person to spell her name

_____ (frequency)

Question #34.

A person asks you for your name. He does not understand your speech. You spell your name.

_____ (frequency)

Question #35.

A stranger spells his name for you. You miss the first two letters. You ask him to say each letter and a word starting with each letter (A as in *apple*, B as in *boy*).

_____ (frequency)

Question #36.

A person tells you his address. You do not understand. You ask him to repeat the street number, one number at a time.

_____ (frequency)

Question #37.

You are talking with one person but are not understanding. You interrupt the person before he finishes to say what you think.

_____ (frequency)

Question #38.

Your friend asks you to buy seven hamburgers. You do not understand how many he wants. You ask him to start counting from zero and stop at the correct number.

_____ (frequency)

Question #39.

You are in a restaurant. The waitress does not understand what you want. You point to the item on the menu.

_____ (frequency)

Question #40.

You are in class. The teacher says something you do not understand. You pretend to understand and hope to get the information from the book later.

_____ (frequency)

Question #41.

You are at the dinner table with your family. Someone does not understand you. You say the same thing a different way.

_____ (frequency)

Question #42.

Someone who does not sign asks you for your phone number. You say each number and show the correct number of fingers as you speak.

_____ (frequency)

Question #43.

Two people are talking. You do not understand the conversation. You ask them to tell you the topic.

_____ (frequency)

Question #44.

You are talking with one person in a restaurant. His face is in the shadows. You know you could understand better if you changed seats with him. You ask to change seats.

_____ (frequency)

Question #45.

You are at the airport. You want to buy a ticket for a flight home. The clerk does not understand you. You write the information.

_____ (frequency)

Question #46.

You are visiting the doctor. He tells you what to do for your sickness. You do not understand his speech. You ask him to write.

_____(frequency)

Question #47.

You are at a meeting. The speaker does not look at you when he talks. You feel angry but do nothing about it.

_____ (frequency)

Question #48.

You meet a deaf friend who is with another person. The other person talks to you but does not sign. You ask her to sign.

_____ (frequency)

Question #49.

You are at a meeting. You realize you are too far from the speaker to understand. There are empty seats in the front of the room. You change your seat.

_____ (frequency)

Question #50.

You are at a meeting at work. You are the only deaf person. You are afraid that you will not understand but you do not ask for help. You do the best you can.

_____ (frequency)

Question #51.

You are talking to the dentist. He speaks very fast. You cannot lipread him. You ask him to slow down.

_____ (frequency)

Question #52.

You are in class. The teacher talks while she writes on the board. You talk to her after class. You explain that you need to see her face in order to speechread.

_____ (frequency)

Question #53.

Your teacher likes to move around the room while she teaches. You have problems reading her signs. You ask her after class to lecture from one place so you can understand her signing.

_____ (frequency)

Question #54.

You are going to a series of meetings or lectures. The speaker does not sign. You ask the speaker to use the slides, pictures, or the overhead projector whenever possible.

_____ (frequency)

Question #55.

You are going to a series of meetings or lectures. The speaker does not sign. You ask him to find a person to take notes for you.

_____ (frequency)

Question #56.

You are going to a series of meetings or lectures. The speaker does not sign. You ask for an interpreter.

_____ (frequency)

Question #57.

You are going to a series of meetings or lectures. The speaker does not sign. You ask for an outline or a reading list.

_____ (frequency)

Question #58.

You are going to a play. It will not be signed. You read the play or reviews of the play before you see it.

_____ (frequency)

Question #59.

You are going to a job interview. You act out the situation in advance with a friend to prepare yourself for the experience.

_____ (frequency)

Question #60.

You are talking with a clerk at the bank. A fire truck goes by. You ask him to stop talking until the noise stops.

_____ (frequency)

Question #61.

You ask a person to repeat because you don't understand. He seems annoyed. You stop asking and pretend to understand.

_____ (frequency)

Question #62.

You ask a stranger for directions to a place. You really want to understand his speech. You ask very specific questions like, "Is this place north or south of here?" "Do I turn left or right at the corner?"

_____ (frequency)

Question #63.

You need to ask directions. You avoid asking a stranger because you think you will have trouble understanding him.

_____ (frequency)

Question #64.

You must make a phone call to a hearing person. The person does not have a TDD. You ask a hearing friend to make the call and interpret for you.

_____ (frequency)

Question #65.

You are at a store. You have trouble hearing the clerk because his voice is soft. You explain you are hearing impaired and ask him to talk louder.

_____ (frequency)

Question #66.

You are at home. You ask your family to get your attention before they speak to you.

_____ (frequency)

Question #67.

You are with five or six friends. No one is signing. You miss something important. You ask the person next to you what was said.

_____ (frequency)

Question #68.

You have trouble understanding a man who is chewing gum. You explain that you need to speechread. You politely ask him to remove the gum when he talks.

_____ (frequency)

Question #69.

You try to avoid people when you know you will have trouble hearing them.

_____ (frequency)

Question #70.

You hate to bother other people with your hearing problem. So, you pretend to understand.

_____ (frequency)

Question #71.

I avoid wearing my hearing aid because it makes me feel different.

_____ (frequency)

SECTION III: Attitudes

Please read each situation. Decide if the situation is true:

1. Almost always,
2. Sometimes, or
3. Almost never.

If you have not experienced this situation _do not_ answer the question. Go on to the next question.

Question #72.

I feel embarrassed when I don't understand someone.

_____ (frequency).

Question #73.

I get upset when I can't follow a conversation.

_____ (frequency)

Question #74.

I become angry when people do not speak clearly enough for me to understand.

_____ (frequency)

Question #75.

I feel stupid when I misunderstand what a person is saying.

_____ (frequency)

Question #76.

It's hard for me to ask someone to repeat things. I feel embarrassed.

_____ (frequency)

Question #77.

Most people think I could understand better if I paid more attention.

_____ (frequency)

Question #78.

I get angry when people speak too softly or too fast.

_____ (frequency)

Question #79.

Sometimes I can't follow conversations at home. I still feel a part of family life.

_____ (frequency)

Question #80.

I feel frustrated when I try to communicate with hearing people.

_____ (frequency)

Question #81.

Most hearing people do not understand what it is like to be deaf. This makes me angry.

_____ (frequency)

Question #82.

I am ashamed of being hearing impaired.

_____ (frequency)

Question #83.

I get angry when someone speaks with his mouth covered or with his back to me.

_____ (frequency)

Question #84.

I prefer to be alone most of the time.

_____ (frequency)

Question #85.

I am uncomfortable with people who communicate differently than I do.

_____ (frequency)

Question #86.

My hearing loss makes me nervous.

_____ (frequency)

Question #87.

My hearing loss makes me feel depressed.

_____ (frequency)

Question #88.

My family understands my hearing loss.

_____ (frequency)

Question #89.

I get annoyed when people shout at me because I have a hearing loss.

_____ (frequency)

Question #90.

People treat me like a stupid person when I don't understand their speech.

_____ (frequency)

Question #91.

People treat me like a stupid person when they don't understand me.

_____ (frequency)

Question #92.

Members of my family don't get annoyed when I have trouble understanding them.

_____ (frequency)

Question #93.

People who know I have a hearing loss think I can hear when I want to.

_____ (frequency)

Question #94.

Members of my family don't leave me out of conversations.

_____ (frequency)

Question #95.

Hearing aids don't always help people understand speech, but they can help in other ways.

_____ (frequency)

Question #96.

I feel speechreading (lipreading) is helpful to me.

_____ (frequency)

Question #97.

I feel the only useful communication system for a deaf person is sign language.

_____ (frequency)

Question #98.

Even though people know I have a hearing loss, they don't help me by speaking clearly or repeating.

_____ (frequency)

Question #99.

My family is willing to make telephone calls for me.

_____ (frequency)

Question #100.

My family is willing to repeat as often as necessary when I don't understand them.

_____ (frequency)

Question #101.

Hearing people get frustrated when I don't understand what they say.

_____ (frequency)

Question #102.

Hearing people get embarrassed when they don't understand my speech.

_____ (frequency)

Question #103.

Hearing people pretend to understand me when they really don't.

_____ (frequency)

Question #104.

I feel the only useful communications system for a deaf person is speech and lipreading.

_____ (frequency)

Question #105.

I feel embarrassed when hearing people don't understand my speech.

_____ (frequency)

Question #106.

I do not mind repeating when people have trouble understanding my speech.

_____ (frequency)

Question #107.

I prefer to write when I communicate with hearing people because I am ashamed of my speech.

_____ (frequency)

Question #108.

I feel that most hearing people try to understand my speech.

_____ (frequency)

Question #109.

I feel that my family tries to understand my speech.

_____ (frequency)

Question #110.

I feel that strangers try to understand my speech.

_____ (frequency)

Note. From "Communication Skill Scale," by H. Kaplan, S. J. Bally, and F. D. Brandt, 1990. Washington, DC: Gallaudet University. Reproduced with permission.

The CSS is not reproduced here in its entirety, but rather as an example of the scale.

The Scale, Scoring Form, and Norms can be obtained from Department of Audiology, Gallaudet University, Washington, DC 20002.

APPENDIX N

The Shortened Hearing Aid Performance Inventory

1. You are sitting alone at home watching the news on TV.

2. You are involved in an intimate conversation with your partner.

3. You are watching TV and there are distracting noises such as others talking.

4. You are at home engaged in some activity and the telephone rings in another room.

5. You are at home in conversation with a member of your family who is in another room.

6. You are listening to a speaker who is talking to a large group and you are seated toward the rear of the room. The speaker's back is partially turned as he or she makes notes on a blackboard.

7. You are starting to cross a busy street and a car horn sounds a warning.

8. You are walking in the downtown section of a large city. There are the usual city noises and you are in conversation with a friend.

9. You are driving your car and listening to a news broadcast on the radio. You are alone and the windows are closed.

10. You are in a crowded grocery store checkout line and are talking with the cashier.

11. You are at home watching TV and the doorbell rings.

12. You are taking an evening stroll with a friend through a quiet neighborhood park; there are the usual environmental sounds around (e.g., children playing, dogs barking, birds singing).

13. You are at home alone listening to your stereo system (instrumental music).

14. You are in whispered conversation with your partner at an intimate restaurant.

15. You are in the kitchen in conversation with your partner during the preparation of the evening meal.

16. You are at home in face-to-face conversation with one member of your family.

17. You are shopping at a large, busy department store and are talking with a sales clerk.

18. You are in church listening to the sermon and sitting in the front pew.

19. You are listening to a speaker who is talking to a large group and you are seated towards the rear of the room. There is occasional noise in the room (e.g., whispering, rattling papers, etc.).

20. You are having a conversation in your home with a salesperson and there is background noise (e.g., TV, people talking, etc.) in the room.

21. You are in church listening to a sermon and sitting in the back pew.

22. You are talking with a friend outdoors on a windy day.

23. You are driving your car with the windows up and radio off and are carrying on a conversation with your partner, who is in the front seat.

24. You are ordering food for the family at a fast-food restaurant.

25. You are at home reading the paper. Two family members are in another room talking quietly and you want to listen in on their conversation.

26. You are talking with a bank teller at the bank.

27. You are in conversation with a neighbor across the fence.

28. You are in a crowded reception room waiting for your name to be called.

29. You are in your backyard gardening. Your neighbor is using a noisy power lawnmower and yells something at you.

30. You are listening in a small, quiet room to someone who speaks softly.

31. Someone is trying to tell you something in a small, quiet room while you have your back turned.

32. You are driving your car with the windows down and are carrying on a conversation with others riding with you.

33. You are in a quiet conversation with your family doctor in an examination room.

34. You are talking to a large group and someone from the back of the audience asks a question in a relatively soft voice. The audience is quiet as they listen to the question.

35. You are at a large, noisy party and are engaged in conversation with one other person.

36. You are at the dinner table with your whole family and are in conversation with one other person.

37. You are one of only a few customers inside your bank and are talking with a teller.

38. You are riding in a car with friends. The windows of the car are wound down. You are in the back seat carrying on a conversation with them.

Note. From "Evaluation of Hearing Aid Benefit Using the Shortened Hearing Aid Performance Inventory," by J. Jerram and S. Purdy, 1997, *Journal of the American Academy of Audiology, 8*, pp. 18–26. Reprinted with permission.

APPENDIX O

Communication Scale for Older Adults (3-Point Response Format)

Communication Strategies

Please read each situation. Decide if the situation is true (1) almost always, (2) sometimes, or (3) almost never; please circle the appropriate answer. *Please respond to each question.*

Question #1

You are talking with someone you do not know well. You do not understand. You ask her to repeat.

    (1) almost always   (2) sometimes   (3) almost never

Question #2

You are talking with two people. You are not understanding. You change the topic so that you can control the conversation.

    (1) almost always   (2) sometimes   (3) almost never

Question #3

You ask a stranger for directions. You understand part of what he says. You tell him the part you understand and ask him to repeat the rest.

    (1) almost always   (2) sometimes   (3) almost never

Question #4

A friend introduces you to a new person. You do not understand the person's name. You ask the person to spell her name.

    (1) almost always   (2) sometimes   (3) almost never

Question #5

A stranger spells his name for you. You miss the first two letters. You ask him to say each letter and a word starting with that letter (a as in *apple*, b as in *boy*).

    (1) almost always   (2) sometimes   (3) almost never

Question #6

A person tells you his address. You do not understand. You ask him to repeat the street number, one number at a time.

  (1) almost always   (2) sometimes   (3) almost never

Question #7

You are talking with one person but are not understanding. You interrupt the person before he finishes to say what you think.

  (1) almost always   (2) sometimes   (3) almost never

Question #8

Your friend asks you to buy seven hamburgers. You do not understand how many he wants. You ask him to start counting from zero and stop at the correct numbers.

  (1) almost always   (2) sometimes   (3) almost never

Question #9

You are at a meeting. The speaker says something you do not understand. You pretend to understand and hope to get the information later.

  (1) almost always   (2) sometimes   (3) almost never

Question #10

Two people are talking. You do not understand the conversation. You ask them to tell you the topic.

  (1) almost always   (2) sometimes   (3) almost never

Question #11

You are talking with one person in a restaurant. His face is in the shadows. You know you could understand better if you changed seats with him. You ask to change seats.

  (1) almost always   (2) sometimes   (3) almost never

Question #12

You are visiting the doctor. He tells you what to do for your illness. You do not understand his speech. You ask him to write it down.

  (1) almost always   (2) sometimes   (3) almost never

Question #13

You are at a meeting. The speaker does not look at you when he talks. You feel angry but do nothing about it.

  (1) almost always   (2) sometimes   (3) almost never

Question #14

You are at a meeting. You realize you are too far from the speaker to understand. There are empty seats in the front of the room. You change your seat.

    (1) almost always   (2) sometimes   (3) almost never

Question #15

You are at a meeting. You are the only hard-of-hearing person. You are afraid that you will not understand but you do not ask for help. You do the best you can.

    (1) almost always   (2) sometimes   (3) almost never

Question #16

You are talking to the dentist. He speaks very fast. You cannot lipread him. You ask him to slow down.

    (1) almost always   (2) sometimes   (3) almost never

Question #17

You are taking a class. The teacher talks while she writes on the board. You talk to her after class. You explain that you need to see her face in order to speechread.

    (1) almost always   (2) sometimes   (3) almost never

Question #18

A speaker likes to move around the room while she lectures. You have problems reading her lips. You ask her after class to lecture from one place in the room.

    (1) almost always   (2) sometimes   (3) almost never

Question #19

You are going to a series of meetings or lectures. You ask the speaker to use slides, pictures, or the overhead projector whenever possible.

    (1) almost always   (2) sometimes   (3) almost never

Question #20

You are going to a series of meetings or lectures. You ask the speaker to find a person to take notes for you.

    (1) almost always   (2) sometimes   (3) almost never

Question #21

You are going to a series of meetings or lectures. You ask for an outline or a reading list.

    (1) almost always   (2) sometimes   (3) almost never

Question #22

You are going to a play. You read the play or the reviews of the play before you see it.

    (1) almost always   (2) sometimes   (3) almost never

Question #23

You are talking with a clerk at the bank. A fire truck goes by. You ask him to stop talking until the noise stops.

    (1) almost always   (2) sometimes   (3) almost never

Question #24

You ask a person to repeat because you don't understand. He seems annoyed. You stop asking and pretend to understand.

    (1) almost always   (2) sometimes   (3) almost never

Question #25

You ask a stranger for directions to a place. You really want to understand his speech. You ask specific questions like, "Is this place north or south of here?"

    (1) almost always   (2) sometimes   (3) almost never

Question #26

You need to ask directions. You avoid asking a stranger because you think you will have trouble understanding him.

    (1) almost always   (2) sometimes   (3) almost never

Question #27

You are at a store. You have trouble hearing the clerk because his voice is soft. You explain you are hearing impaired and ask him to talk louder.

    (1) almost always   (2) sometimes   (3) almost never

Question #28

You ask your family or friends to get your attention before they speak to you.

    (1) almost always   (2) sometimes   (3) almost never

Question #29

You are with five or six friends. You miss something important. You ask the person next to you what was said.

    (1) almost always   (2) sometimes   (3) almost never

Question #30

You have trouble understanding a man who is chewing gum. You explain that you need to speechread. You politely ask him to remove the chewing gum when he talks.

(1) almost always   (2) sometimes   (3) almost never

Question #31

You try to avoid people when you know will have trouble understanding them.

(1) almost always   (2) sometimes   (3) almost never

Question #32

You hate to bother other people with your hearing problem. So you pretend to understand.

(1) almost always   (2) sometimes   (3) almost never

Question #33

You avoid wearing your hearing aid because it makes you feel different.

(1) almost always   (2) sometimes   (3) almost never

Question #34

You are at a lecture on a subject of great interest. There is a microphone but the speaker does not use it. You raise your hand and request that the speaker use the microphone.

(1) almost always   (2) sometimes   (3) almost never

Question #35

You are at a lecture on a subject of great interest. There is a microphone but it is not set loud enough for you to understand. You leave the meeting angry to complain to someone "in charge."

(1) almost always   (2) sometimes   (3) almost never

Question #36

You are at a lecture on a subject of great interest. The speaker is talking too fast for you to understand. You leave the lecture because it has become a waste of time.

(1) almost always   (2) sometimes   (3) almost never

Question #37

You are at a lecture on a subject of great interest. The speaker moves around so much that you have trouble understanding her. You complain to the organizers of the lecture after it is over.

(1) almost always   (2) sometimes   (3) almost never

Question #38

You are at a holiday dinner. You can't understand the conversation because everyone is talking at once. You promise yourself you will not go back next year.

(1) almost always   (2) sometimes   (3) almost never

Question #39

You are at a holiday dinner. You can't understand the conversation because everyone is talking at once. You ask for everyone's attention, explain the problem, and ask people to take turns so you can understand.

(1) almost always   (2) sometimes   (3) almost never

Question #40

You are at a holiday dinner. You can't understand the conversation because everyone is talking at once. You explain the problem to the host so that he can handle the situation.

(1) almost always   (2) sometimes   (3) almost never

Question #41

You are at a holiday dinner. You can't understand the conversation because everyone is talking at once. However, you don't say anything because you are glad to be at the party.

(1) almost always   (2) sometimes   (3) almost never

Communication Attitudes

Please read each situation. Decide if the situation is true (1) almost always, (2) sometimes, or (3) almost never; please circle the appropriate answer. *Please respond to each question.*

Question #1

I feel embarrassed when I don't understand someone.

(1) almost always   (2) sometimes   (3) almost never

Question #2

I get upset when I can't follow a conversation.

(1) almost always   (2) sometimes   (3) almost never

Question #3

I become angry when people do not speak clearly enough for me to understand.

(1) almost always   (2) sometimes   (3) almost never

Question #4

I feel stupid when I misunderstand what a person is saying.

    (1) almost always   (2) sometimes   (3) almost never

Question #5

It's hard for me to ask someone to repeat things. I feel embarrassed.

    (1) almost always   (2) sometimes   (3) almost never

Question #6

Most people think I could understand better if I paid more attention.

    (1) almost always   (2) sometimes   (3) almost never

Question #7

I get angry when people speak too softly or too fast.

    (1) almost always   (2) sometimes   (3) almost never

Question #8

Sometimes I can't follow conversations at home. I still feel part of family.

    (1) almost always   (2) sometimes   (3) almost never

Question #9

I feel frustrated when I try to communicate with people.

    (1) almost always   (2) sometimes   (3) almost never

Question #10

Most people do not understand what it is like to be hard of hearing. This makes me angry.

    (1) almost always   (2) sometimes   (3) almost never

Question #11

I am ashamed of being hearing impaired.

    (1) almost always   (2) sometimes   (3) almost never

Question #12

I get angry when someone speaks with his mouth covered or with his back to me.

    (1) almost always   (2) sometimes   (3) almost never

Question #13

I prefer to be alone most of the time.

    (1) almost always   (2) sometimes   (3) almost never

Question #14

My hearing loss makes me nervous.

(1) almost always   (2) sometimes   (3) almost never

Question #15

My hearing loss makes me depressed.

(1) almost always   (2) sometimes   (3) almost never

Question #16

My family does not understand my hearing loss.

(1) almost always   (2) sometimes   (3) almost never

Question #17

I get annoyed when people shout at me because I have a hearing loss.

(1) almost always   (2) sometimes   (3) almost never

Question #18

People treat me like a stupid person when I don't understand their speech.

(1) almost always   (2) sometimes   (3) almost never

Question #19

Hard-of-hearing and hearing people often have difficulty communicating. It is only the responsibility of the hearing person to improve communication.

(1) almost always   (2) sometimes   (3) almost never

Question #20

Hard-of-hearing and hearing people often have difficulty communicating. It is only the responsibility of the hard-of-hearing person to improve communication.

(1) almost always   (2) sometimes   (3) almost never

Question #21

Members of my family get annoyed when I have trouble understanding them.

(1) almost always   (2) sometimes   (3) almost never

Question #22

People who know I have a hearing loss think I can hear when I want to.

(1) almost always   (2) sometimes   (3) almost never

Question #23

Members of my family leave me out of conversations.

    (1) almost always   (2) sometimes   (3) almost never

Question #24

Hearing aids don't always help people understand speech but they can help in other ways.

    (1) almost always   (2) sometimes   (3) almost never

Question #25

I feel speechreading (lipreading) is helpful to me.

    (1) almost always   (2) sometimes   (3) almost never

Question #26

Even though people know I have a hearing loss, they don't help me by speaking clearly or repeating.

    (1) almost always   (2) sometimes   (3) almost never

Question #27

My family is willing to make telephone calls for me.

    (1) almost always   (2) sometimes   (3) almost never

Question # 28

My family is willing to repeat as often as necessary when I don't understand them.

    (1) almost always   (2) sometimes   (3) almost never

Question #29

Hearing people get frustrated when I don't understand what they say.

    (1) almost always   (2) sometimes   (3) almost never

Question #30

Members of my family make it easy for me to speechread them.

    (1) almost always   (2) sometimes   (3) almost never

Question #31

Strangers make it easy for me to speechread them.

    (1) almost always   (2) sometimes   (3) almost never

Note. From "Communication Score for Older Adults (CSOA)," by H. Kaplan, S. Bally, F. Brandt, D. Busacco, & J. Pray, J., 1997, *Journal of the American Academy of Audiology, 8*, pp. 203–217. Reprinted with permission.

Index